A.M. Adelstein

Clinical Neuroepidemiology

Clinical Neuroepidemiology

Edited by
F CLIFFORD ROSE
Consultant Neurologist, Charing Cross Hospital, London
Consultant Neurologist, Medical Ophthalmology Unit,
St Thomas' Hospital, London

PITMAN MEDICAL

First published 1980

Catalogue Number 21 3266 81

Pitman Medical Limited
57 High Street, Tunbridge Wells, Kent

Associated Companies:
Pitman Publishing Pty Ltd., Melbourne
Pitman Publishing New Zealand Ltd., Wellington

British Library Cataloguing in Publication Data
Clinical neuroepidemiology. - (Progress in
    neurological research series).
    1. Nervous system - Diseases - Congresses
    2. Epidemiology - Congresses
    I. Rose, Frank Clifford   II. Series
    614.5'98   RC346

ISBN 0-272-79570-4

Set in 10 on 11 pt IBM Press Roman by
Gatehouse Wood Limited, Cowden
Printed by offset-lithography and bound
in Great Britain at The Pitman Press, Bath

CONTENTS

PART III   MULTIPLE SCLEROSIS

PART IV PAEDIATRIC NEUROEPIDEMIOLOGY

vi

CONTRIBUTORS

Roy M Acheson, MA, MD, ScD, FRCP, FFCM, Professor of Community Medicine, Addenbrooke's Hospital, Cambridge

A M Adelstein, MD, MRCP, Chief Medical Statistician, Office of Population Censuses and Surveys, London

E M Alberman, MD, FRCP, Professor of Clinical Epidemiology, London Hospital Medical College, London

R Angunawela, MD(Ceylon), MRCP, Department of Geriatrics, Cumberland Infirmary, Carlisle

John F Annegers, PhD, Associate Consultant, Department of Medical Statistics and Epidemiology, Mayo Clinic, Rochester, Minnesota

Peter O Behan, MD, FACP, FRCP(Glas), FRCP(Lond), Department of Neurology, Institute of Neurological Sciences, Glasgow

Wilhelmina M H Behan, MB, ChB, MRCPath, Senior Lecturer in Pathology, Institute of Neurological Sciences, Glasgow

M Bellman, MB, MRCP, DCH, Lecturer in Child Health, Middlesex Hospital Medical School, London

Bernard Benjamin, Emeritus Professor, Department of Actuarial Sciences, The City University, London

Rosaleen Brady, LRCP and SI, DSS, Research Assistant, Medico-Social Research Board, Dublin

R Capildeo, MB, MRCP, Senior Registrar, Department of Neurology, Charing Cross Hospital, London

Oliver Chadwick, Department of Child and Adolescent Psychiatry, Institute of Psychiatry, University of London

P L Chin, MB, MRCP, Consultant Geriatrician, Cumberland Infirmary, Carlisle, Cumberland

Geoffrey Dean, MD, FRCP, FRCPI, FFCM, Director, The Medico-Social Research Board, Dublin

Heather M Dick, MB, ChB, MRCP, MRCPath, Consultant in Clinical Immunology, Tissue Typing Department of Bacteriology, Royal Infirmary, Glasgow

Allan Downie, MB, ChB, FRCP, Consultant Neurologist, The Medical School, University of Aberdeen, Scotland

Marta Elian, MD, Consultant Neurophysiologist, Central Middlesex Hospital, London

J B Foster, MD, FRCP, Consultant Neurologist, Newcastle General Hospital, Newcastle upon Tyne

M Garraway, MB, MSc, MFCM, Senior Lecturer, Department of Community Medicine, University of Edinburgh

John Goodall, MRCP, Lewis Hospital, Stornoway, Isle of Lewis

P J Graham, FRCP, FRCPsych, Professor of Child Psychiatry, Institute of Child Health, The Hospital for Sick Children, London

Steven Haberman, MA, FIA, Lecturer in Actuarial Science, The City University, London

J Haine, MB, BS, Department of Geriatrics, Cumberland Infirmary, Carlisle

W Allen Hauser, MD, Associate Professor, Sergiersky Center, Columbia University, New York

W Bryan Jennett, MD, FRCS, FRSE, Professor of Neurosurgery, Institute of Neurological Sciences, Glasgow

Steven M Juergens, MD, Resident in Internal Medicine, Hennipen County Medical Center, Minneapolis, Minnesota

Reginald Kelly, MD, FRCP, Consultant Neurologist, St Thomas' Hospital, and National Hospital, Maida Vale, London

Leonard T Kurland, MD, DrPH, Professor and Chairman, Department of Medical Statistics and Epidemiology, Mayo Clinic and Mayo Medical School, Rochester, Minnesota, USA

J F Kurtzke, MD, Department of Neurology and Community Medicine, Georgetown University, and Chief, Neurology Service, Veterans Administration Medical Center, Washington DC, USA

K M Laurence, DSc, MB, ChB, FRCP, FRCPath, Department of Child Health, Welsh National School of Medicine, Cardiff

Hilda McLoughlin, Research Assistant, Medico-Social Research Board, Dublin

M G Marmot, MB, PhD, MPH, Department of Medical Statistics and Epidemiology, London School of Hygiene and Tropical Medicine, Keppel Street (Gower Street), London

Jørgen Marquardsen, MD, Department of Neurology, Aalborg Sygehus Syd., Aalborg, Denmark

T W Meade, BM, FRCP, FFCM, Director, Epidemiology and Medical Care Unit, Northwick Park Hospital, Harrow, Middlesex

J H D Millar, MD, FRCP, Consultant Neurologist, Royal Victoria and Claremont Stroke Hospitals, Belfast

D Mitchell, MB, BS, DRCOG, Department of Geriatrics, Cumberland Infirmary, Carlisle

Donald W Mulder, MD, Senior Consultant and Professor, Department of Neurology, Mayo Clinic and Mayo Medical School, Rochester, Minnesota

Haruo Okazaki, MD, Consultant, Department of Pathology and Anatomy, Mayo Clinic, Associate Professor of Pathology, Mayo Medical School, Rochester Minnesota

B O Osuntokun, BSc(Lond), PhD, MD, FRCP, FMCP, FWACP, FAS, Professor of Neurology, Department of Medicine, University of Ibadan, Ibadan, Nigeria

Catherine Peckham, MD, MFCM, Senior Lecturer, Department of Epidemiology and Community Medicine, Charing Cross Hospital Medical School, London

Naomi Richman, MB, MSc, MRCPsych, Senior Lecturer, Department of Child Psychiatry, Institute of Child Health, London

D F Roberts, Professor of Human Genetics, University of Newcastle upon Tyne

F Clifford Rose, FRCP, Consultant Neurologist, Charing Cross Hospital, London

Geoffrey A Rose, MA, DM, FRCP, FFCM, Professor of Epidemiology, Department of Medical Statistics and Epidemiology, London School of Hygiene and Tropical Medicine; Consultant Physician, St Mary's Hospital, London

Euan M Ross, MD, MRCP, DCH, Senior Lecturer in Child Health and Community Medicine, The Middlesex Hospital Medical School; Consultant Paediatrician, Central Middlesex Hospital, London

Michael Rutter, MD, FRCP, FRCPsych, Professor of Child and Adolescent Psychiatry, Institute of Psychiatry, University of London

Bruce S Schoenberg, MD, MPH, Head, Section on Neuro-epidemiology, National Institute of Neurological and Communicative Disorders and Stroke, Bethesda, Maryland 20205, USA

Devera A Schoenberg, MS, Research Neuro-epidemiologist, Bethesda, Maryland 20205, USA

David I Shepherd, MD(Hons), MRCP, Consultant Neurologist, North Manchester General Hospital, Crumpsall, Manchester M8 6RB. Formerly Sir Ashley Mackintosh Research Fellow, Department of Medicine, University of Aberdeen

D S Smith, FRCP, Consultant Physician in Rheumatology and Rehabilitation, Northwick Park Hospital, Harrow, Middlesex

Jim Stevenson, Research Fellow, Department of Child Psychiatry, Institute of Child Health, London

Luis Vassalo, MD, FRCP, University of Malta Medical School, Guardamangia, Malta

W E Waters, MB, FFCM, DIH, Professor of Community Medicine, University of Southampton

Jean M Weddell, MD, FFCM, Medical Planner, Allied Medical Group, Formerly Senior Lecturer, Department of Community Medicine, St. Thomas' Hospital Medical School, London

J P Whisnant, MD, Professor and Chairman, Department of Neurology, Mayo Clinic, USA

D R R Williams, MRC Research Fellow in Epidemiology, University Department of Community Medicine, Addenbrooke's Hospital, Cambridge

Foreword

The Medical Society of London was founded in 1773 by Dr John Coakley Lettsom (1744–1814). He was a West Indies-born Quaker who practised in London after apprenticeship to an apothecary in Yorkshire and further training in Edinburgh, Paris, and Leiden. Our elegant meeting-house at 11 Chandos Street, in the centre of London, is appropriately called Lettsom House and is well worth a visit because it is a history-of-medicine treasure trove and its Lettsom Library contains a priceless collection of rare medical books. This has been the central, historic and charming setting for a continuing series of Mansell Bequest Symposia, all of which have been organised by Dr F Clifford Rose.

Mrs Mansell had the harrowing experience of being a helpless but devoted and close witness to her husband's motor neurone disease so she left money to this Society to advance knowledge on neurological disease. Dr F Clifford Rose has certainly fulfilled the late Mrs Mansell's wishes for he has already organised splendid and satisfying symposia on 'Motor Neurone Disease' and on 'Clinical Neuro-immunology'. He now adds yet another dimension with this academic study of Neuroepidemiology. The Medical Society of London owes him a debt of gratitude for he has also been an effective Secretary, Councillor, Vice-President, and the 1980 Lettsom Lecturer.

The Mansell Neurological Symposia are, and will continue to be, major annual academic contributions to a wide international field of neurology and medicine.

D Geraint James
President,
Medical Society of London

Preface

To many people epidemiology suggests the study of infectious diseases. The etymological derivation of the word is the study (logos) among (epi) people (demos): this means it is concerned with populations rather than individuals. Some of its principles were recognised in biblical and Hippocratic times but its scientific value could only have been realised on a statistical basis.

It was in England that this era was initiated. Following an outbreak of Plague in 1603, a custom was established in the City of London to record christenings and burials. John Gaunt, the son of a London draper, in his spare time studied these weekly records and published an analysis in 1662 in a book entitled *Natural and Political Observations made upon the Bills of Mortality*. Gaunt's pioneering work eventually led in the nineteenth century to the proof of an environmental factor as a cause of disease. This, too, occurred in London when John Snow stopped a cholera epidemic by removing the handle from a pump giving sewage-contaminated water.

Since then, the medical practitioner has gradually become aware that the study of groups can help the individual patient, hence the use of the word clinical in the title of this book to emphasise the value of epidemiology at the bedside.

The epidemiology of neurological disease is of more recent origin and, although the contributors to this book are from several countries, it is the first on neuro-epidemiology produced in Britain; if it acts as an incentive to further studies in this field, its purpose will have been well served.

F.C.R.
London, 1979

Part I   General Aspects

Chapter 1

A REVIEW OF STATISTICAL METHODS

Bernard Benjamin

Epidemiology was defined as 'the science of the infective diseases—their prime causes, propagation and prevention and more especially their epidemic manifest-ations' [1]. It is today massively extended in scope from its original concept, which was designed to deal with the great pestilences of the nineteenth century— the crowd diseases arising from emergent industrialisation and growing urbanis-ation. The concept has become extended from the study of the spread of infection from person to person to the study of the distribution of all diseases, whether infectious or not, in terms of their relative prevalence in different segments of the community; this was in order to isolate the demographic or environmental factors so that preventive medicine could benefit and public health policy develop.

Two fundamental aspects, however, have not changed, First, there is still the same objective of preventive medicine, sadly undervalued as it is in the modern health service. Second, though computers have greatly facilitated the application of more recondite and more rigorous mathematical methods, the basic pattern of the statistical methodology remains unchanged, ie the comparison of morbidity or mortality between two groups similar in most (ideally in all) respects other than the involvement of a factor suspected to be of aetiological significance or, in the case of studies of outcome, of prognostic significance.

It was by these methods that Farr [2], as long ago as 1854 (and long before the isolation of the vibrio), demonstrated the water-borne character of cholera.

Table I

Water supply	No. of persons	Cholera deaths	Rate/1000
From the Thames at Battersea — 3.5 grains of organic matter per gallon	266,500	2284	8.57
From the Thames at Thames Ditton — 1.4 grains of organic matter per gallon	173,700	294	1.69

Were the groups comparable? As Farr explained—

'The Lambeth company had, in January 1852, wisely removed its source of supply to a part of the Thames above Teddington Lock; another company lingered on its old site; and the epidemic cholera of 1854, therefore, found parts of the population of London on the south side of the river in very different conditions; the one supplied with very impure water by the Southwark company; the other supplied with water much less impure by the Lambeth company. The companies had been in competition and they often supplied the same streets and districts, so their customers were nearly in all respects in the same sanitary conditions with one exception; a gallon of the Southwark water contained 3.5 grains of organic matter and a gallon of the Lambeth water only 1.4 grains.'

It need only be added that between 1855 and 1857, six of the London Water Companies were compelled by Parliament to improve the quality of their water; a process that was accelerated more by the regular publication of analyses in the weekly tables of the Registrar-General than by any instruction or inspection.

Over one hundred years later, Bradford Hill and Doll [3] demonstrated the link between lung cancer and the smoking of manufactured cigarettes in exactly the same way. They followed up, from 1951, some 40000 men and women medical practitioners, who agreed to keep records of their smoking habits. They were able to demonstrate that mortality from lung cancer (and a number of other diseases) was heavier in smokers than in non-smokers; that the excess mortality was much greater for cigarette smokers than for pipe or cigar smokers and (a very important point) was proportional to the quantity of cigarettes smoked; and that the excess mortality was smaller for those who had smoked but had given up. The groups compared were standardised for age and were similar in occupational and social respects *except* for their smoking habits. The Doll and Hill Report (1964) is a classic for statistical readers for both the careful statistical organisation applied and the thoroughness with which possible sources of bias were eliminated in the final analyses.

These epidemiological investigations usually begin because something happens to stimulate the enquiring mind. This may be provoked by a sudden rise in deaths from a particular disease, an excessive mortality from a particular disease in a particular occupation or social group (as shown for example, by the periodical occupational mortality investigations of the Registrar-General), an increased reference to hospital out-patient departments, a rise in national insurance sickness claims, or reports from general practitioners of a cluster of cases with the same new complex of symptoms. Or it may be that someone in general or hospital practice notices a recurring pattern in the medical histories of patients presenting with a particular abnormality.

The first reaction to this stimulus may be to look retrospectively at the differences in environment, culture or inheritance (in the case of a suspected genetic factor) between those affected by the disease and those who have not been affected. Sometimes the association is so overwhelmingly strong as to leave no doubts as to

3

the influences of a particular aetiological prognostic factor. Over 150 years ago John Snow [4] looked at the water drinking habits of those who died from cholera in the locality of the Broad Street well and those who escaped. The result of this enquiry was, to quote his own words, that 'there had been no particular outbreak or increase of cholera except among the persons who were in the habit of drinking the water of the Broad Street pump-well.' As a result, without further ado, the pump handle was removed, even though there was still an unwillingness generally to accept that the disease was water-borne. (All this occurred long before bacteriology had developed and before the vibrio had been isolated.)

Even today there are quick convictions, as in the case of some industrial carcinogens, and immediate preventive action is taken. However, retrospective studies are more often not conclusive, simply because they are retrospective, ie they are concerned with patients who *have already* exhibited disease and whose past experience has to be examined for exposure to the suspected environmental factor. This approach has three main defects. First, the requisite data may not have been recorded or, even if recorded, indifferently so. As the factor at the time of documentation had not come under suspicion of being aetiologically important, there would have been no incentive to record its presence nor to expend much effort in recording it carefully or in a standard manner. Even if carefully recorded, the data are unlikely to be in the form specific to some, at that time, unconceived experiment. Secondly, since the retrospective study group is identified by disease and not by free selection it is difficult to find an appropriate group for comparison; for example, a test group may be taken from hospital patients diagnosed as suffering from disease X and their occupational experience may be examined. This experience may then be compared with hospital patients admitted for diseases other than X. Will this latter group be representative of *all* those who do not suffer from disease X whether or not admitted to hospital for some other reason? Hospital patients are 'sick' people and are unlikely to be representative of the general population. If, alternatively, an attempt is made to select controls from the general population there is the problem of identifying those who have *not* suffered disease X. A third defect of the retrospective study is that observation is taking place late in the chain of events leading to frank disease. This is particularly true of studies based upon death. It is difficult at such a late stage to establish the time of onset of disease and even more difficult to establish the environmental conditions specifically antecedent to onset [5].

The prospective study, ie a follow-up of a representative population sample in respect of which environmental conditions are concurrently observed, provides the opportunity of observing the emergence of the first symptoms of disease in those initially free of disease; the point of observation is close to the intervention of the actual environmental condition associated with the onset of disease. It is further possible not only to establish the facts of occurrence of disease and of the concurrent level of risk factors but also the prognostic effect of medical intervention and of environmental changes. But although it is important to stress the superiority of the prospective study, it is also necessary to bear in mind that the retrospective method has often provided valid results and that, given the resources available, it may be the only method available. If a retrospective study *can* give

4

sufficient results it is to be preferred as being very much cheaper and quicker than a prospective study. The basic statistical method—the comparison of groups—is the same in both the retrospective and the prospective study. The main difference in the method is not statistical; it is simply that the prospective study is more controllable and is likely to be more rigorous while, on the other hand, it entails a great deal of administrative organisation.

Multivariate Analysis

There is a statistical problem involved in all investigations of the influence of environmental conditions and various risk factors. It is extremely difficult to distinguish the separate operation of the social, economic and cultural factors that make up the whole complex of the human environment. The better-off people are also those who are well-educated, in managerial or professional occupations, and in high-class housing. They can afford to avoid atmospheric pollution, and inclement weather conditions, to take long holidays, to eat well, to retire at an early age, to get better medical treatment. All these advantages operate simultaneously, eg it is difficult to find people in good housing who are not also well-nourished, so that every factor is confounded by the effects of others. It would ideally be desirable to replicate in the human population the plot experimentation of agricultural scientists but human beings are not like plants and cannot be allocated to precisely defined conditions permitting the clear separation of the different effects. One has to take a population that is to be analysed as it is found, with groups chosen to exhibit a particular condition but with other attributes present to an extent which cannot be predetermined.

Considerable advance has been made in the development of mathematical techniques of multivariate analysis, especially because computers have made much more manageable the calculations involved. Techniques of principal component analysis and cluster analysis do enable us now to discern patterns of social conditions. These patterns represent the simplest descriptions possible of the social and economic stereotype clusters in the population.

Such methods are basically taxonomic but they are enormously effective in isolating risk groups. They enable to be set up longitudinal studies that are as analogous as is practicable to the plot experimentation of the agricultural scientists. The real touchstone is whether action based on the tested hypothesis effectively removes the risk that is being attacked; for example, the removal of the handle of the Broad Street pump which ended a cholera outbreak, or the insistence of daily baths for chimney sweeps, which drastically reduced the incidence of cancer of the scrotum.

These sophisticated methods are directed to the simple objective outlined at the outset of this paper, namely, to attempt to so classify data that it is possible to make comparisons in which all factors are standardised except for the one effect that is under investigation. It follows that we must seek data that *are* so classifiable. Failure properly to take account of other variables can produce misleading results, and results that can never be reproduced by later workers. At one time it was shown that, in a typical urban area, cases of tuberculosis were not randomly distributed but showed a tendency to occur in closely neighbouring houses, indicating a high risk of infection 'over the garden wall'. However, a study of the home addresses of workers employed in the same factory showed that they were not randomly distributed but tended to live adjacent to others. It then appeared more likely that the disease was spread over the work bench, and little more was heard of the garden wall scare.

The Raw Materials

As already noted, most epidemiological investigations begin with macroscopic observation based on population statistics of morbidity and mortality. The mortality statistics based upon death registration in the United Kingdom have reached a high level of refinement, but the availability of morbidity statistics still leaves much to be desired; they are patchy and their use calls for much medical and statistical insight. The widest base is provided by national sickness insurance records, which are claims on insurance during absence from work on account of sickness certified by a medical practitioner. Their use is subject to a number of statistical reservations. When a man decides to absent himself from employment and whether or not he claims depends not only on his physical state but also on a number of economic and psychological considerations. The frankness of the medical practitioner in certifying the cause of absence is inhibited by awareness that the employee *and* his employer will read it. Nevertheless, the Department of Health and Social Security do produce regular analyses of samples of these certificates and skilled handling enables a tremendous amount of epidemiological information to be extracted at least as a starting point. A special enquiry into the incidence of incapacity for work in different areas and occupations was published in 1965 [6] and this quarry is still being mined [7].

Although there are statistics of general practice, they are not as yet on a comprehensive and continuing basis, though the Royal College of General Practitioners is working effectively to this end. The last extensive survey [8] was published in 1974 and was based on the clinical records of 140 general practices in England and Wales in the year May 1970 to April 1971; this was a joint venture of the College of General Practitioners and the Department of Health and Social Security and its object was to measure the amount and pattern of sickness dealt with in general practice. The population covered was nationally representative in sex, age, and geographical distribution. The most important measure calculated was the patient-consulting rate, ie the proportion of patients consulting at least once during the year, and this rate was calculated specific to disease, sex, age, region and occupation. There has, in addition, been a succession of studies from individual practices. The earliest of these, which still makes fascinating reading, was that of William Pickles in 1939 [9], and another pioneer study was that by Fry in 1952 [10].

Information about sickness treated in hospital is provided by the Hospital Activity Analysis [11] maintained routinely by the Department of Health and Social Security. This is a continuing total analysis of in-patient discharge summaries. For specific diseases, discharge rates (virtually admission rates) can be provided for broad sex and age groups even down to hospital level. Information is also gathered about operations performed and about occupation.

There is a national cancer register based on voluntary notification from treatment centres and maintained by the Office of Population Censuses and Surveys, and also a national psychiatric register based on admissions to psychiatric beds and maintained by the Department of Health and Social Security.

An important new development has been the creation of the General Household Survey (GHS), a continuing periodical sample survey of the general population resident in private households, carried out by the Office of Population Censuses and Surveys. The survey aims to provide a means of examining relationships between the most significant variables with which social policy is concerned and of monitoring changes in these relationships over time [12]. Since its inception, very little use has been made of the GHS for morbidity measurement as such, although it has been used to measure demands on the health services and also, by providing information on possession of cars, telephones, central heating and consumer durables, to give more definition to the socio-economic groups used in mortality analysis. It has also been used to provide information on smoking habits. We may yet see a revival of the Sickness Survey which ran so successfully during and after the Second World War only to be abandoned hastily as an economy measure in the early 1950s. But none of these sources of data could be more than a starting point. Only rarely would these records contain a sufficient range of information to provide the multivariate classification for which we have stressed the need. There would be much wrong if it were otherwise, for it would mean that records designed primarily for limited health administration purposes were being loaded, like a Christmas tree, with a goody for everybody. This would be wasteful and it would not even work. The records would be of poor quality since they would not be there for any specific purpose and no one would be interested in seeing that they were properly maintained; moreover, even if the data were wastefully there 'just in case they might be needed', they would be unlikely to be in the right format for a particular enquiry. At least it has never yet happened. It really is essential to design records specifically directed to the hypothesis that is to be tested. The secret of designing good research records is to prepare in skeleton the statistical tables that will be required and to work backwards from there, taking due account of data processing requirements.

Time and numbers are both problems that test the patience of the epidemiologist. If, as is often the case, the disease to be investigated is of medium or low frequency of occurrence, then it may be some considerable time before the test group can produce sufficient occurrences to support the degree of cross-classification that may be necessary. It is better to wait until the data are sufficient than to rush out with findings that are statistically unreliable and may be invalidated by later work on larger numbers, especially if in the meantime an unnecessary scare has been caused. This would not be a problem if there were limitless numbers of subjects available for follow-up, but numbers are usually severely limited. In a prospective study the cost of keeping in touch with, and of arranging examinations of people, ten per cent of whom change their address every year, are high. Moreover, with-

7

drawals are selective and an attempt has to be made to discover just how selective they are. Again, it is necessary to guess the order of size of the risks that are to be measured, and from there to work backwards to the minimum size of population that will produce reliable results. It has to be remembered that computers and sophisticated statistical techniques add nothing to either the quality or the quantity of the original data.

Computers are helpful, and may even be essential, in handling the sheer drudgery of multifactorial analysis. But a well-planned study hardly needs much in the way of mathematics, often no more than what Sir Austin Bradford Hill used to call 'arithmetic with logic'. William Farr, no mean mathematician, would have agreed.

References

1 Stallybrass, CO (1931) *The Principles of Epidemiology*. S. Routledge and Son, London
2 Farr, W (1855) Appendix to 17th Report of Registrar-General for England and Wales. HMSO
3 Doll, R and Bradford Hill, A (1964) *Brit. Med. J., 1899,* 1460
4 Snow, J (1855) *The Mode of Communication of Cholera.* London
5 Benjamin, B (1965) *Social and Economic Factors effecting Mortality.* Mouton & Co., The Hague
6 Ministry of Pensions and National Insurance (1965) Report on an Enquiry into the Incidence of Incapacity for Work. HMSO
7 Daw, RH (1971) *J. Inst. Act., 97,* 17
8 Royal College of General Practitioners and the Department of Health and Social Security (1974) *Morbidity Statistics from General Practice. A Second National Study 1970-71.* HMSO
9 Pickles, WB (1939) *Epidemiology in a Country Practice.* John Wright, Bristol
10 Fry, J (1952) *Brit. Med. J., 2,* 249
11 Benjamin, B Ed (1977) *Medical Records.* William Heinemann Medical Books, London
12 Office of Population Censuses and Surveys (1974) *The General Household Survey 1975.* HMSO

Chapter 2

A MATHEMATICAL APPROACH TO THE INCIDENCE
AND PREVALENCE OF DISEASE

Steven Haberman

Although the concepts of incidence and prevalence of disease are widely discussed in the literature of epidemiology and vital statistics, there has been little attempt at a unified, mathematical presentation of the basic definitions and their inter-relationships. We have attempted to remedy this deficiency and have reported detailed results and proofs elsewhere [1-3]. In this chapter we propose to summarise the principal findings and indicate how they may be applied to actual incidence and prevalence data, with particular reference to cerebrovascular disease.

1. Introduction

We shall consider the morbidity of a single disease X.

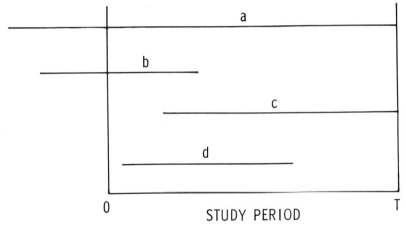

Figure 1 Flow of cases of Disease X in a follow-up study

Consider a population that is observed for an arbitrary period from $t = 0$ to $t = T$. Then the cases of X identified may be classified with respect to time into four groups (Figure 1), namely:

(*a*) those existing before $t = 0$, continuing throughout the interval and still existing at $t = T$;

9

(b) those existing before $t = 0$, and terminating during the interval;
(c) those arising during the interval and still existing at $t = T$;
(d) those arising during the interval and terminating before the end of the interval.

The incidence rate for X over this period may be determined from (c) and (d). To compute any of the prevalence rates necessitates all four categories, unless preexisting cases are specifically excluded from the investigation, as it often is with epidemiological studies [4]. It should be noted that a description of these four categories requires a full knowledge of the types of decrement (eg death, recovery) to which the group of persons currently sick with X is subjected.

2. Definitions

For convenience, we shall assume in our illustrations below that cases of X existing before $t = 0$, ie groups (a) and (b), have been excluded from study. The definitions of the four main morbidity measures, expressed in terms of a single disease X, are given below. Accompanying each measure is a pictorial representation of the flow of cases of X that are of interest. The definitions are as follows [5, 6]:

(i) *the central incidence rate:* the number of persons who start at least one episode of sickness due to X during a defined period, divided by the average number of persons exposed to the risk of sickness during the period (Figure 2);

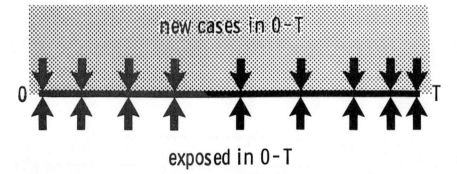

Figure 2 Calculation of incidence rates

(ii) *the point prevalence rate:* the number of persons who are sick from X at a given point in time divided by the number of persons exposed to risk at that time (Figure 3);
(iii) *the period prevalence rate:* the number of persons who are sick from X some time during the defined period divided by the number of persons exposed to the risk of being sick during that period (Figure 4);
(iv) *the cumulative prevalence rate:* the number of persons who are sick from X some time during a defined period and are alive at the end of the period,

10

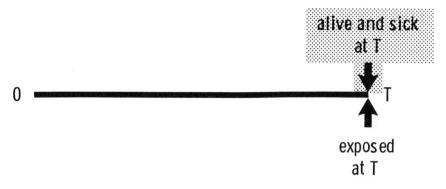

Figure 3 Calculation of point prevalence rates

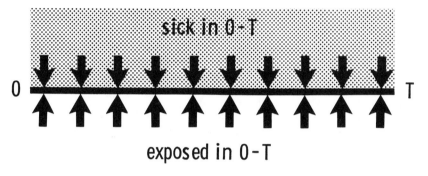

Figure 4 Calculation of period prevalence rates

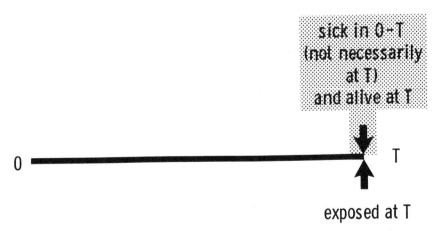

Figure 5 Calculation of cumulative prevalence rates

11

divided by the number of persons exposed to risk at the end of the period (Figure 5).

These four indices are the measures of incidence and prevalence in most common use in epidemiological studies.

3. Comments

The numerators of the above rates may be defined in terms of episodes of sickness, rather than persons.

If the restriction of considering only one disease, X, is waived, then the numerators may, alternatively, be defined in terms of diseases or episodes.

Thus, consider a person who suffers in one calendar year from disease X twice, and from disease Y three times (each attack being at separate points of time). Then he contributes to measures based on—

persons   1 unit
diseases 2 units
episodes 5 units

With the rates defined in section 2 above, persons who begin more than one episode of sickness due to X during the period of observation must be counted only once in the incidence rate. The same is true for persons who experience more than one spell of sickness due to X during the observation period and their contribution to the period and cumulative prevalence rates.

An alternative form of incidence measure is the *initial* incidence rate defined as in section 2 above, except that the denominator is the number of persons exposed to the risk of sickness at the beginning of the study period.

The cumulative prevalence rate is a hybrid in that it effectively uses the numerator of the period rate, with recoveries excluded, together with the denominator of the point rate. It has been used in longitudinal studies of chronic diseases [7] and investigations into infectious diseases [8]. It is considered a legitimate measure for those diseases where the incidence of sickness sets into motion an irreversible train of events [8].

All the rates, except the point prevalence rate, explicitly refer to a time interval, which must be precisely specified if the rates are to be correctly interpreted.

Great care must be taken with the definition of an episode of sickness—in particular with the points of time that mark the beginning and termination of the episode, eg admission and discharge from hospital, or cessation and resumption of full-time work. Exact specification of the endpoints is crucial to making valid rate estimates and to comparing the results of studies where these endpoints may be defined differently.

The point prevalence is often called 'the proportion of persons sick from X at a point of time'. This is not a valid interpretation of the cumulative prevalence rate. However, the complement of the cumulative prevalence rate is widely employed, namely the proportion of persons alive at the end of the period who were never sick from X during the period.

A list of the possible uses of these rates is given in [9].

4. Prevalence and Incidence

From these definitions, we see that the notion of incidence relates to the emergence of new cases of the disease, whereas prevalence relates to the number of persons who are sick at a point of time or over a period. Thus, the former is a 'flow' statistic, whereas the latter is a 'stock' statistic, to use the nomenclature of demography [10]. A comparison between prevalence and incidence is thus similar to a comparison between modes of data collection in demography (the census and vital registration of events) and in accountancy (the balance sheet and revenue account).

Despite the well-defined distinction between the concepts of incidence and prevalence, and between the types of prevalence rate, it is not uncommon for epidemiological papers to develop prevalence rates without stating which type they are using, and also to confuse incidence and prevalence. (For example, Kurtzke [11], reviewing stroke incidence rates, directly referred to the period prevalence rates derived by Logan and Cushion [12] as though they constituted incidence rates, and mentioned no assumptions made nor errors thereby introduced.)

5. Morbidity Measurement of Chronic Diseases

Chronic diseases (for example, cerebrovascular disease) are characterised by being present for long periods, but having intermittent, acute episodes of illness. Thus, longitudinal studies, which aim to follow a community over a long period, are an important source of information about the progress of these conditions. Although incidence rates are the more fundamental concept, it may be easier to determine one of the prevalence rates for a chronic disease being studied longitudinally. But the interpretation of prevalence rates, and any attempt to qualify relationships between these rates and clinical and demographic attributes (for example, sex, age, race, socioeconomic status, geographical region) may be seriously affected by the dynamic course of the chronic disease. In addition, the use of prevalence rates for inferring relationships between the underlying incidence rates and such variables will be affected. Sartwell and Merrell [13] have identified cases where such sources of bias have arisen or may arise. The following are three examples—

(a) A disease may have a more rapidly fatal course in one group relative to another. Prevalence rates may be approximately equal, although the incidence rates are higher for the first group (eg, tuberculosis in Negroes and whites in US).
(b) Improvements in therapy may shorten the course of a disease by producing a more rapid recovery, or they may lengthen the course by controlling rather than curing the disease. In both cases, prevalence rates and not incidence rates will be affected. This effect often hinders the study of time trends.
(c) Two groups may have the same incidence rates, but an external factor operating in one group to make the disease more benign and hence of longer duration would push up the prevalence rates.

13

It would seem preferable to consider incidence rates and avoid these sources of bias. However, the interpretation of incidence rates may also be hindered since one may be observing a 'detection rate', lower than the genuine incidence rate. Of the cases with onset in the time period under consideration, some will be discovered early, others late (perhaps at death) and others escape detection. So the detection rate for a period will include cases with onsets spread over a long time span and will depend on the clinical level at which the cases are discovered. In addition, hospital-based studies may fail to recognise all the incident cases of the disease unless there is in use a medical record indexing and retrieval system similar to that used for several decades in the vicinity of Rochester, Minnesota [7].

6. Mathematical Approach

We shall now consider some of the relationships that may be derived by representing the occurrence of a disease in a population by a simple mathematical model.

It is possible [1] to find expressions for each of the three prevalence rates in terms of the underlying incidence rates.

We shall consider a disease X and persons aged y in a population that has been followed prospectively for years since birth (at time zero). The results can be generalised to incorporate an age at entry greater than zero [1]. We shall need the following definitions—

Let B_y be the number of persons aged y (at time y) alive who are suffering from X at that age.

Let C_y be the number of persons who become sick from X at some time during the y year period.

Let D_y be the number of persons aged y (at time y) alive who were sick from X at some time during the previous y years.

Let E_y be the number of persons aged y (at time y) who are exposed to the risk of catching X during the y year period.

Let N_y be the total number of persons in the community aged y (at time y).

Then, from the definitions of section 2 above (p. 10) the point prevalence rate at time y is R_y, where

$$R_y = B_y/N_y \qquad \text{(eqn 1)}$$

The period prevalence rate at time y is S_y where

$$S_y = C_y/N_y \qquad \text{(eqn 2)}$$

The cumulative prevalence rate at time y is T_y, where

$$T_y = D_y/N_y \qquad \text{(eqn 3)}$$

It may be proven that [1]

C_y = number of days of sickness occurring in the population during the y year period $\qquad \text{(eqn 4)}$

We shall call the right-hand side of (eqn 4) d_y. Then the period prevalence rate S_y is given by

$$S_y = d_y/E_y \qquad \text{(eqn 5)}$$

14

Without altering the value of this expression, we may introduce F into both the numerator and denominator of the above, namely

$$S_y = F(d_y)/FE_y \qquad \text{(eqn 6)}$$

If F is chosen to be the average proportion of persons falling sick during the period, then FE_y represents the average number of persons who are sick during the period, and the term in brackets is clearly the average period of sickness for those who are sick during the y year period. We have, therefore, factorised the period prevalence rate into
(a) the average proportion of persons falling sick during the period, and
(b) the average period of their sickness.
This corresponds to the often quoted result of H Dorn [14] that the period prevalence rate is the product of average incidence and average duration in the sick population.
We have shown that, under certain assumptions about the nature of the community under study, simple integrals may be derived for both the period prevalence rate, R_y, and the cumulative prevalence rate, T_y [1]. An alternative approach would be to use the differential calculus.
If we assume that:
(i) the recovery rate from X may be taken as zero,
(ii) the survival rate for persons without X is equal to the survival rate for persons of the same age and is taken at random from the total population
then, it may be proved [1] that

$$R_y = T_y = 1 - \prod_{s=0}^{y-1}(1 - j_s) \qquad \text{(eqn 7)}$$

$$\text{i.e. } R_y = T_y = 1 - \left\{ (1 - j_0)(1 - j_1)\dots(1 - j_{y-1}) \right\}$$

where j_s is the initial annual incidence rate for age s.
These formulae are similar to some basic compound interest formulae [15] relating discount rates to present values, and to some basic life table formulae. The analogy between prevalence and the life table is being explored further.
If j's are small relative to unity then (eqn 9) may be approximated by

$$R_y = T_y = \sum_{s=0}^{y-1} j_s$$

This approximate relationship (ie, that point or cumulative prevalence is equal to the sum of the underlying incidence rates) has an intuitive appeal. The importance of the derivation in (eqn 1) is to focus on the assumptions needed for the approximation to be a reasonable one.
A numerical example furnishes some idea of the accuracy of this approximation. If $y = 5$, and the j's are 1.0, 1.1, 1.2, 1.3, 1.4 per 1000 pa, then the exact formula gives $R_5 = 5.99$ per 1000, and the approximate one gives $R_5 = 6.00$ per 1000. If the j's are 10, 20, 30, 40, 50 per 1000 pa then the exact formula gives $R_5 = 141.72$ per 1000, and the approximate one gives $R_5 = 150.00$ per 1000 (an error of about 6 per cent).

15

The assumption that the recovery rate may be taken as zero is justified as a first approximation where the onset of illness constitutes an irreversible event. This may be realistic for serious chronic conditions. Thus, the Joint Committee for Stroke Facilities [16] suggested that only 10 per cent of the survivors of acute cerebrovascular disease 'would be able to return to work virtually without impairment'.

7. Mathematical Representation of Incidence Rates

The source of incidence data for this section is the continuing investigation of the natural history of cerebrovascular disease being carried out at Rochester, Minnesota [7, 17]. Annual age-specific incidence rates are shown in Table I, for ages over 35.

A graphical examination of the rates in Table I and analysis of their first differences suggested that an exponential model of the Gompertz [18] or Makeham [19] type would provide a reasonable representation.

$$\text{The Gompertz model for } j_s \text{ is } j_s = Bc^s \qquad \text{(eqn 8)}$$

$$\text{The Makeham model for } j_s \text{ is } j_s = A + Bc^s \qquad \text{(eqn 9)}$$

where A, B and c are constants to be determined by the fitting process. An illustration of a Makeham-type is given in Figure 6.

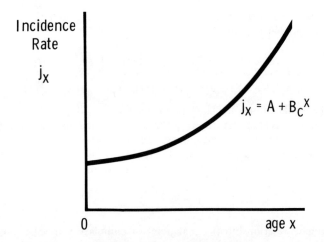

Figure 6 Curve for incidence rates

If Gompertz's model is suitable, then the ratio of incidence rates at successive ages is constant, and equal to c, ie

$$\frac{j_{x+1}}{j_x} = c$$

c is usually greater than unity. This corresponds to the wearing out of the human body being paralleled by an exponential increase in incidence of disease X. Such a feature is particularly apt for chronic, degenerative diseases.

16

These curves were fitted to the j_s values given in Table I. The Gompertz equation was fitted by using the method of least squares applied to $\log_{10} j_s$, and the Makeham equation was fitted by using the graduation method proposed by Benjamin and Haycocks [20]. The values of the constants are shown in Table II and the expected incidence rates in Table III. All eight curves provide a statistically significant fit to the data ($p < 0.05$).

TABLE I: Incidence Rates (per 1000 pa) for Rochester Study

Study period	Sex	Race	Age group	All strokes	Cerebral infarction only
1945–54 [17]	Both	White	35–44	0.34	0.08
			45–54	1.59	1.08
			55–64	3.69	2.47
			65–74	10.81	8.20
			Over 75	24.94	20.84
1955–69 [7]	Both	White	35–44	0.35	0.17
			45–54	1.10	0.72
			55–64	3.64	2.77
			65–74	7.91	6.32
			Over 75	21.56	17.86

TABLE II: Curve Fitting of Rochester Incidence Rates

No.	Study period	Disease	Curve	Value of constants		
1	1945–54	All strokes	Gompertz	B=0.006429	c=1.1108	
2	1945–54	Cerebral infarction	Gompertz	B=0.000768	c=1.1405	
3	1945–54	All strokes	Makeham	A=0.03828	B=0.01376	c=1.1029
4	1945–54	Cerebral infarction	Makeham	A=0.003665	B=0.00761	c=1.1110
5	1955–69	All strokes	Gompertz	B=0.006518	c=1.1075	
6	1955–69	Cerebral infarction	Gompertz	B=0.002045	c=1.1237	
7	1955–69	All strokes	Makeham	A=0.6196	B=0.02811	c=1.0868
8	1955–69	Cerebral infarction	Makeham	A=0.5678	B=0.01821	c=1.0899

TABLE III: Expected Incidence Rates (per 1000 pa)

No of fit	Age group				
	35–44	45–54	55–64	65–74	Over 75
1	0.43	1.23	3.52	10.06	28.76
2	0.15	0.55	2.05	7.65	28.49
3	0.55	1.48	3.86	9.94	25.53
4	0.32	0.91	2.61	7.46	21.37
5	0.39	1.08	2.99	8.30	23.06
6	0.21	0.65	2.06	6.54	20.70
7	0.16	1.17	3.48	8.79	20.96
8	0.01	0.79	2.64	7.02	17.39

Work is in progress which involves the fitting of models (eqn 8) and (eqn 9) to all the sets of incidence rates for cerebrovascular disease reported from community-based and hospital-based studies, and then a comparison of the values of the parameters A, B and c resulting from this procedure.

8. Mathematical Representation of Prevalence Results

We shall use the results of the previous section to represent the cumulative prevalence rates reported by the Rochester stroke investigation [7] and presented in Table IV. In order to proceed further, we shall need to define the following probabilities:

P_s is the probability that a person aged s in the community will not die between ages s and $s + 1$

$\widetilde{P}_s$ is the probability that a person aged s with X will not die from X between ages s and $s + 1$

Each of these is a probability of survival over one year. We shall assume that the one-year probability of survival for a person with X aged s is proportional to the one-year probability of survival for a person of the same age and taken at random from the whole community. We shall assume that the proportionality factor, α, is constant, that is, α is independent of s [2]. Of course, $0 < \alpha < 1$. So our assumption may be written:

$$\widetilde{P}_s = \alpha \cdot P_s \qquad \text{(eqn 10)}$$

This assumption has been investigated in detail by Cutler and Axtell [21], who suggested that a value of α close to unity indicates that some subgroup of the patient cohort have been 'cured' (eg, localised cancer of the cervix) but a value of $\alpha < 1$ is a feature of a true chronic disease (eg, regional cancer of the breast where $\alpha = 0.93$).

From the survival experience of the Framingham study [2], sex-specific survival rates are available, and it is possible to compute values of α for use in (eqn 10) [2]. The values to be used are 0.867 for white men and 0.931 for white women.

TABLE IV: Cumulative Prevalence Rates for all Strokes from Rochester [7] (per 1000)

Age group	Year			
	1955	1960	1965	1970
35–44	0.96	1.32	1.58	1.98
45–54	4.69	3.32	3.79	4.41
55–64	14.11	20.11	13.37	8.08
65–74	29.38	36.99	43.44	35.60
Over 75	57.84	79.15	81.80	59.69

18

If we assume that the initial incidence rate j_s may be represented by a Makeham (eqn 9), then we may obtain the following expression for T_y:

$$T_y = \frac{A(1 - \alpha^n)}{\log_e(1/\alpha)} + Bc^y \frac{(1 - (\alpha/c)^n}{\log_e(c/\alpha)} \qquad \text{(eqn 11)}$$

where n refers to the period of follow-up.

The Rochester study began in 1945, and did not specifically follow longitudinally a group of births. The prevalence rates shown in Table IV were computed after 10, 15, 20 and 25 years of follow-up, so the value of n in (eqn 11) is 10, 15, 20 and 25 respectively.

Over the 25-year period of the study, the incidence rates decreased with time. However, in order to simplify the calculations this trend was not allowed for, the A, B, c values being those applicable to the 1955-69 experience for all strokes as fitted by the Makeham model (number 7 in Tables II and III).

TABLE V: Computed Cumulative Prevalence Rates (per 1000) for Rochester Study (Method 1)
(From Haberman [2] with permission)

Age group	Prevalence Date			
	1955 (n=10)	1960 (n=15)	1965(n=20)	1970(n=25)
35–44	0.9 (94)	0.8 (165)	0.6 (263)	0.6 (330)
45–54	4.8 (102)	5.1 (65)	5.2 (73)	5.1 (86)
55–64	14.4 (98)	15.6 (129)	16.0 (84)	16.1 (50)
65–74	37.3 (79)	41.0 (90)	42.3 (103)	42.7 (83)
75–84	92.6 (62)	102.0 (78)	105.4 (78)	106.7 (56)

(Figures in parentheses denote 100 X the ratio of the actual prevalence rates to those computed.)

The results are shown in Table V. The figures in parentheses denote the percentage ratios between the actual and computed rates. The representation of the actual prevalence rates is fair, the difference being caused probably by the smallness of the data base and the stringent assumptions made in the development of the theory [2]. In addition, the omission of the downward time trend in incidence rates causes the computed rates to overstate the prevalence rates at the end of the period.

An alternative way of relating cumulative prevalence rates to incidence rates is to use (eqn 7), namely

$$1 - T_y = \prod_{s=0}^{y-1} (1 - j_s) \qquad \text{(eqn 7)}$$

The data in Table I constitute the j_s. In order to allow for the downward trend in incidence rates, the age-specific rates quoted for the period 1955-69 were adjusted by the factors given below to provide age-specific rates for each of the constituent

19

quinquennia. The factors were calculated from the crude incidence rates for the three quinquennia [7].

Period	Trend Factor
1955–59	1.117
1960–64	1.026
1965–69	0.903

The results, from the above compounding process, are given in Table VI, in the same form as Table V. The fit of the resulting calculated prevalence rates was poorer than that of the rates in Table V.

TABLE VI: Computed Cumulative Prevalence Rates (per 1000) for Rochester Study (Method 2) (From Haberman [2] with permission)

Age group	1955 (n=10)	Prevalence Date 1960 (n=15)	1965(n=20)	1970(n=25)
35–44	1.8 (53)	2.0 (68)	2.3 (70)	2.3 (88)
45–54	9.6 (49)	8,9 (37)	7.6 (50)	7.2 (61)
55–64	26.1 (54)	33.7 (60)	27.2 (49)	23.8 (34)
65–74	70.2 (42)	74.4 (50)	72.3 (60)	61.5 (58)
75–84	165.3 (35)	195.6 (40)	172.3 (47)	159.1 (38)

(Figures in parentheses denote 100 X the ratio of the actual prevalence rates to those computed.)

The poor fit of the models (in particular, of Table VI) may indicate the presence of errors in the prevalence data of Table IV under analysis. Despite an increasing length of study, the actual cumulative prevalence rates in later periods are lower than in earlier quinquennia. N Matsumoto and his colleagues [7] suggest that the cause is probably the secular downward trend in incidence rates and the improvement in long-term survivorship rates. Thus, Garraway and associates [22] have reported a 45 per cent fall in the age-adjusted incidence rate over the period 1945 to 1974 in the Rochester study, and an increase in the 5-year survival rate from 0.33 (1945–9) to 0.49 (1970–4).

9. Stochastic Approach

We have used the Poisson Process [22] to represent the flow of incident cases for a disease X [3]. The Poisson Process has been used with great success to represent random, rare events; for example, the disintegration of nuclear particles, incoming telephone calls, chromosome breakages under harmful irradiation, falling of bombs in wartime. The details will not be discussed here. Broadly, the results show that if the incidence of a disease forms a Poisson Process then so does the prevalence of the disease.

20

10. Conclusions and Summary

Four measures of the intensity of disease in a community are defined and discussed, namely, the incidence rate, the point, cumulative and period prevalence rates. Attention is focused on the errors that can arise from a misunderstanding of these definitions. In general, prevalence rates are more readily available for chronic diseases, but their use for making inferences about incidence of disease can lead to difficulties.

A mathematical approach to the problem of relating incidence rates to the three types of prevalence rates is described. It is proved that the period prevalence rate is the product of average incidence and average duration in the sick population. An approach based on the differential calculus produces, under certain simplifying assumptions, a simple (compound interest-type) result linking the cumulative and point prevalence rates to the underlying annual incidence rates.

The equations derived above were applied to the results of the Rochester community-based study investigating the natural history of cerebrovascular disease. In addition, simple Gompertz and Makeham type curves were fitted to the incidence rates of this study, and the accuracy of fit discussed. The computed prevalence rates were compared with the actual, published rates, and the accuracy of the fit was discussed.

It is suggested that simple models such as those described herein may be used to test the consistency of incidence and prevalence data, to provide insight into the flow of new cases of a disease into a community, to examine more closely the shape of incidence rates and prevalence rates, to provide information about subsidiary variables like the average duration in the sick population, and to add to one's understanding of the effect of certain epidemiological assumptions on incidence and prevalence rates.

The application of these models need not be restricted to chronic diseases. Thus, prevalence rates for infectious diseases have been discussed by Nyboe [8, 23].

References

1 Haberman, S (1978) *Social Science and Medicine, 12,* 147
2 Haberman, S (1978) *Social Science and Medicine, 12,* 153
3 Haberman, S (1978) *Social Science and Medicine, 12,* 159
4 Lilienfeld, AM (1976) *Foundations of Epidemiology,* Chapter 9. Oxford University Press, London
5 *GRO Studies on Medical and Population Subjects* (1954) No. 8
6 WHO Technical Report Series (1959) No. 164
7 Matsumoto, N, Whisnant, JP, Kurland, LT and Okazaki, H (1973) *Stroke, 4,* 20
8 Nyboe, J (1957) *Bull. WHO, 17,* 319
9 WHO Technical Report Series (1952) No. 53
10 Cox, PR (1976) *Demography,* 5th edn, Chapters 3 and 18. Cambridge University Press, Cambridge
11 Kurtzke, JF (1969) *Epidemiology of Cerbrovascular Disease,* pp 24, 149. Springer Verlag, New York

12 Logan, W and Cushion, A (1958) *GRO Studies on Medical and Population Subjects, 1,* No. 14
13 Sartwell, P and Merrell, M (1952) *Amer. J. Publ. Hlth., 42,* 579
14 Dorn, H (1951) *Amer. J. Publ. Hlth., 41,* 271
15 Donald, DWA (1970) *Compound Interest and Annuities Certain,* 2nd edn, Chapter 2. Cambridge University Press, Cambridge
16 Stallones, R, Dyken, M, Fang, H, Heyman, A, Seltser, R and Stamler, J (1972) *Stroke, 3,* 360
17 Whisnant, JP, Fitzgibbons, J, Kurland, LT and Sayre, G (1971) *Stroke, 2,* 11
18 Gompertz, B (1825) *Phil. Trans., 115,* 513
19 Makeham, W (1867) *J. Inst. Act., 13,* 325
20 Benjamin, B and Haycocks, HW (1970) *Analysis of Mortality and Other Actuarial Statistics,* chapter 14. Cambridge University Press, Cambridge
21 Cutler, SJ and Axtell, LM (1963) *J. of Amer. Stat. Ass., 58,* 701
22 Garraway, WM, Whisnant, JP, Furlan, AJ, Phillips, LH, Kurland, LT and O'Fallon, WM (1979) *New Eng. J. Med., 300,* 449
23 Feller, W (1968) *Introduction to Probability Theory and its Applications,* 3rd edn. Vol. 1, chapter 17. Wiley, New York

Chapter 3

NEUROEPIDEMIOLOGY: SOME GENERAL PRINCIPLES

Geoffrey A Rose

Neurologists have long been aware of the relevance of epidemiology. It was epidemiological techniques that identified the cause and modes of spread of anterior poliomyelitis and led to the splendid achievement of eradication. The relation of encephalitis lethargica to its sequelae was partly elucidated by epidemiology, although this story is not yet completed. More recently, in 1959, an epidemic outbreak of acute peripheral neuropathy in Morocco, involving about 1000 people, was traced to orthocresyl phosphate in aviation oil which had been sold falsely as 'olive oil'. In 1971, an even more disastrous epidemic occurred in Iraq, due to imported grain dressed with methyl mercury and mistakenly ingested: it is said that 100000 suffered neurological damage, often permanent, and that 10000 died.

Until recently, less use was made of epidemiology in the study of non-epidemic diseases of the nervous system. The methods are particularly appropriate to natural history and aetiological enquiries.

Study of Natural History

Unless the natural history of a condition is known, it is not possible to give a true prognosis to patients and their families, and it is difficult to assess the effects of treatment. Any one physician sees only those cases that have been referred to him. His picture of the disease is incomplete and biased by the selective factors that determined referral. Similarly, his experience of the outcome is liable to bias by incomplete and selective follow-up. A task of epidemiology is to stand farther back, to attempt description of the totality of cases, and to follow them all up. In this way it offers the hope of a complete and balanced account of natural history and outcome. As a medical student I was taught that multiple sclerosis was inevitably a progressive and fatal disease, which was a correct summary of neurological experience at the time. Now it has been suggested that in as many as one-third of patients there is an isolated, non-recurring episode of the same disease process.

Search for Causes

The search for causes has particular relevance to the neurologist, who has to deal with certain diseases that are incurable. Aetiology, as distinct from pathogenesis, is largely the domain of epidemiology. Though surrounded by technical accretions

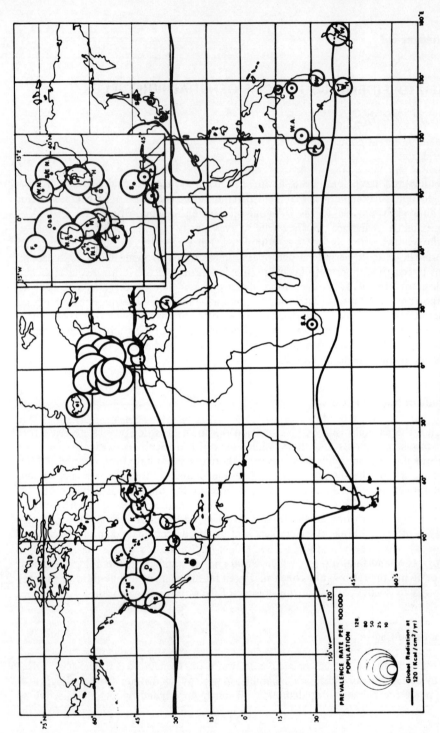

Figure 1 Apparent distribution of multiple sclerosis, based on prevalence estimates [1]

and a certain amount of jargon, at heart it is no more than organised common sense and logical reasoning, further grounds for commending it to neurologists.

The first task is to describe the distribution of disease, conveniently accomplished under three headings: *Where* does it occur? *When* does it occur (trends, seasonal effects, etc)? And *who* gets it? (At one particular place and time, what are the differences between the affected and the unaffected?) Each of these questions implies a comparison. No epidemiological result has much meaning if considered in isolation, but if comparisons are to be valid they must be free of bias. This need for definition and standardisation is the first distinction between the methods of surveys and those of clinical practice, where the individual physician is not usually troubled if colleagues in other places follow different diagnostic practices.

A second difference arises from the particular objective of diagnosis. In clinical practice the aim is, as far as possible, to arrive at the correct decision on management for each patient, whereas in epidemiology the overriding requirement is to come to the right management policy for a group (for purposes of prevention or in management of future patients); thus, in epidemiology errors in individual subjects can usually be tolerated. This is fortunate since in surveys the use of simple and often crude methods is the necessary price of standardisation and the need to study large numbers. However, the corollary of using simple methods for comparisons is the need for quality control of data: it is a help to know the size of the errors.

If a condition is relatively common, such as migraine or hypertension, it is possible to undertake a survey based on personal examination, and one can then insist on the all-important standardisation of criteria and methods of examination, recording and coding. But the population frequency of most neurological disorders is so low as to make such surveys impracticable and, unfortunately, the enumeration of cases has then to be based on routine clinical services. These, as we have seen, are not at all designed with the purpose of standardised comparisons in mind.

Some of the resulting problems can be illustrated by an example. Figure 1 shows a world map of the distribution of multiple sclerosis. (Its aetiological interpretation is discussed in Part III of this volume.) Distributions should always be described by rates rather than simply by numbers of cases, so that the number of cases can be related to the defined population at risk. In this instance, distribution has been described by prevalence rates, which measure the proportion of a population affected at one particular time: the area of each circle is proportional to the estimated prevalence of multiple sclerosis in that locality. An interesting pattern seems to emerge, but before attempting an explanation it is as well to question its reality. The use of existing clinical data rather than standardised examinations raises a number of doubts—

1 Do Doctors in Different Places use the Same Criteria for Defining a Case?

Some require evidence of recurrent episodes and progression, others accept the first episode, some even remain uncertain until there is pathological proof.

2 Are the Chances of Case Identification Equal?

Apart altogether from varying diagnostic criteria, it seems unlikely that two patients, one in Mexico and one in London, would have an equal chance of referral to hospital, seeing a neurologist, and being recorded in the diagnostic index.

3 Are the Related Populations Adequately Defined?

Neurological catchment areas often have uncertain boundaries, since some patients may travel a long way to see a specialist. Populations vary in structure, for example, with regard to age, and such factors must be known and taken into account in the comparison. Sometimes estimates of population structure are unreliable (this has been a particular problem in studying disease in migrant groups). Sometimes no population estimates at all may be available, and results must be reported as proportions of all admissions or consultations. Differences in such proportionate estimates reflect not only the varying frequency of the disease being studied but also the varying frequency of competing causes of admission.

4 Is Prevalence an Adequate Measure of Incidence?

In searching for aetiological explanations of the distribution of a disease we should always prefer, if possible, to study incidence, that is, the rate of occurrence of new cases in defined populations. This can be difficult, requiring larger numbers and agreement both on what constitutes 'a new case' and on its appropriate date of onset. Prevalence rates are an attractive alternative. Unfortunately, the size of the prevalence pool depends not only on the rate of inflow (incidence) but also on outflow (mortality and recovery rates). It is doubtful whether the average duration of a case of multiple sclerosis will be the same in Mexico and London, and to that extent the difference in prevalence provides a distorted measure of any difference in incidence rates.

In practice, it is usually impossible to answer any of these questions at all confidently and, to that extent, this sort of comparative epidemiological exercise must be viewed with much caution. It should not, however, be dismissed. So far as possible, the implied assumptions should be tested, and it should be asked whether the possible biases are reasonably likely, by their size and distribution, to account for observed patterns of disease.

Interpreting Results

Having satisfied ourselves adequately on the trustworthiness of the data, the next difficulty is to explain them. In a laboratory study in animals there is no such problem. Two groups of litter-mates are housed and fed identically, while one receives a treatment and the other serves as a control. Any differences in outcome can reflect only chance or the effect of the treatment: all true associations are causal. This is far removed from an observational epidemiological study, where the groups to be compared may differ in all kinds of ways in addition to exposure to the supposed cause. Some of these confusing ('confounding') variables are easily recognised and measured, such for example as age and sex, and these can then be taken into account in the analysis. Others, such as social class, are known to be important but may be hard to characterise adequately. Worst of all, the presence of others may be quite unsuspected. Simply to exclude all the alternative explanations one can think of does not mean that the remaining suspect is indeed guilty: one can never exclude the unconsidered explanation. This is why conclusions from observational studies can at best be tentative. The conclusion will be strengthened, however, if it can be shown to be consistent in a number of studies, or in different types of study (descriptive prevalence studies, case-control, longitudinal cohort, or experimental trial). The inherent uncertainties are such that one single epidemiological report is rarely adequate. The evidence needs to be wider and to be considered as a whole.

Reference

1   McAlpine, D, Lumsden, CE and Acheson, ED (1972) *Multiple sclerosis: a re-appraisal.* Churchill Livingstone, Edinburgh

Chapter 4

THE CLASSIFICATION AND CODING OF NEUROLOGICAL DISEASE

Rudy Capildeo, Steven Haberman and F Clifford Rose

Introduction

The 1958 Committee on the Medical Certification of Causes of Death listed 8 main uses for the classification of diseases, namely:

1 Medicolegal
2 General public health
3 Location of cases for clinical investigation
4 Retrospective studies
5 Supplying end-points to prospective studies
6 Actuarial and underwriting purposes
7 Demographic analyses
8 General statistical

Since it was originally introduced for mortality statistics, the WHO's *Manual of International Classification of Diseases, Injuries and Causes of Death* does not meet all these requirements. In the field of neurology particularly, the WHO classification is unsuitable since neither the 7th revision (1957), 8th revision (1967), or 9th revision (1974) has kept up with advances in the specialty.

The classification and coding of diseases produce considerable problems for the clinician. Not only does he have to consider the clinical features for each disease, but he also has to give consideration to primary as opposed to secondary factors, aetiological and prognostic factors and also how the clinical features of the disease have been altered by advances in medicine, eg, the use of L-dopa in Parkinson's disease. It also makes the clinician consider the medical and social implications of the disease itself, eg, in using the term 'epilepsy' as a diagnostic label. To this could be added the value of investigations in establishing the diagnosis and the means by which he can assess improvement following the introduction of treatment. In all these ways, the clinician studying disease uses the methods of an epidemiologist.

Aim and Methods of Classification

The aim of classification of disease is to *'define a homogeneous patient group as accurately as possible'*. Although clinicians view disease particularly from a diag-

28

nostic angle, it can be considered from other viewpoints using, for example, functional scales, social scales, 'total illness profiles', each of which can form the basis of a different type of classification. A single measure may correlate sufficiently for practical purposes, eg, loss of mobility as part of a functional scale incorporating 'activities of daily living' (ADL), or loss of earnings due to illness could be included in a social assessment profile. The different approaches might indicate social needs which could lead to appropriate ancillary aid being provided.

Diseases can be classified under a 'single disease' index or 'disease categories', but these are not mutually exclusive, eg, multiple sclerosis could be classified as an individual disease or under 'demyelinating diseases'. Dystrophia myotonica might be classified individually rather than under the 'muscular dystrophies'. For some diseases, it is difficult to think of meaningful categories, particularly when the aetiology is unknown, eg, motor neurone disease and syringomyelia.

A single disease approach implies that each disease can be easily defined, but this is clearly not always the case; for example, epilepsy, dementia or head injury. If Parkinson's disease is considered as a 'single disease' entity, how would a Parkinsonian patient with dementia be classified?

Although a classification incorporating groups of diseases indicates that each has the same aetiological basis, it can still produce problems, eg, all cerebrovascular diseases have a vascular basis but should *migraine* be included? Similarly, the 'epilepsies' is an unsatisfactory category since aetiology varies enormously. An aetiological classification, although ideal, is not always practicable so that the easiest way is to use a clinical approach.

Clinicians in different centres, regions or countries may use different criteria when applying the same diagnostic label. If variations in diagnostic practice could be excluded, differences in the patterns of disease between regions or countries may prove to be apparent rather than real. When using a diagnostic label, it would be inaccurate to discuss 100 stroke patients without further qualifying them. It is for this reason that the basis on which diagnostic labels are given must be indicated, and this is one of the underlying principles for our new classification of stroke [1].

Cumulative Numbering System

The basis of this system is that for any table used for the classification of a disease, a numerical total is derived that can be easily coded and which is unique. '0' is always used for 'unknown' information and 9, or serial 9s, used to indicate 'none', eg, 'no investigation carried out' or 'autopsy not performed'. Coding should be carried out using all possible information, eg, in hospital, when the patient is discharged or dies. Consider the following simple anatomical table:

0 Unknown
1 Cerebellum
2 Brain stem
4 Right hemisphere
8 Left hemisphere

TABLE I: Stroke Assessment Form using Cumulative Numbering System

Name	Duration C.X.H. ....
Hosp. No.	Duration W.L.H. ....
Sex M:1 F:2	Total Duration ....
Age (years)	

	TABLE I			TABLE V	
	Anatomical			*Admission : Disability*	
0	Unknown		0	Unknown	
1	Cerebellum		1	Speech	– Independent
2	Brain Stem		2	Arm	– Useful
4	Right Hemisphere		4	Leg	– Useful
8	Left Hemisphere		8	Speech	– Dependent
	Score		16	Arm	– Useless
			32	Leg	– Useless
	TABLE II		64	Conscious	– Drowsy
	Pathological		128	Unconscious	– Reacting
0	Unknown		256	Unconscious	– No reaction
1	A-V Malformation		999	None	
2	Aneurysm			Score	
4	Haematoma/Haemorrhage				
8	Intracranial arterial lesion				
16	Extracranial arterial lesion			TABLE VI	
32	Infarction Score			*Discharge : Disability*	
			0	Unknown	
	TABLE III		1	Speech	– Independent
	Investigations		2	Arm	– Useful
0	Unknown		4	Leg	– Useful
1	ECG		8	Speech	– Dependent
2	EchoEG		16	Arm	– Useless
4	EEG		32	Leg	– Useless
8	Brain Scan		64	Dead	
16	LP		99	None	
32	Angio			Score	
64	EMI Scan				
128	Neurosurgery				
256	Autopsy				
999	None			TABLE VII	
	Score			*Outcome*	
			0	Unknown	
	TABLE IV		1	At work	
	Associated Conditions		2	At home	
0	Unknown		4	Family at home	
1	Periph. Vasc. Disease		8	Outside support–family/friends	
2	Diabetes		16	Social Services support	
4	Previous TIA		32	Other causes for disability	
8	Previous Stroke		64	Chair or bed-bound	
16	Ischaemic Heart Disease		128	Institutionalised	
32	Hypertension		256	Dead	
99	None			Score	
	Score				

C.X.H. = Charing Cross Hospital
W.L.H. = West London Hospital

A patient with a left cerebral hemisphere lesion will be coded 8. A patient with a left cerebral hemisphere lesion (8) and a brain stem lesion (4) will be coded 12 (8 + 4). It can be seen that no other possible combination adds up to this number, which is therefore unique.

The series can be built up further (16, 32, 64, 128, 256 and 512). In practice, a table up to 512 will contain 12 statements (since it will include '0' and '999'). Adding one further digit for coding means that three more statements can be added, eg, after 64, the next three numbers are 128, 256 and 512.

When devising tables it is frequently very difficult to construct 'league tables', ie, the higher the score, the more important the item. Since each item is easily identified its position in the table is unimportant. Further, new items can be added with subsequent revisions and these will not invalidate the previous codings as they are instantly recognised from the cumulative numbering code.

To decode a cumulative number, the highest significant number below is traced and then subtracted from it. This process is continued until the cumulative number is reduced to zero. Consider the following table of investigations:

   0 Unknown
   1 ECG
   2 EchoEG
   4 EEG
   8 Brain scan
  16 LP
  32 Angiography
  64 CAT scan
 128 Neurosurgery
 256 Autopsy
 999 None

Examples

  48 = 32 + 16 = angiography + LP
196 = 128 + 64 + 4 = neurosurgery + CAT scan + EEG
243 = 128 + 64 + 32 + 16 + 2 + 1 = neurosurgery + CAT + angiography
     + LP + echoencephalography + ECG

It is suggested that the diagnosis is indicated by a rubric, the digits before the decimal points indicating the code numbers for each table, eg:

Cerebral Infarction	10.00
Cerebral Haemorrhage	11.00
Subarachnoid Haemorrhage	12.00
Transient Ischaemic Attack	13.00

This method was used for a new classification of stroke [1, 2] and can be adopted for other neurological diseases.

Stroke

Seven tables were originally used but three further tables have been added for assessing: (1) premorbid ability, (2) maximum level of disability, (3) other causes of disability [3]. 'Premorbid ability' is assessed by using the 'outcome' table, and 'maximum disability' by using the 'admission disability' table: if 'maximum disability' occurs on day 2 or later following admission, an 'evolving stroke' will be indicated. A new table for 'other causes of disability' is necessary to qualify 'outcome' table.

All these data can be incorporated in a computerised summary of the patient.

Transient Ischaemic Attacks (TIAs)

The same tables that are used for 'stroke' can be used for TIAs. By definition, there should be no residual neurological disability after 24 hours. Therefore, (a) the 'initial' or 'admission disability' can be recorded, as well as the time interval between this and (b) the 'minimum level of disability'. The 'discharge disability' will be 'none' if the patient has had no further attacks; if this is not so, either the patient has not had a TIA or the patient suffered a completed stroke during hospitalisation. The 'investigations' table will indicate whether the patient underwent angiography, and for the specific purposes of, say, a multicentre study, a table can be added defining medical and surgical management.

Reversible Ischaemic Neurological Deficit (RIND)

Some patients have neurological signs for only a short time after a completed stroke, recovering fully within days. In these patients the signs persist longer than 24 hours and since the natural history of this condition may be different from TIA, the term RIND has been coined. If 'discharge disability' shows no deficit, eg, on day 4, but there was continuing deficit after 24 hours, then a patient in the RIND category will be shown.

Therefore, by using a second score for measuring disability (maximum or minimum) after admission but prior to discharge, it is possible to indicate

1 a completed stroke (due to cerebral infarction or haemorrhage);
2 an evolving stroke;
3 a transient ischaemic attack (TIA);
4 reversible ischaemic neurological deficit (RIND).

Subarachnoid Haemorrhage

A subarachnoid haemorrhage is defined as 'blood in the subarachnoid space'. The term should not be used synonymously with intracerebral aneurysm, although this is the commonest cause. Confusion in terminology occurs when the patient is found to have developed a hemiplegia because this indicates either that bleeding has extended into the brain (ie, cerebral haemorrhage) or that infarction has occurred, possibly due to prolonged vasospasm. The same tables as for stroke can be used to indicate subarachnoid or cerebral haemorrhage due to either an aneurysm or a vascular malformation. If the main rubric shows 'subarachnoid haemorrhage' but 'aneurysm' is not coded this means that it was not identified, particularly if 'angiography' is coded. If 'aneurysm' is coded, but 'investigations' have not been carried out, then the pathological diagnosis is clearly 'presumed' as opposed to 'proven'.

Cerebrovascular Disease in Children

This has recently been reviewed [4]. It should be possible to devise simple tables to cover the same main areas as in adults.

1 *Premorbid health.* This would provide a general idea of the health of the child prior to the cerebrovascular disease. Categories might include: premature delivery, birth trauma, low birth weight, malnutrition, normal health. Other physical disabilities, eg, orthopaedic, hearing, etc, can be included.

2 *Anatomical classification.*

3 *Pathological classification* would include cerebral venous thrombosis, subdural and extradural haematoma, intracranial and extracranial arterial occlusions (eg, 'moyamoya').

4 *Investigations*

5 *Associated conditions.* In view of the larger number of possible associated conditions only the main categories need be classified. Categories might include: congenital heart disease, acquired heart disease, blood dyscrasias (congenital, acquired and bleeding disorders), diabetes, hypertension.

6 *Presentation* relates to the onset of the cerebrovascular disease. Categories might include: febrile illness, epilepsy, ENT infection, unconsciousness, acute hemiplegia.

7 *Disability*

8 *Outcome.* Other physical disabilities that may have been present before the onset of the cerebrovascular disease will be indicated in the table for 'Premorbid Health'. Disabilities arising later as a result of the cerebrovascular disease require classification: mental retardation, behaviour disturbance, epilepsy, visual, hearing and orthopaedic problems.

Outcomes in social terms include: at home, or institution, attending a normal or 'special' school and must also be seen in the context of the home situation, eg, both parents at home, number of siblings, if any other children are handicapped. Family socioeconomic problems may be difficult to classify, but a social network diagram that can be tabulated for computerisation has been devised [5].

Multiple Sclerosis (MS)

There are a number of well-known classifications [6-9] the basis for which is essentially clinical—a history of remitting and relapsing episodes and two or more sites of injury in the central nervous system—but there are problems, eg, the classification of optic neuritis or progressive spastic paraparesis. McDonald and Halliday suggest the following categories to include the clinical picture of progressive spastic paraparesis, accepting optic neuritis only if one other CNS lesion is present. (The classification of optic neuritis is considered in the monograph by Perkin and Clifford Rose, 1979 [10].)

1 Proved—autopsy evidence only accepted.
2 Clinically definite—2 or more clinical episodes and
                     2 or more separate CNS lesions.
  Also age of onset between 10 and 50 years is considered essential (a debatable point) and duration of symptoms and signs for more than 1 year.
3 Early probable or latent—for 1 clinical episode but at least 2 separate CNS lesions.
4 Progressive probable—progressive history of paraplegia and 2 separate CNS lesions.
5 Progressive possible—progressive history of paraplegia and only 1 CNS lesion.
6 Suspected—single episode suggestive of MS or single lesion only or recurrent optic neuritis with one other CNS lesion.

Using the terms clinically definite, progressive, probable, etc, although qualifying the degree of certainty, does not indicate the actual basis for diagnosis in each individual case since investigations are not included. For this reason, separate tables devised to indicate the data base should be used. A 'league' table has been adopted so that items with the higher scores are thought to be more significant.

TABLE II: Classification of Multiple Sclerosis

(a)	Age at Presentation (0-9)	(c)	Clinical Findings
	0 Under 10 yrs		1 Optic neuritis
	1 Over 10 yrs		2 Brain stem lesion
	2 Over 20 yrs, etc.		4 Spastic paraplegia
(b)	History	(d)	Investigations
	1 Single episode		0 None
	2 Symptoms/signs for 1 yr or more		1 IgG oligoclonal band in CSF
	4 Progressive		2 VER delay
	8 Several episodes with remissions		512 Autopsy

VER = Visual evoked delay

(a) Age at Presentation

Categories 'under 10 years', '10 years-50 years' and 'over 51 years' could be used, but a simple 0-9 score will actually measure the appropriate decade, or the age can be recorded separately. The difference between the patient's age when coding is carried out and the 'age at presentation' gives the duration of the disease in years.

(b) History

'Several episodes with remissions' is the most important item (8). A score of 8-10, taken with the clinical findings, is equivalent to 'clinically definite'.

(c) Clinical Findings

Only the most important findings have been included. A score of 3 would indicate two separate CNS lesions and a score of 7, three separate CNS lesions.

(d) Investigations

In the absence of a definite diagnostic test, only the more important investigations have been included. Autopsy is purposely given a very high number in the series since this is the only category accepted for a diagnosis of multiple sclerosis 'proved'.

Analysing the scores from tables *(b)*, *(c)* and *(d)*, a total score of over 512 is equivalent to 'proved' and over 11 as 'clinically definite'. 'Progressive probable', and 'progressive possible', 'suspected' and a single episode of optic neuritis will also be accurately identified.

(e) Disability Tables

These can be constructed in the same way as suggested for the cerebrovascular diseases (*see* Table I) and can be used to monitor the clinical progress of the disease for each patient. Similarly, the social situation relating to the patient's 'needs' can be indicated by using the 'outcome' table (*see* Table I).

Other Neurological Diseases

For *Parkinson's disease,* an anatomical and pathological table would have little meaning, and an aetiological table might be more appropriate, eg, idiopathic, drug-induced, post-encephalitic. A clinical table indicating the major problem, eg, tremor, rigidity, bradykinesia could be simply constructed. Duration of disease, overall disability and social situation can be coded as previously suggested. Although the type of medication, how long the patient has been on a particular drug, side-effects, and so on are important, the coding of this information must be related to the needs for which the classification is going to be used.

Head injury patients can be coded in much the same way. Tables showing the extent of injury, disability and outcome can be added to the Glasgow Coma Scale.

Summary

The purpose of this chapter has been to propose methods of classification for the commoner neurological diseases. There is a need for multidisciplinary international teams to consider the broad issues, namely the purposes of any new classification, and to devise a new system that should operate for a defined period *before* further revisions. The methods suggested have been successfully adopted in the field of cerebrovascular disease and could be considered for other neurological diseases.

References

1 Capildeo, R, Haberman, S and Clifford Rose, F (1978) The Definition and Classification of Stroke. *Quart. J. Med., 186,* 177
2 Capildeo, R, Haberman, S, and Clifford Rose, F (1977) A New Classification of Stroke: Preliminary Communication. *Brit. Med. J., 2,* 1578
3 Capildeo, R, Haberman, S and Clifford Rose, F (1979) Towards a computer-based data bank for stroke patients. In *Progress in Stroke Research* (ed RM Greenhalgh and F Clifford Rose). Pitman Medical Publications, 1979
4 Capildeo, R (1979) Cerebrovascular Disease. In *Paediatric Neurology* (ed F. Clifford Rose). Blackwell Scientific Publications, Oxford
5 Capildeo, R, Court, Christine and Clifford Rose, F (1976) Social Network Diagram. *Brit. Med. J., 1,* 143
6 Allison, RS and Miller, JHD (1954) Prevalence and familiar incidence of disseminated sclerosis. *Ulster Med. J., 23,* suppl No. 2
7 Schumacher, GA, Beebe, G, Kibler, RF et al (1965) Problems of experimental trials of therapy in multiple sclerosis. *Ann. New York Acad. Sci., 122,* 552
8 McAlpine, D (1972) In *Multiple Sclerosis—A Reappraisal* (ed D McAlpine, CE Lumsden and ED Acheson) Churchill Livingstone, London and Edinburgh
9 McDonald, WI and Halliday, AM (1977) Diagnosis and classification of multiple sclerosis. *Brit. Med. Bull., 33,* 4
10 Perkin, GD and Clifford Rose, F (1979) In *Optic Neuritis and its Differential Diagnosis.* Oxford University Press, London

Chapter 5

THE CONTRIBUTION OF THE MAYO CLINIC CENTRALISED DIAGNOSTIC INDEX TO NEUROEPIDEMIOLOGY IN THE UNITED STATES*

Leonard T Kurland

Introduction

On 16 December, 1976, the Assistant Secretary of Health in Washington DC, announced a moratorium on the national swine flu vaccination programme. The expected swine flu epidemic had not materialised, but the major reason for his dramatic action was the impression that, among vaccinees, an unusual number of cases of Guillain-Barré syndrome (GBS) had developed a few weeks after immunisation. An important factor in that decision was the report by Lesser and his associates [1] which provided the only population-based rates for GBS in the United States that could serve for comparison with the experience among the vaccinees.

We now know that the risk of GBS among the vaccinees was only 1 in 120 000 during the first few weeks after vaccination, but this small risk was greater than expected on the basis of our experience over a 30-year period in Rochester, Minnesota.

It is worthy of note that the descriptive epidemiological study of GBS in Olmsted County was completed by a medical student during a brief clerkship. That paper is among more than 125 published since the Rochester Epidemiology Program Project began in 1966, of which about 30 relate to diseases of the nervous system. Internists and surgeons on the Mayo staff, dozens of medical students and visiting scientists have participated in these projects.

The major data resource for the population of Olmsted County, Minnesota (which includes the city of Rochester) is the set of detailed and largely handwritten records of the Mayo Clinic, about 20 per cent of which are for people from Olmsted County. The system originated in 1889; a dossier-style records linkage system was developed in 1907; and a detailed diagnostic and surgical index to facilitate retrievals was developed in 1910 and automated in 1935 with a specific identifier for local residents. The records over the past 90 years are available for retrieval in their original form and record loss rarely occurs. This unique system is maintained by the Mayo Clinic as a national resource and is available to all responsible investigators for any appropriate research effort.

The system that links demographic, clinical, laboratory and follow-up data into a single file composed of records from physician encounters at the clinic, the

*This investigation was supported in part by Research Grant GM 14231, National Institutes of Health, Bethesda, Maryland, USA.

hospital and even at home was organised at the Mayo Clinic 70 years ago, not because of any concern for epidemiology but because it was considered a logical means of assuring the best care of the patient. For the Olmsted County population, it is complete in the sense that for each individual, for his period of residence in the county, it contains a record of nearly every medical contact. The community, with the Mayo Clinic and the Olmsted Medical Group and their affiliated hospitals, is remarkably self-contained from a medical standpoint, and few residents seek outside care according to long-standing evidence most recently documented by a sample survey of households in this county.

The accurate description of the incidence and clinical course of a disease or syndrome in a defined population requires the following: (1) the availability and acceptance by the population of refined diagnostic and therapeutic methods; (2) a records linkage system that documents the delivery of quality medical care and a detailed centralised disease classification system which ensures retrievability of pertinent medical data; (3) a thorough follow-up capability; (4) a highly motivated staff, with clinical expertise, who can initiate and carry out the studies; and (5) the epidemiology and statistical backup to support the clinical staff in research design, data handling, and data analysis. The recognition that all these were present at Mayo Clinic led to the systematic development of such research through the Rochester Epidemiology Program Project.

Examples of the development and phenomenal productivity of the small part of the records linkage system pertaining to a circumscribed population will constitute the greater part of this chapter. Benefits derived from this resource extend far beyond the local community. For dozens of neurological disorders other than the Guillain-Barré syndrome, this resource has provided the first available incidence of prevalence rates and meaningful survivorship statistics, and these have often served as a basis for national and international comparisons and for manpower and resource planning in neurology. I shall cite a few examples to illustrate the variety of topics and research designs utilised in this programme. Several other papers with new results based on this data resource will be found in this volume.

Description of the Resource

In a records linkage system, social and medical data for members of a community or other populations are identified from various sources. This implies identification of the medical records of each person so that they can be united physically or through a centralised automated (or computerised) system for later retrieval.

Each year about half the local population is seen at one of the facilities covered by the Mayo Clinic. In addition, the independent Olmsted Medical Group and the Community Hospital attend many others in the county, and the diagnostic indices for all such encounters are maintained in our department. The data base for Olmsted County residents also includes information abstracted from records in other medical institutions in the adjacent counties for those infrequent instances in which such facilities are used by local residents. About two-thirds of all deaths in the community come to autopsy in our Department of Pathology and Anatomy.

38

A centralised and largely automated diagnostic index allows us to retrieve a listing of the institutional identification numbers of all local residents whose histories contain a given diagnosis for any period from 1935 to the present. If cases prior to 1935 are to be included, the earlier Mayo Clinic manual diagnostic index is reviewed.

The listed series of original medical records is then retrieved and assembled, and the information required by the study protocol is abstracted on a precoded form developed specifically for the study in question. The abstracting from the medical records is done by a staff of trained and experienced history readers under the close supervision of the clinician directing the study. The resulting record (written abstract, punch cards, magnetic tape, etc) for each patient in each study is on permanent file and is available for subsequent study.

Examples of Neuroepidemiological Studies
Utilising Rochester Data Base

Multiple Sclerosis (MS)

My first exposure to the Rochester resource occurred 30 years ago when I attended a conference on multiple sclerosis (MS) in New York City. At the time, I was at the Harvard School of Public Health designing a national study on the epidemiology of MS and was tremendously impressed when I learned that Mayo physicians, through a single data resource, could easily conduct a most comprehensive study on MS incidence, prevalence and outcome. Rochester, Minnesota, thus has the distinction of being the site of the first morbidity study of MS in North America [2]. The report revealed that the prevalence rates were more than twice those reported anywhere before, and the prognosis, based on the experience of the community, was far more optimistic than contemporary estimates, which had been derived largely from series of hospitalised patients. In later years, MS surveys conducted at great expense in other populations in the northern United States and Canada corroborated the high prevalence and better survivorship of MS as reported from Rochester [3].

A few years ago the study was extended to answer the question of whether or not MS incidence has been increasing. Repeated prevalence studies in other communities had suggested an increase, presumably due to environmental changes, although improving record systems and case ascertainment provided an alternative explanation. It was decided to measure the incidence rates in the Rochester population over as long a period as possible, that is, 1903 through 1964 and, for this volume, that study has now been updated through 1974. To my knowledge, compilation of incidence rates for any chronic disease over 70 years from medical records is unprecedented. The mean annual incidence rates were, on the whole, somewhat higher than those reported in other cities in the northern United States and Canada, presumably because of superior case ascertainment; but there was no indication of an increase in the incidence rate over time (Table I) [4].

Survivorship among the MS patients of Rochester was compared with that of the normal Minnesota population of similar age and sex. At 25 years after onset,

TABLE I: Multiple Sclerosis in Rochester, Minnesota, 1903–1974

Years	Male	Female	Total	Rate/10^5
1903–14	0	4	4	4
1915–24	2	3	5	4
1925–34	0	11	11	5
1935–44	2	4	6	2
1945–54	3	5	8	3
1955–64	7	6	13	3
1965–74	2	15	17	3
1903–74	16	48	64	3.2*

*Weighted average

survival was 64 per cent for the MS patients and 87 per cent for the general population. Ambulation was still possible for 50 per cent of patients surviving 25 years after onset. This relatively favourable outcome suggests that essentially complete case ascertainment in a community identifies a higher proportion of milder cases with better prognoses than are recognised in the usual hospital series [5].

Parkinsonism

A study of Parkinsonism in the Rochester population over a 32-year period provided an annual incidence of about 1 in 5000 persons in the total population and about 1 per 1000 for those aged 50 years and older. The mean age at onset of Parkinsonism was stable at about 65 years over the entire 30-year study period. If the age-adjusted rate for Rochester is applied to the present US population, approximately 40 000 persons are newly affected in the United States each year. The cumulative incidence rates indicate that about 2.5 per cent of the population may be expected to develop Parkinsonism during their lifetime.

Several years ago Poskanzer and Schwab (1963) [6] reported that between 1920 and 1960 there had been a steady increase in the mean age at which Parkinsonism was diagnosed at the Massachusetts General Hospital, and they reasoned that this was due to a 'cohort effect' of common exposure to the various 'flu' epidemics of 1918 to 1926. They postulated that new cases of Parkinsonism would decline in number after 1980 and the disease would disappear after 1985.

Among referral patients at the Mayo Clinic also, the mean age at diagnosis of Parkinsonism had increased (although only from 51 years in 1935 to about 63 years in 1967), but a similar increase was also noted for referral patients with herpes zoster and stroke. However, among the resident population of Rochester the mean age at *onset* of Parkinsonism has remained essentially unchanged since 1935 [7].

The increase in mean age over time noted by Poskanzer and Schwab [6] can be explained as well, and perhaps better, as a reflection of the increasing frequency with which elderly patients in recent years have been using medical facilities and particularly specialty services. Since the care usually provided by the general practitioner, as well as specialty services, for the elderly population of Rochester is provided in facilities that index all medical records, the Rochester experience was

40

free of the type of selection bias that presumably accounted for the age shift of the Parkinsonism patients observed at the Massachusetts General Hospital [7].

Epilepsy

An ambitious study of epilepsy in Rochester by Hauser, Annegers and others covers a 40-year period. By means of the central data file, essentially all local patients with diagnosed or suspected epilepsy after 1934 were identified, evaluated, and followed. Incidence, prevalence and outcome (including a remarkable level of spontaneous remission of idiopathic epilepsy) were reported [8]. The identification of the cohort of local patients with epilepsy then facilitated a series of analytic (aetiological) studies [9-11].

Perhaps the most dramatic of those studies began when the identification numbers of females in the cohort were collated against diagnoses of pregnancy between 1939 (the clinical advent of diphenylhydantoin) and 1972. The incidence of congenital anomalies and infant mortality in their offspring was derived from the newborn and paediatric records and follow-up. Four groups of mothers with a history of epilepsy were identified: (1) those whose epilepsy and remission had preceded the pregnancy; (2) those whose pregnancies antedated the epilepsy; (3) those in which epilepsy and pregnancy were concurrent but in whom no anticonvulsants were taken during the first trimester of pregnancy; and (4) those with concurrent epilepsy and pregnancy who were on anticonvulsants during the first trimester. In only the last group was there an excess of malformations and these were primarily cleft palate or septal defect of the heart [9]. The value of the long-term follow-up capability in a records linkage system is again demonstrated in this

TABLE II: Approximate average annual incidence per 100 000 population for various neurological disorders in the western hemisphere and the estimated number in the United States

Disorder	W. Hemisphere rate/100000	United States No.
Herpes zoster	400	880 000
Cerebrovascular disease	200	440 000
Convulsive disorders	40	88 000
Bell's palsy	20	44 000
Parkinsonism	20	44 000
Primary brain tumour	10	22 000
Trigeminal neuralgia	4	8 800
Dorsolateral sclerosis	3	6 600
Multiple sclerosis	2	4 400
Guillain-Barré syndrome	1	2 200
Motor neurone disease	1	2 200
Polymyositis	0.5	1 100
Huntington's chorea	0.5	1 100
Myasthenia gravis	0.4	880
Syringomyelia	0.3	660
Wilson's disease	0.2	440

Source: Kurtzke JF and Kurland LT (1973) [22]

41

study, since most ventricular septal defects were not identified until years after the infant was born—in one case at the age of 23 years.

The children of fathers with epilepsy in analogous groups did not demonstrate an increase in congenital malformations. Among the children of mothers taking anticonvulsants (but in none of the other groups, including children of fathers with epilepsy) there may also be an increased risk of epilepsy or mental retardation. Other recent studies pertaining to epilepsy are presented elsewhere in this volume, as are an update on stroke, primary brain tumour and the results of new studies on amyotrophic lateral sclerosis and head trauma.

Although the Rochester Project lends itself best to studies of incidence and outcome of serious, progressive or recurrent diseases, it has been possible to determine incidence and prevalence rates on a large number of neurological and neuromuscular disorders; extrapolation of some of these results and data collection from other sources provides the estimates in Tables II and III. These tables do not include a number of common problems such as headache, major infections of the nervous system, acute or chronic trauma of the neuraxis, the common polyneuropathies and radiculopathies or dementia and retardation *per se*. Studies currently under way should provide information regarding trauma and dementia and plans are being developed for future study of mental retardation. The major sources that provided the basis for the estimates in these two tables are those from Rochester, Minnesota, and surveys in Iceland [12–15] and Carlisle, England [16]. The incidence and prevalence rates are based on the best estimates, taking into account the seeming accuracy and representativeness of the various studies. The tabulated

TABLE III: Approximate average prevalence per 100 000 population for various neurological disorders in the western hemisphere and the estimated number in the United States

Disorder	W. Hemisphere rate/100 000	United States No.
Cerebrovascular disease	500	1 100 000
Convulsive disorders	500	1 100 000
Parkinsonism	200	440 000
Blindness	100	220 000
Cerebral palsy	60	132 000
Multiple sclerosis	50	110 000
Brain tumour	40	88 000
Dorsolateral sclerosis	20	44 000
Syringomyelia	8	17 600
Muscular dystrophy	6	13 200
Polymyositis	6	13 200
Huntington's chorea	6	13 200
Motor neurone disease	5	11 000
Myasthenia gravis	4	8 800
Myotonic dystrophy	2	4 400
Charcot-Marie-Tooth disease	2	4.4
Friedreich's ataxia	1	2.2
Wilson's disease	1	2.2

Source: Kurtzke JF and Kurland LT (1973) [22]

rates have been rounded off, and they refer to the population of all ages, even though the disorder favours one sex or age group. Furthermore, the information is largely applicable to the whites of economically developed countries, predominantly those of North America and Northern Europe. The estimated numbers in the United Kingdom would be approximately one quarter of that estimated for the US. A few words are in order on some of the less serious illnesses in this list.

Herpes zoster is noted for its preponderance in the elderly population; the results of a study with long-term follow-up reported 20 years ago suggested that elderly patients with herpes zoster may also have an increased incidence of some types of malignant neoplasm [17]. Bell's palsy reaches its peak incidence in the 4th decade and remains relatively stable thereafter. No geographical or seasonal clustering of cases was noted in our study. A higher age at onset was associated with greater residual facial weakness; but in general only about 1 in 5 patients had residual facial weakness [18].

When the study on GBS was recently updated to cover the period 1935 through 1976 [19] it was noted that the incidence rates did not vary significantly over time and the rate was higher in those 40 years of age and over. An attempt was also made to identify from the records immunisations, upper respiratory and gastrointestinal infections preceding the onset of neurological symptoms. The basis for comparison, the 'control' for these items was the information recorded in the records for the patients with Bell's palsy. On the basis of that small study no association was noted for immunisations, although there was a significant association between antecedent infections and GBS.

Several other types of studies have been carried out in recent years. In one, the utilisation of computerised axial tomography (CAT) in the population of Olmsted County was evaluated [20]. In our practice, the CAT scan with rare exceptions was ordered by a neurologist or neurosurgeon. In two-thirds of those examined, the scan revealed some abnormality. The benefits of the CAT scan in reducing invasive and more dangerous diagnostic procedures seems clear; our studies are expected to demonstrate how valuable the judicious use of this remarkable technique is in the practice of neurology in our community. Extrapolation from our population's experience indicates that, when used with discretion, one CAT scan unit can provide for the diagnostic needs of a population of 500 000 persons.

In another study [21] we have attempted to estimate neurosurgical needs within the USA on the basis of the operations and diagnostic procedures performed by neurosurgeons on residents of Olmsted County, Minnesota, in a recent 5-year period. The record system enabled us to identify the variety of procedures and their frequencies; it appeared that one neurosurgeon with appropriate neurological support could provide for the neurosurgical needs of a population of 100 000. The problems of expertise needed for the variety of procedures a neurosurgeon might be called upon to perform is alluded to in that paper [21].

It is clear that the Rochester-Olmsted data source has been a major contributor to the available estimates on the incidence and prevalence rates for neurological disorders in the United States [22]. Extrapolations from this source alone are risky because the population of the community is small (60 000 in the city; 90 000 in the County), and the assumption that for some diseases the Rochester rates may

43

be representative of the country as a whole has not been tested. Fortunately, additional population-based studies have been forthcoming in the past few decades and they provide some basis for comparison with those of this mid-American community. A series of descriptive epidemiological studies is available from Carlisle, England [16], from Guam [23, 24], Iceland [12–15], Israel [25, 26] and recently from Fukuoka and Niigata in Japan [27]. However, most of these are special surveys which do not arise from nor result in a resource with an established and continuing records linkage.

In addition to the obvious economy in effort in providing data for almost any disorder in the disease classification, a major advantage of a total community resource lies in its ability to identify existing co-morbidity (multiple diagnoses in the same persons) and to integrate information from general sources as well as specialty areas. The study of malformations among patients with epilepsy demonstrates the value of combining data from records of neurologists, paediatricians, obstetricians, pathologists, cardiologists and so on. An aetiological study utilising the Rochester data resource does not have to contend with limitations of information in the practice of a particular specialty, which offers an immense advantage over special retrospective surveys or disease registries. Since individual physicians only occasionally see in their practice a sufficient number of patients with a specific illness to enable them to pursue new ideas, nearly all clinical investigators are dependent on the existence and availability of a system of medical records indexed in a manner to permit retrieval by demographic features of the patients, by diagnosis, or by surgical or other treatment. Furthermore, it is generally impractical for a clinical researcher to organise, in advance, a system for follow-up of his patients that will ensure continual data on outcome (quality of life or survivorship) after a particular diagnosis or treatment. Despite its relatively high cost, it is sometimes necessary to organise and conduct special prospective studies such as those in Tecumseh, Michigan; Framingham, Massachusetts; and the Harvard alumni studies. The ingenuity of the epidemiologists responsible for these projects has often enabled them to extend their findings well beyond the original clinical area of interest.

But in addition to these, there are only a few medical record resources that are applicable to an enumerated and identifiable population such as the Oxford records linkage study, the records of the military and veterans services, the Health Insurance Plan of Greater New York, and the Kaiser-Permanente medical care plan. Furthermore, the availability of most of these resources is seriously limited by the difficulties in assembling records on families or by rules restricting investigations to those affiliated with the hospital or data centre.

The size and the diversity of the population of the United States (ethnic, occupational, socio-economic), and the high calibre and uniform training programme for physicians, provide a basis for the establishment of medical research archives in selected centres. To develop such a system for a specified locality would require that most medical encounters in the local population be recorded and indexed so that for any chosen entity the incidence rates, secular trends and outcome could be measured. If centralised records facilities were organised in relatively stable communities with good medical facilities and populations of between 50 000 and 150 000, immense opportunities would open for comparison of incidence and for surveillance of changes over time, which would help identify causes of disease or new threats to the public health. Ideally, such communities would be sufficiently distant from other medical centres to insure local diagnosis and treatment initially, if not throughout the course of illness. If such a plan were successful in the United States, it would encourage development of additional medical records archives in other countries. Perhaps the records facility at Mayo Clinic may serve as a model for such an endeavour.

Among the problems that would have to be met locally are the organisation of a system of medical records with prompt entry of data from medical encounters, development of a standardised indexing and retrieval process, uniform procedures of follow-up on preselected sets of patients (by diagnosis and treatment) and provision for any qualified research worker to review and abstract such records following appropriate committee approval of research plans.

However, a major threat to such a plan, if not to existing registries and records linkage systems, is the well-intentioned but grossly misdirected legislation on privacy of medical records.

If the concern for confidentiality that should be levied at some of the non-medical users of records is carried to excess and impinges on legitimate health care research, it could jeopardise the potential benefit of such national archives as I have recommended. We must monitor and assist in the development of sensible privacy legislation, but we should also encourage legislation that will readily permit the transfer of data for clinical studies, the establishment of a system of national archives and the use of collective records in research and education that should benefit the population of the future.

References

1 Lesser, RP, Hauser, WA, Kurland, LT and Mulder, DW (1973) *Neurology (Minneap.), 23,* 1269
2 MacLean, AR, Berkson, J, Woltman, HW and Schionneman, L (1950) *Res. Publ. Assoc. Res. Nerv. Ment. Dis., 28,* 25
3 Kurland, LT, Kurtzke, JF and Goldberg, ID (1973) *Epidemiology of Neurologic and Sense Organ Disorders,* Cambridge, Harvard University Press
4 Scarlett, J, unpublished data
5 Percy, AK, Nobrega, FT, Okazaki, H, Glattre, E and Kurland, LT (1971) *Arch. Neurol., 25,* 105
6 Poskanzer, DC and Schwab, RS (1963) *J. Chronic Dis., 16,* 961
7 Kurland, LT, Hauser, WA, Okazaki, H and Nobrega, FT (1968) In *Third Symposium on Parkinson's Disease,* Edinburgh, E & S Livingstone
8 Hauser, WA and Kurland, LT (1975) *Epilepsia, 16,* 1
9 Annegers, JF, Elveback, LR, Hauser, WA and Kurland, LT (1974) *Arch. Neurol., 31,* 364
10 Annegers, JF, Elveback, LR, Labarthe, DR and Hauser, WA (1976a) *Epilepsia, 17,* 11
11 Annegers, JF, Hauser, WA, Elveback, LR, Anderson, VE and Kurland, LT (1976b) *Epilepsia, 17,* 1
12 Gudmundsson, KR and Gudmundsson, G (1962) *Acta Neurol. Scand. (Suppl), 2,* 1
13 Gudmundsson, G (1966) *Acta Neurol. Scand. (Suppl), 25,* 1
14 Gudmundsson, KR (1969) *Acta Neurol. Scand., 45,* 114
15 Gudmundsson, KR (1970) *Acta Neurol. Scand., 46,* 538

16 Brewis, M, Poskanzer, DC, Rolland, C and Miller, H (1966) *Acta Neurol. Scand. (Suppl)*, *24*, 1
17 Kurland, LT (1958) *J. Chron. Dis.*, *8(4)*, 378
18 Hauser, WA, Karnes, WE, Annis, J and Kurland, LT (1971) *Mayo Clin. Proc.*, *46*, 258
19 Kennedy, RH, Danielson, MAK, Mulder, DW and Kurland, LT (1978) *Mayo Clin. Proc.*, *53*, 93
20 Kennedy, RH, Baker, Jr, HL, Houser, OW, Whisnant, JP and Kennedy, MA (1979) *Radiology*, *130(1)*, 153
21 Glista, GG, Miller, RH, Kurland, LT and Jereczek, ML (1977) *J. Neurosurg.*, *46(1)*, 46
22 Kurtzke, JF and Kurland, LT (1973) *Clinical Neurology*, Vol 3 (ed AB Baker, LH Baker and MD Hagerstown) Harper and Row
23 Chen, K, Brody, JA and Kurland, LT (1968) *Arch. Neurol.*, *19*, 573
24 Mathai, KV, Dunn, DP, Kurland, LT and Reeder, FA (1968) *Epilepsia, 9*, 77
25 Alter, M, Antonovsky, A and Leibowitz, U (1968) In *The Epidemiology of Multiple Sclerosis* (ed M Alter and JF Kurtzke) Springfield, Ill: Charles C Thomas
26 Kahana, E, Alter, M, Braham, J and Sofer, D (1974) *Science, 183*, 90
27 Kuroiwa, Y and Kondo, K (ed) (1976) *Neuroepidemiology: Its Principal and Clinical Applications,* Tokyo, Igaku Shoin

Chapter 6

HLA ANTIGEN ASSOCIATIONS IN NEUROLOGICAL DISORDERS

Heather M Dick

Prompted by the finding that certain diseases of inbred mouse-strains were closely associated with specific mouse histocompatibility antigen (H-2) types, there has been a search for similar associations between human disease and the HLA (Human Leucocyte Antigen) system. The findings in the mouse were of linkage between specific H-2 types and susceptibility to infection by some leukaemogenic viruses but, in human disease studies, the malignant disorders have proved a disappointing field for study of HLA antigen associations. Most positive findings have been detected in the autoimmune disorders, and in some diseases of unknown aetiology, but often with an immunological basis. In neurological studies, multiple sclerosis was one of the first diseases in which an alteration in the HLA antigen frequencies between patients and controls was demonstrated. Myasthenia gravis has also been extensively studied, showing similar HLA association patterns to several other disorders (e.g. juvenile onset diabetes, Graves' disease, coeliac disease). Less extensive studies have been carried out in such disorders as motor neurone disease, Landry-Guillain-Barré syndrome and chronic relapsing polyneuritis, also demonstrating deviations from the normal of certain HLA antigen frequencies: for review, *see* Fog and his associates, 1977 [1].

It is pertinent at this time to examine the concepts that are being applied in such HLA and disease studies, particularly those factors that may affect the performance and interpretation of this kind of study and also review the possible mechanisms by which the possession of specific HLA antigens could predispose an individual to develop a neurological disorder such as multiple sclerosis.

HLA Antigens

The HLA antigen system is a highly polymorphic group of cell membrane products. The antigens are genetically determined by a series of at least five closely linked genes which occur together on chromosome 6 of the autosomal chromosomes. The HLA loci, named A, B, C, D and DR are included in a chromosomal region that is often given the general name of the major histocompatibility complex or system (MHC or MHS), in recognition of the fact that these antigens are important in graft recognition and rejection. Each of the HLA loci has many possible alleles, and each gene product is apparently fully expressed by the cell. Thus, an individual cell will express two each of the A, B, C, D and DR antigens (one derived from each of the pair of autosomes inherited from the parents).

TABLE I HLA Antigens

HLA - A	HLA - B		HLA - C	HLA - D	HLA - DR
HLA - A1	HLA - B5	Bw42	HLA - Cw1	HLA - Dw1	HLA - DRw1
A2	B7	Bw44	Cw2	Dw2	DRw2
A3	B8	Bw45	Cw3	Dw3	DRw3
A9 (Aw23, 24)	B12	Bw46	Cw4	Dw4	DRw4
A10 (A25, 26)	B13	Bw47	Cw5	Dw5	DRw5
A11	B14	Bw48	Cw6	Dw6	DRw6
A28	B15	Bw49		Dw7	DRw7
A29	Bw16	Bw50		Dw8	
Aw30	B17	Bw51		Dw9	
Aw31	B18	Bw52		Dw10	
Aw32	Bw21	Bw53		Dw11	
Aw33	Bw22	Bw54			
Aw36	B27				
Aw43	Bw35	B5 is split into Bw51, 52			
	B37	B12 is split into Bw44, 45			
	Bw38	Bw16 is split into Bw38, 39			
	Bw39	Bw22 includes Bw54			
	B40				
	Bw41				

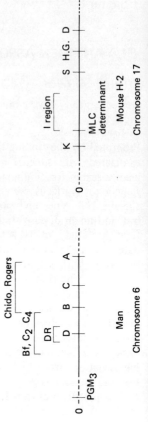

Figure 1 The Major Histocompatibility Complex in mouse and man

Note: In mouse H-2 region, the S locus products are the equivalent of C_2 in man, and H-2G is a red cell alloantigen

In the same chromosomal region are genes for several other polymorphic products, including at least three components of the complement cascade (C2, C4 and Factor B of the alternate pathway). There is a remarkable degree of similarity between the arrangement of genes in the MHC of most mammalian species studied, including mouse, rat, chimpanzee, rhesus monkey, dog, and pig (Figure 1) mouse and man. HLA antigens are expressed on nucleated cells and platelets, but are apparently not present on mature red cells, although they have been detected on reticulocytes. Mature human red cells do express an antigen system, Bg, which appears to have some serologically detectable relationship to HLA. At least two other distinct red cell groups, Chido and Rogers, are also defined by genes in the MHC region. The easiest source of cells for detection and characterisation of HLA antigens is peripheral blood leucocytes, and it is these cells that are used for the technique of tissue typing.

Identification of HLA Antigens

HLA-A, B, C antigens are identified by relatively simple serological procedures using preparations of purified viable lymphocytes. Because of the complexity of the HLA system, many selected antisera are required to define the known A, B and C antigens. HLA antibodies for tissue typing purposes are derived from the sera of ante- or post-natal women, who develop anti-HLA antibodies during pregnancy by a process analogous to Rhesus D immunisation. HLA antibodies, however, are not harmful to either mother or infant, but are an invaluable source of reagents for tissue-typing purposes. It has not proved possible to prepare specific HLA antisera by animal immunisation, apparently because the species antibody is preferentially produced, without isoantigenic specificity. HLA antisera must therefore be identified and carefully characterised by laboratory workers specialising in the techniques, and with the relevant experience of the interpretation of the serological tests.

HLA-D antigens require an even more sophisticated laboratory procedure, the mixed leucocyte culture, for their detection. To determine HLA-D specificities individually, it is necessary to use a panel of highly selected lymphocytes as 'typing' cells. To allow specificity to be identified, these typing cells must be derived from individuals who are homozygous for an HLA-D specificity. Such homozygous typing cells (HTC) are naturally rare, and it is a tedious and complex process to identify them (see Bradley and Festenstein, 1978) [2]. Because of the stringent requirements for this technique there are relatively few laboratories where HLA-D antigens can be accurately identified. Only a few HLA and disease studies have included the HLA-D antigens in the analysis. HLA-DR antigens have only recently been characterised (Histocompatibility Testing, 1977) and have an interesting restricted tissue distribution. Unlike HLA-A, B, C and D antigens, the HLA-DR series are expressed mainly on the B-lymphocyte sub-population, on monocytes, spermatozoa and a few other cells. The DR antigens are detected using serological tests similar to those for HLA-A, B, C but using purified populations of B-lymphocytes. Antisera to define the HLA-DR series are still relatively scarce, and there is some way to go towards the full identification of the DR series.

49

Genetics of HLA

HLA antigens are expressed on tissue cells, as the product of alleles of each of the A, B, C, D and DR series. Inheritance follows Mendelian patterns, with segregation of the genes in offspring, depending on which of the pair of autosomal 6 chromosomes is inherited en bloc with the other genes in the MHC region. Recombination (i.e. breakage and reassortment of the genes) is a relatively rare event in this chromosomal region, occurring with a frequency of less than 1 per cent. It is possible to follow the inheritance of the MHC (including HLA antigens) in succeeding family generations, providing convenient markers when diseases with hereditary or familial patterns of inheritance are considered (Figure 2). If susceptibility to a disease is in any way related to genes in the MHC, then HLA antigen associations might be detectable, even if an HLA antigen itself is not the primary 'cause' of the disease. However, diseases which have a polygenic background (i.e. in which several genes are implicated) or with a multifactorial origin may not show HLA associations, even when one or more of the relevant factors is linked to genes in the MHC or their products.

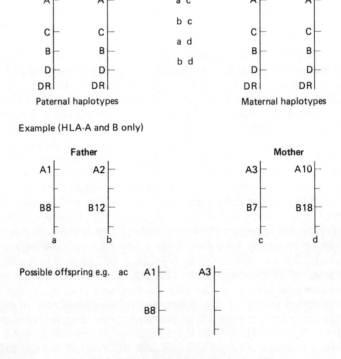

Figure 2 HLA antigen inheritance in families

50

Linkage Disequilibrium

In the study of the frequency with which the individual HLA genes are distributed in a population, it is possible to detect certain unusual patterns. A highly polymorphic system like HLA might be expected to show entirely random associations of individual HLA genes, where generations of outbred mating should have led to a state of equilibrium. However, when HLA gene frequencies are determined, it is clear that certain specific genes occur together in MHC haplotypes more often than would be expected if random distribution was occurring.

Thus, in Northern European Caucasian populations, the presence of HLA-A1 and B8 *together* on the same haplotype is about four times more frequent than would be expected for randomly distributed genes. The calculation is made using the known individual gene frequencies, and the observed A1, B8 haplotype association in an actual population study.

Example

Gene frequency : A1   0.11
              B8   0.17

Expected A1, B8 haplotype frequency (if no association exists)

$$= \quad 0.11 \times 0.17$$
$$= \quad 0.018$$

Observed A1, B8 haplotype frequency

$$= \quad 0.088$$

Difference between observed and expected frequency is denoted as D (or delta), the linkage disequilibrium value. In this illustration:

$$D = 0.088 - 0.018 = 0.07$$

Linkage disequilibrium occurs between several pairs of A and B alleles in most populations thus far studied, and is also detectable between B and C and B and D alleles. It is possible that linkage disequilibrium is also present between HLA genes and other genes within the MHC, including postulated disease susceptibility genes.

Several explanations have been suggested to explain the existence of linkage disequilibrium, and its persistence within population groups. There are good statistical reasons for accepting that the likeliest explanation is the existence of a selective survival advantage for specific gene combinations. This advantage need not necessarily be a direct result of the HLA gene, but might have arisen because of the presence of another (unidentified) gene, in linkage disequilibrium with HLA genes. The phenomenon of genes inherited in company with other genes which have a survival advantage, simply by being carried along, has been named 'hitch-hiking' [3]. Thus, the persistence of the A1, B8, or A3, B7 linkage disequilibria may reflect the presence of a third, as yet unidentified locus, which has been selected for by having a survival advantage [4].

Immune Response (Ir) and Immune Associated (Ia) Genes

In studies on the murine homologue of HLA, the H-2 system, it has been shown that the ability of certain strains of mice to respond to defined antigens is closely related to the H-2 type of the mouse strain. One H-2 type will accompany an ability to make a good antibody response, while another, different H-2 type may show a poor response. Using carefully designed breeding programmes, it has been possible to determine that these responses, and several other immunologically determined responses, are the result of the presence of specific genes within the MHC, separate from those responsible for the serologically determined H2K and H2D antigens (the equivalents of HLA-A and B). These immune response (Ir) genes have been shown to occur at several loci, within the MHC region, and close to the mouse equivalent of the HLA-D locus and between the H2K and H2D loci. The presence of specific Ir genes has been correlated with susceptibility or resistance to certain diseases, particularly some of the mouse leukaemia virus infections. Other functions related to the MHC and I region include those which are important in specific antigen recognition, and in restricting the interaction between different kinds of lymphocytes when an immune response is developed. Ir genes also control differences in response to a wide variety of antigens, including both synthetic and foreign protein antigens. Two particularly interesting responses controlled by genes in the MHC region in rodents are differences in susceptibility to autoimmune thyroiditis induced by injection of thyroglobulin and to experimental autoimmune encephalomyelitis after injection of basic myelin protein: for reviews see Katz and Benacerraf, 1976 [5], and Munro and Waldmann, 1978 [6]. High response or susceptibility is generally dominant in the mouse.

Using antisera produced by selective immunisation between mouse strains identical for H2K and H2D, it has proved possible to identify a further series of cell membrane antigens which have a close genetic relationship to the I region. These immune associated (Ia) antigens are expressed on B-lymphocytes, monocytes, sperm and epidermal cells. They are glycoproteins and there are at least four discrete molecular products, each controlled by I region genes. Many of the functions of Ia antigens are closely related to immune responsiveness, and most particularly to the self-recognition mechanism. Interactions between lymphocytes of the T and B cell series, and other forms of helper and suppressor activity are involved. It has been suggested that the mouse Ia antigens have their equivalent in the human DR antigen system, an analogy which has important implications for any hypothesis applied to explain HLA and disease associations.

The MHC region has many functions that are crucial in response to infection or related to the development of normal and abnormal immune responses, whether antibody or cell-mediated. The presence of genes for complement components also implicates this region in possible abnormal forms of response to antigen.

HLA and Disease Association Studies

With this background information on the MHC and its relevance to immune responses, we may examine some of the important prerequisites for the proper design of studies aimed at identifying the relationship between this region, including the HLA system, and disease susceptibility or resistance. HLA and disease association studies may take two main forms in the choice of patient material studied.

Population Studies

A group of unrelated patients suffering from a selected disease can be selected, often retrospectively, or perhaps prospectively (at the time of diagnosis). Factors that can influence the outcome of such group studies include the precision with which the disease may be diagnosed, early mortality leading to selective loss in retrospective studies, selection effects of hospital clinic attendances, and the choice of appropriate controls. In some diseases there may be racial differences to consider, both in susceptibility and in the frequency of HLA antigens within different racial groups.

Family Studies

A second approach (which may follow on from a population study) is to determine the HLA antigen inheritance patterns in patients and their families. Problems of selection and the degree of ascertainment of relatives (e.g. how wide a kinship should be studied) can arise from family studies. It is often useful to determine some of the other polymorphic characters known to be determined by genes in the MHC to give a more complete picture of the inheritance, and even to allow mapping of possible disease susceptibility genes to a specific region of the MHC.

Serological Problems

Selection of appropriate antisera, and the ability to detect a full range of the known HLA alleles, will be critical to accuracy. Low frequency antigens can be difficult to identify, and imperfect typing may produce misleading results. Many HLA antigens show marked cross-reactivity with each other, and it can be difficult to distinguish some antigens in the homozygous and heterozygous state. In general, HLA antigen expression is not markedly affected by disease or treatment, but there are some reported exceptions to this, e.g. in malignant disease, immune deficiency etc: for review, *see* Dick, 1978 [7].

Statistical Problems

The phenomenon of linkage disequilibrium has already been mentioned, and other factors that must be taken into account include selection of appropriate controls, ascertainment of true gene frequencies, and various methods used to determine truly significant differences in HLA antigen frequencies. Increased frequency is easier to detect than reduced frequency, particularly for antigens which have a low normal frequency. It should be remembered that many HLA alleles fall into this category, with frequencies of 5 per cent or less.

The increasing amount of information about the MHC region products and their function in the experimental mouse model has led to the extrapolation of the Ir region concept to human HLA. Early studies showed correlations between B or A and B antigens (e.g. A3, B7 in multiple sclerosis) but more recently attention has

53

been focused on HLA-D and now HLA-DR, which may represent the human MHC equivalent of the Ir/Ia products in the mouse. The highest association for HLA is, of course, that between B27 and ankylosing spondylitis. In most other diseases, there are many patients lacking the associated antigen but with the disease. This may be because the antigen we can detect is not the specific disease-related product, but is rather the product of a gene in close linkage disequilibrium with the critical gene. Preliminary work does not clearly implicate the DR antigens, e.g. there is not 100 per cent correlation between the presence or absence of DRw2 and multiple sclerosis.

Multiple Sclerosis (MS)

The association between MS and HLA-B7, Dw2 and DRw2 is now well-defined in Northern European studies. The initial finding was of an increased frequency of the A3, B7 antigens in MS patients, with an increased risk of developing the disease (calculated as relative risk—RR, see below) in B7 positive individuals of approximately 1.7 compared to the chance for B7 negative individuals. More detailed work has demonstrated that HLA-Dw2 and DRw2 are also increased in frequency in MS patients. In non-Caucasian patients, there is incomplete evidence that other HLA antigens may be implicated, with the B7 association becoming weaker and eventually non-significant in Southern Europe, and in other racial groups, e.g. Japanese: for details, see Batchelor and associates, 1978 [8]; Jersild, 1978 [9].

A statistical device to quantify the relationship between the HLA antigen (or any other marker) and disease is the calculation of relative risk, which reflects the increased chance of developing the disease when the antigen under study is present, compared to the risk in its absence.

$$\text{Relative risk (RR)} \quad = \quad \frac{pd\,(1-pc)}{pc\,(1-pd)}$$

where pd is the frequency of the antigen in patients and pc is the frequency of the antigen in controls.

Further interesting information may be derived from the observation that in those rare cases where MS is accompanied by complement deficiency, the HLA association is with B18, not B7, suggesting that there may be at least two subdivisions of the disease. Optic neuritis seems to show the association with B7, Dw2, DRw2, giving an increased risk of 2.9 in Northern Europeans for Dw2 positive individuals.

Correlations have also been sought between HLA and raised titres of measles antibody, but the results have been contradictory (see Batchelor et al., 1978) [8] and it remains to be shown what the real connection is between viral infection, MS and the HLA system. The presence of HLA-B7 has rather been suggested to correlate with a tendency not to develop high titres of antibody, e.g. to gluten, islet cells, or thyroglobulin. The correlation may be between HLA and Ir, genes determining what type of antigen recognition and kind of antibody is produced, rather than with individual response to a specific antigen such as measles virus.

It is tempting to postulate that MS is the result of a predisposing gene, in linkage

54

disequilibrium with HLA, more especially HLA-D or DRw2. This would be true only if the association between MS and these antigens were found in almost all cases, within all racial groups. It is possible that the MS 'susceptibility' gene is in linkage disequilibrium with different HLA markers in different racial groups, which would still be acceptable in genetic terms, with a selective effect influencing the persistence of the two alleles.

The role of MHC products in many immunological defence mechanisms suggests a second possibility, where the HLA antigens themselves are relevant to the development of the disease state. Recognition of MHC products in close relationship to microbial antigens is known to be relevant to cellular interaction, and defective or abnormal responses to infection might stem from the physiological role of HLA gene products in this process. Family studies of HLA inheritance in MS suggest strongly that this is not a single gene-related disorder: either two or more genes must be postulated to explain the lack of correlation with HLA in family cases, or the disease must be multifactorial in origin, with genetic elements, including HLA, forming only one of the relevant predisposing factors.

The lack of an absolute correlation for any of the HLA products so far studied and the development of MS means that HLA typing does not yet have much to offer as a diagnostic tool. The very real problems associated with accurate clinical diagnosis of MS, and the long natural history of the disease also reduce the value of HLA antigens as prognostic aids. Even within family groups, the presence or absence of the B7, Dw2 or DRw2 antigens does not correlate well with disease. There is some suggestive evidence that DRw2 in optic neuritis may have a correlation with the subsequent development of MS, but the association is not absolute. With the chance of both false positive and false negative results, the use of HLA typing in diagnosis or management is to be deprecated at this stage in our knowledge.

Myasthenia Gravis (MG)

Most of the comments on the statistical evaluation and proper interpretation of HLA antigen frequencies in MS are also applicable to the discussion of myasthenia gravis and HLA. The B8, Dw3, association for MG in Caucasian patients is replaced in Japanese by an association with B12, and family studies do not support a primary role for B8 in aetiology.

Myasthenia gravis belongs to a group of disorders most of which are, or could be, explained as autoimmune disorders. The HLA-B8, Dw3 associated diseases include coeliac disease, thyroiditis and Addison's disease. The peculiar feature these patients may have in common could be an increased tendency to develop autoantibodies, and possibly to have some imbalance in their cell-mediated immune response. There is good correlation between antibody titres to several autoantibodies and the HLA-B8 phenotype, e.g. anti-adrenal, anti-gluten, anti-islet cell, and smooth muscle antibody titres are significantly higher in B8 positive patients with the relevant diseases than in B8 negative patients. In view of the relevance of the MHC region to antigen handling and to the type and amount of immune response, it may be that it is these controlling influences exerted by an Ir-like region which are abnormal in patients with myasthenia gravis. Evidence for abnormal immune responses (e.g. lymphocyte function tests, antibody production, skin responses) in myasthenia is conflicting but suggestive. It is likely that the kinds of test for measuring immune responsiveness which we are currently able to apply are either too insensitive or lack specificity and do not enable us to discriminate with sufficient accuracy between different types of responder. In autoimmune disorders, the primary antigen stimulus is likely to be complex, including perhaps microbial as well as tissue antigens. It is clearly more difficult to apply analytical processes to such polyspecific and polyclonal responses, than to conduct the same type of study in highly selected inbred mouse strains with well-defined genetic traits. However, the application of knowledge gained in the experimental model can be most fruitful in expanding our knowledge of the pathology of disease.

References

1 Fog, T., Schuller, E, Jersild, C, Engelfriet, CP and Bertrams, J (1977) In *HLA and Disease*. (ed J Dausset and A Svejgaard). Munksgaard, Copenhagen, p. 108
2 Bradley, BA and Festenstein, HF (1978) *Brit. Med. Bull., 34,* 223
3 Thomson, Glenys (1977) *Genetics, 85,* 753
4 Bodmer, WF and Thomson, Glenys (1977) In *HLA and Disease*. (ed. J Dausset and A Svejgaard). Munksgaard, Copenhagen, p. 280
5 Katz, DH and Benacerraf, B (1976) (ed). *The Role of Products of the Histocompatibility Gene Complex in Immune Responses.* Academic Press, Inc., New York
6 Munro, A and Waldmann, H (1976) *Brit. Med. Bull., 34,* 253
7 Dick, Heather M (1978) *Brit. Med. Bull., 34,* 271
8 Batchelor, JR, Compston, A and McDonald, WI (1978) *Brit. Med. Bull., 34,* 279
9 Jersild, C (1978) In *Birth Defects* (Original article series) Vol. 14, No. 5. A.R. Liss, p. 123

Chapter 7

NEUROEPIDEMIOLOGY IN AFRICA

B O Osuntokun *

Introduction

Neurology in the tropics, and especially in Africa, is still largely at the stage in which neurology was a century ago: mainly that of recognition, description, and analysis of disorders of the nervous system and their correlation with the underlying pathological lesions. Neuroepidemiology, the study of the frequency and distribution of disease in populations and communities and correlation with social and biological variables, which is regarded by many as the key to the natural history of diseases of the nervous system and of great value in elucidating aetiology and pathogenesis in many neurological disorders, has received very little attention in Africa. The manpower available for health care delivery and research in neurology is, as with other disciplines in Africa, severely limited; for example, Nigeria with an estimated population of nearly 100 million has fewer than 5000 doctors, a dozen neurologists, half a dozen neurosurgeons and one or two neuropathologists. Yet Nigeria is better endowed in terms of trained and skilled personnel for management of neurological disorders than any other black African country. Most of the information available on the pattern and frequency of neurological disorders in Africa is based on hospital data which constitutes only the 'tip of the iceberg' and in fact may not necessarily reflect the true picture in the community. Extrapolation of such data to entire communities or to the population as a whole is highly conjectural. In many parts of Africa, diagnostic methods are inadequate and insufficient, so that in many neurological disorders, the causative and contributing factors are not correctly identified.

There is great need and urgency for accurate epidemiological data in Africa, to enhance the planning and execution of effective health care delivery. It is salutary that neuroepidemiological studies similar to those carried out in the USA [1] and Britain [2] are now being planned for execution in a few countries in black Africa as part of the efforts of the World Health Organisation to stimulate world-wide interest in the prevention and management of common neurological diseases of public health importance [3]. The following account of the pattern of neurology in Africa is based on published information from hospital statistics and the few epidemiological studies carried out in a limited area of black Africa.

---

*Currently for the 1978/79 academic year, Commonwealth Visiting Professor of Medicine (Neurology), University of London, Royal Postgraduate Medical School, and Honorary Consultant Neurologist, Hammersmith Hospital, London, UK.

Infections of the Nervous System

As a group, infections of the nervous system constitute the commonest neurological problem in black Africa [4--10] accounting, for example, for over 40 per cent of neurological diseases seen at Ibadan, Nigeria [6]. Apart from aseptic meningitis (usually of viral aetiology), pneumococcal, meningococcal, and *Haemophilus influenzae* meningitis especially in children are the commonest forms. *Escherichia coli* meningitis also occurs in young children.

Pneumococcal meningitis seems to be more prevalent in the forest belts than in the drier savannah areas of Africa and afflicts all age groups. Pregnancy and sickle cell disease increase the susceptibility to the disease [11, 12]. In sickle cell disease the increased susceptibility is due to interference with the production of antibody to pneumococcal antigen, functional autosplenectomy, defective opsonising function of polymorphs against pneumococci, and low C3 levels. Pneumococcal meningitis in the absence of an obvious primary focus is rather frequent in the African Negroes who appear to be peculiarly susceptible to pneumococcal infections [13, 14].

Sporadic cases of meningococcal meningitis afflicting some 50 000 patients every year in West Africa [3] are seen in the forest belts of Africa in which epidemics are virtually unknown. More commonly, recurrent violent and unpredictable outbreaks of cerebrospinal meningitis caused by *Neisseria meningitidis* occur in countries situated in the meningitis belt of Africa. This belt corresponds to the Sahel between the Sahara to the north and the equatorial forest to the south stretching from the Atlantic Ocean to the Red Sea. Epidemics usually begin in November-December reaching a peak in February-March and die out in April-May with the first rains [3]. Epidemics of meningococcal meningitis have been reported in other parts of Africa, especially Zambia [15]. Meningitis caused by *H. influenzae* and *Esch. coli* predominantly afflicts children.

Aseptic meningitis, the commonest form of meningitis according to most of the reports from Africa [4--7], is presumably due to viral infection. In most cases the viruses identified are poliomyelitis, coxsackie, mumps, influenza, adenovirus although in many cases no virus is isolated. Most, over 70 per cent, of the patients are children. Lymphocytic pleocytosis with normal CSF sugar content are hallmarks. It is possible some of the cases could have been caused by *Mycobacterium tuberculosis*. Other organisms known to cause acute bacterial meningitis in Africa include Salmonella, Pseudomonas, Proteus and Staphylococcus.

Tuberculous meningitis appears to be as common as pneumococcal meningitis [6] and two-thirds of the patients are under the age of ten years. Unusual presentations include absence of characteristic changes in the CSF and the presence of polymorphonuclear pleocytosis [4, 16, 17]. Other causes of subacute meningitis include torulosis (due to *Cryptococcus neoformans*), very rarely amoebic (*Entamoeba histolytica*) [7] infections and malignancies including Burkitt's lymphoma which may present as primary neurological illness [18].

Cerebral abscess, encountered in Africans less commonly than meningitis, is usually a complication of infections of the paranasal (especially frontal) sinuses, middle ear, septicaemia and head injuries and, very rarely, may be complications of intestinal amoebiasis.

Tetanus is still commonly seen in all parts of black Africa. In Ibadan, Nigeria, it is as a nosological entity the commonest neurological disease, accounting for 20 per cent of neurological admissions [6] and one of the commonest causes of death in the adult wards of the University College Hospital, Ibadan, Nigeria [19]. Neonatal tetanus is a common cause of death in children [5].

Neurosyphilis is uncommon in areas of Africa where the prevalence of yaws is at a high level due to cross immunity conferred by infection with *Treponema pertenue* (the causative agent of yaws) against *Treponema pallidum* infection. In the experience of most physicians in black Africa, tabes dorsalis is a rare manifestation of neurosyphilis in the African in whom it usually manifests as dementia, myelopathy, deafness, epilepsy and occlusive cerebrovascular disease [4, 6]. Cerebrovascular syphilis is responsible for 3.5%, 5%, 5.4%, 19%, and 27% of stroke in Dakar, Senegal [4], Ibadan, Nigeria [6], Kampala, Uganda [7], Rhodesia [9] and in Natal [10] respectively. In most countries in black Africa, there has been considerable decrease in the prevalence of neurosyphilis over the past two decades.

Evidence relating to the pattern of encephalitides in Africa is fragmentary, and incomplete. In Southern Nigeria, Ghana and Senegal, the most frequently isolated viruses in patients (two-thirds of whom are usually in the first decade of life) with encephalitis are the arboviruses, herpes group of viruses, and the enteroviruses [4, 5, 20, 21]. Postinfectious encephalopathy as a sequela to measles infection has been reported as occurring in high frequencies among the Senegalese [4] in whom subacute sclerosing panencephalitis (SSPE) as a complication of measles has also been documented. By contrast, SSPE is rare in other parts of black Africa [5-7], in spite of the high prevalence of measles infection. Cerebral complications during the course of varicella, hepatitis and cytomegalovirus infections have been reported [4]. Occasional epidemics of yellow fever have also occurred in the past two decades—one in Senegal in 1965 [4]. A rare epidemic of encephalitis by a Marburg-like virus caused several hundred deaths in Central Africa in 1976. The virulent Lassa virus, the cause of a disease with high mortality in non-indigenous and non-immune, and which characteristically presents with myositis, hepatitis, myocarditis, nephritis, haemorrhagic diathesis and encephalitis and transmitted by a rodent, seems confined mainly to certain areas of Nigeria and Sierra Leone [6].

Animal rabies is endemic in most parts of black Africa. Human deaths from rabies are reported annually from most of the countries [4-7] in black Africa.

Paralytic poliomyelitis, essentially a disease of indigenous children under the age of 5 years, is common and has been widely reported from all parts of black Africa with a frequency of 1 per 1000 in hospital populations at Ibadan, Nigeria [6], and an estimated 90 000 cripples from poliomyelitis in Uganda [7]. Epidemics of poliomyelitis are rare in the tropics although they have occasionally occurred in Tanzania [22] and Kenya [23]. Acquired immunity to polio viruses in African children occurs early in populations with a low standard of hygiene, reaching nearly 100 per cent by the age of 10 years [24].

Neurological manifestations of whooping cough, either as convulsions or acute toxic-anoxic encephalopathies, are said to occur more commonly in subtropical Africa than in the temperate countries of northern hemispheres.

Typhoid fever often presents as a primarily acute neurological, encephalitic and neuropsychiatric illness, e.g. acute encephalitis, especially in children in Senegal [25], schizophrenic-like psychosis, Parkinsonism, acute confusional states and post-typhoid symmetrical peripheral polyneuropathy [26].

Malarial infection is the commonest cause of a febrile illness in children in most parts of tropical Africa. In children suffering from malaria three-fifths have some cerebral involvement [4]. Cerebral malaria in the indigenous African is usually a disease of very young children. Of 121 Nigerians with cerebral malaria, 98 per cent were in the first decade and 90 per cent were less than 2 years of age; it was not encountered within the first 3 months of life and is very rare, although reported, in patients homozygous for the haemoglobin S gene [6].

There are endemic foci for trypanosomiasis in various parts of Africa. In West Africa, the infective agent is *Trypanosoma gambiense* transmitted by *Glossina palpalis* and *G. tachinoides* which in chronic infections involves the brain. It is common in parts of Senegal and northern parts of Ghana and Nigeria: in the last-named, patients suffering from cerebral trypanosomiasis once accounted for 60 per cent of the asylum population [27]. Neuropsychiatric syndromes caused by gambiense cerebral infection occur late in *T. gambiense* infections and include schizophrenic-like psychosis, fluctuating but persistent disturbances of consciousness, slowly progressive personality changes, progressive dementia, disorders of affect, sometimes acute symptoms with hallucinations, delirium and mania, inversion of sleep rhythms, speech difficulties, aggressive tendencies and various forms of psychomotor retardation including coma, especially in children [28-30]. The mortality is high, at about 30 per cent, under modern treatment even with suramin, pentamidine, and arsenical compounds. In East Africa, trypanosomiasis is commonly due to infection with *T. rhodesiense* (transmitted mainly by *G. morsitans* and to a lesser extent by *G. pallidipes* and *G. swynnertoni*) and causes more acute illness and cerebral involvement than in *T. gambiense* infection which has also been reported in some parts of Kenya, Uganda, and the former French Equatorial Africa. Trypanosomiasis from *T. rhodesiense* infections occurs in foci in Uganda, Kenya, Rhodesia, Zambia, Angola, and Tanzania. Involvement of the nervous system occurs early in the disease, commonly in the form of acute or insidious onset, but there is progressive encephalopathy with deterioration in personality and consciousness. A meningovascular stage with signs of meningeal irritation, especially in children, may precede a more diffuse meningocerebral involvement. The mortality rate is higher than *T. gambiense* infections.

Helminthic infections of the brain are rare in the Africans. Cerebral cysticercosis is rare in Senegal, Ghana, Nigeria, Uganda, and Kenya, but appears to be a common cause of epilepsy (6%-16%) among the Bantus in South Africa (Natal) and Rhodesians [30, 31]. In schistosomal infections the brain and the spinal cord may rarely be involved. In an autopsy survey in Nigerians the frequency of schistosomal granuloma in the brain was 2 per 10 000 [32]. Schistosoma granuloma was a cause of epilepsy in 2 out of 1923 Nigerian epileptics [33]. It is possible that schistosomal infections may cause an acute reversible encephalopathy as well as widespread granulomatous deposits in the brain and spinal cord mimicking space-occupying lesions, but such manifestations are rare in the black Africans [34] although transverse myelitis and radiculitis due to schistosomal infections have been reported from Nigeria [6], Sudan, Uganda, Rhodesia and South Africa by a few authors [34].

Cerebrovascular Disorders

Although cerebrovascular disease (CVD) is the third commonest cause of death (after coronary artery disease and cancer) in developed countries, some held until recently that CVD like coronary artery disease was rare in the African Negro [35].

In the last two decades, however, several reports though based on hospital data have indicated that CVD has become a major cause of mortality and morbidity in Africans [36]. CVD accounts for about 4 per cent of deaths in the African adult, 4 per cent of total admissions to hospitals and about 16 per cent of neurological admissions. In published series from Senegal, Ghana, Nigeria, Kenya, Uganda, Rhodesia and South Africa, nonembolic cerebral infarction accounted for 60 per cent of patients with stroke, cerebral haemorrhage for 20 per cent, subarachnoid haemorrhage (SAH) for 15 per cent and embolic infarction for 5 per cent. In SAH, the cause is more commonly due to a ruptured aneurysm although angiomas and arteriovenous malformations are seen. The sources of emboli are usually valvular disease in endomyocardial fibrosis, rheumatic heart disease, heart muscle disease and in atrial fibrillation and sickle cell crisis. Males predominated in most series with the male to female ratios varying from 3 to 2, to 3 to 1, although the male predominance was probably artefactual because in most hospital populations, as in most African communities, as breadwinners, males receive more attention than females. Compared with Caucasians, a higher proportion of relatively young Africans (under the age of 40) appear to suffer from stroke although this is also probably artefactual because in most African countries the mean expectation of life is still less than 40 years: the only community study of stroke so far reported from Africa in fact showed no unusually high age-specific incidence rate for stroke in Africans under the age of 40 compared with Caucasians [36]. However, a non-haemorrhagic nonatherosclerotic stroke, found in young people in Ceylon and India [37, 38], has been described among young nondiabetic normotensive Africans with normal serum lipids in Senegal and Nigeria [4, 6] and is probably infective in origin. Non-embolic ischaemic stroke seemed to have a high predilection for those in the upper socio-economic classes. The identifiable major predisposing factors to stroke are hypertension (in 80 per cent of patients with cerebral haemorrhage and 60 per cent of those with ischaemic stroke), diabetes mellitus (in 5 to 10 per cent of patients with ischaemic stroke), sickle cell and sickle-cell-haemoglobin-C disease, especially in children and pregnant women, infections (including the meningitides), anaemia, dehydration and congestive heart failure. Undernutrition predisposes to infection. The role of undernutrition and infection as risk factors in stroke in the African has recently been reviewed [15]. Transient ischaemic attack (TIA) is relatively uncommon in Africans, indicating the rarity of severe atherosclerosis of large vessels. TIA has been found mainly in patients in the upper socio-economic groups who were also hypertensive and diabetic [36]. As in Caucasians, hyperlipidaemia is not a risk factor in stroke in Africans.

61

In one cardiovascular survey in Uganda, the prevalence rate of stroke in 412 middle-aged and elderly persons was 7 per 10,000: the prevalence rate of hypertension was 33.7 per cent [39]. In the only reported community study of stroke in a developing country, the male to female ratio was 5 to 2, incidence rates were higher in males than in females in all age groups, and the incidence rate in an urban area (Ibadan, Nigeria) was 26 per 100,000, which is much less than the incidence rates of 50 to 400 per 100,000 for Western countries and Japan. Table I which shows the age-specific incidence rates in Ibadan, Nigeria, indicates that stroke is *not* frequent in young people and that it is a disease of the elderly (as in Caucasians) with peak incidence rates in the 8th decade in the male and in the 7th decade in the female. The atypical fall in the 9th decade in male and 8th and 9th decades in females is probably an artefact due to inadequate medical facilities and epidemiological data. The age-specific incidence rates are comparable with those recorded in Caucasians and Japanese populations except in those under the age of 40 in which age-specific incidence rates are considerably lower. Hypertension and diabetes mellitus were the main risk factors found. Mortality and recurrence rates were similar to those described in Caucasians.

TABLE I   Age-specific incidence rate of stroke in Ibadan, Nigeria [36]

Age Group (years)	Incidence rate per 1000 population	
	Males	Females
10–19	0.03	0.01
20–29	0.01	0.01
30–39	0.12	0.08
40–49	0.9	0.4
50–59	2.5	1.4
60–69	5.4	2.9
70–79	7.8	1.3
80+	2.0	2.0

From the evidence available, the pathology and pathogenesis of CVD in the African may be different in degree and kind compared with Caucasians and black Americans. It has been shown that atherosclerosis of cerebral vessels is less severe and occurred less frequently in Nigerians than in American Caucasians and blacks [40]. Nigerians who suffered from hypertension and diabetes mellitus showed a more severe and higher frequency of cerebral atherosclerosis compared with normal Nigerians, but showed a lower frequency and less severe cerebral atherosclerosis compared with Caucasian and Negro populations in the USA with the same or lower frequency of hypertension [41].

Hypertension in Africans predisposes to a high frequency of cerebrovascular disease other than through mainly cerebral atherosclerosis. Hypertension of course, is a factor in accelerating the formation of atherosclerosis, but it also predisposes to hyalinosis of small blood vessels in the brain, with resultant formation of microaneurysms which may rupture or become occluded, resulting in small haemorrhages and deep cerebral infarcts. Hence, hypertension predisposes to CVD even in the absence of cerebral atherosclerosis [42]. Hypertension impairs cardiac function, causing diminished cerebral perfusion. In the Nigerian, the commonest complication of hypertension is heart failure [43].

Subdural haematoma, hypertensive encephalopathy, intracranial venous thrombosis, vascular myelopathy, haematomyelia and intermittent claudication of the spinal cord have been reported in the same frequencies in the African as in Caucasian populations [6]. It should be borne in mind, however, that hypertensive encephalopathy may occur in the black African in the absence of severe hypertensive retinopathy [43].

Sickle cell anaemia is a recognised cause of subarachnoid haemorrhage in young Africans [44]. Other neurological manifestations of sickle cell disease as encountered in Africans include mental changes, disturbance of consciousness, convulsions, meningism, cranial nerve palsies, retinopathy, monocular blindness with optic atrophy, ischaemic infarction, massive intracerebral haemorrhage, dural sinus thrombosis and increased susceptibility to pneumococcal meningitis. Subjects heterozygous for haemoglobin A and S during attacks of migraine are especially prone to develop transient neurological deficit of 'complicated migraine' [44].

Epilepsy and other Paroxysmal Disorders of the Nervous System

Epilepsy

No study on the incidence rate of epilepsy in the African has been reported so far. Prevalence rates in Africans, based on surveys of defined communities (distinct from hospital populations) varied from 4 per 1000 in Congolese, Ghanaians and Ugandans, to 7 to 8 per 1000 in Rhodesians and Senegalese, 13 per 1000 in Nigerians, and 20 per 1000 among the Wapogoro tribe in Tanzania [33]. Overall, epilepsy appears to be more common in some African populations than in Caucasians with a prevalence rate of 4 to 6 per 1000. Apart from infections affecting the nervous system, epilepsy is the commonest disease of the nervous system in the Africans.

The age distribution in epilepsy is similar to that described in Caucasian populations; for example, in the largest series of epileptics in the African ever reported, that of 1923 [33], 85 per cent of the patients were aged 30 or less: in 67 per cent of the series the onset age was in the first and second decades of life. Males predominate among African epileptics in the ratio of 3 males to 2 females in most reported series. Again, this may be an artefact for reasons previously stated, although Orley [45] from Uganda and Hurst and his colleagues [46] from South Africa reported a female preponderance in two small series of 83 (38 males and 45 females) and 50 (21 males and 29 females).

Idiopathic epilepsy is the commonest form of epilepsy in all age groups below 40 years, beyond which the frequency of symptomatic epilepsy rises sharply to reach 100 per cent in the 8th decade in most reported series [33]. Excluding the report of Piraux [47], in which symptomatic epilepsy accounted for 75 per cent in 209 patients, idiopathic epilepsy constitutes about 60 per cent of epilepsy reported in Africans. Major aetiological factors in symptomatic epilepsy include sequelae of infections (10% to 20%), vascular lesions (6% to 20%), trauma (4% to

12%) cerebral tumours (3% to 10%), metabolic derangements (1% to 2%) and birth injury (1% to 2%), The commonest cause of symptomatic epilepsy in the African is infective and infectious disease of the central nervous system. Epilepsy followed recovery from meningitis, encephalitis, cerebral abscess or was associated with tuberculoma of the brain or neurosyphilis. Parasitic infection such as cysticercosis appeared to be a common cause of epilepsy in the Bantus and Southern Rhodesians but not in West Africans [51] ; very rarely, schistosomal granuloma of the brain is found as a cause of epilepsy [33]. Other parasitic infections such as toxocariasis, ascariasis and filariasis have not been shown to cause epilepsy in Africans [48]. An important 'infective' factor presaging epilepsy in Africans is febrile convulsions, usually a concomitant of malaria, bronchopneumonia and gastrointestinal infections; for example, in University College Hospital, Ibadan, Nigeria, 5 per cent of all children under the age of 10 attending the hospital suffer from febrile convulsions, which constitutes 20 per cent of the 4000 paediatric emergencies seen annually. Followed up for 5 years more than 30 per cent of the patients with febrile convulsions developed recurrent seizures in the absence of fever [33]. Febrile convulsion is very common in childhood among the Wapogoro tribe of Tanzania which apparently has one of the highest prevalence rates of epilepsy in the world [49]. In the African child, who is likely to be malnourished, febrile convulsions do not carry a good prognosis—unlike the Caucasian child—with a mortality rate of 29 per cent [50]. The convulsions may also result in damage to the brain and predispose to recurrent seizures in childhood or later in life. Febrile infantile convulsions occurred significantly more commonly in Nigerian epileptics, especially those who suffered from temporal lobe epilepsy, than in matched controls [51].

In some parts of Nigeria, crude 'resuscitative' measures such as thrusting patients' limbs into fire, causing severe burns and contractures, rubbing pepper into the eyes and face, causing severe conjunctivitis and subsequent blindess, or forcing down the throat of the unconscious child a concoction containing, as the main ingredient, cow's urine, produce a high mortality and morbidity due to induced hypoglycaemia and aspiration bronchopneumonia [50]. Severe burns were reported as frequent complications of epilepsy in the Wapogoro tribe of Tanzanians and in Rhodesians [49, 52] as a result of patients falling on domestic fires around which families gather every evening. Apparently, staring into flames precipitates seizures by photic stimulations, and relations will not pull patients away from the fire for fear of contacting the disease through the foaming saliva. In almost all parts of Africa the morbidity and social problems of epilepsy are tremendous [33, 53].

In developing countries in Africa, poor antenatal and obstetric care is responsible for the high frequency of birth injury to infants due to prolonged labour. Prolonged labour is believed to predispose to epilepsy, especially of the temporal lobe type, which is common in Africans, by producing sclerosis of Ammons's horn in the temporal lobe. Post-traumatic epilepsy is becoming increasingly common in the developing countries in Africa [5, 54].

So far, there is no evidence of any racially determined predisposition to epilepsy among Africans and neither are traits such as haemoglobinopathy and glucose-6-phosphate dehydrogenase deficiency of any aetiological significance. A positive family history of epilepsy was obtained in 6 to 18 per cent of African patients who suffered from centrencephalic epilepsy compared with 10 per cent in symptomatic epilepsy [33]. Some authors have reported a high familial tendency in some African populations—20 per cent in urban and 85 per cent in rural black Rhodesians [55] and 20 to 28 per cent in Bantu patients with epilepsy [46, 56].

In most published series of African epileptics, based mainly on clinical evidence, grand mal attacks constituted 60 to 92 per cent and petit mal attacks were relatively uncommon, 2 to 5 per cent, while partial epilepsy with complex symptomatology (temporal lobe epilepsy) accounted for about 10 to 20 per cent [33]. However, electroencephalographic (EEG) findings presented a different type of EEG change in the African, with focal and diffuse abnormalities predominating [57, 58]. In a series of 1180 patients seen at Ibadan, Nigeria, who had EEG examinations, 40 per cent showed focal abnormalities in the temporal lobe; in 26 per cent, focal abnormalities with or without secondary centrencephalic discharges were present in sites other than temporal lobes; in 8 per cent, primary centrencephalic discharges were present (half these showed petit mal features), diffuse and nonspecific abnormalities were found in 16 per cent and the examination was normal in 10 per cent [58]. It is possible that the rarity of petit mal in the Africans is due to symptoms or manifestations being not readily recognised as significant or serious enough to make the patients or parents seek help in a hospital.

Other Paroxysmal Disorders

Headache and Migraine. Although some authors claim that migraine is uncommon among Africans in Rhodesia and in South Africa [9, 10], from hospital practice in Kenya and Nigeria migraine is seen in hospital as frequently as in Caucasian populations [6, 59, 60]. In the Nigerian, migraine and polymyositis constitute the only two nongynaecological diseases in which there is an outstanding predominance of females, the male to female ratio being 2 to 5. Thirty per cent of the Nigerian patients belonged to the upper socioeconomic classes which formed only about 10 per cent of the population, but, as in the Caucasian, they were more likely than not to attend a hospital and complain of headache. In 95 per cent of Nigerian patients, the onset of migrainous headaches began before the age of 20, 85 per cent of them in the 2nd decade: 1 per cent of the patients suffered from idiopathic epilepsy. The variant of migrainous headache referred to as periodic migrainous neuralgia (cluster headaches, Horton's syndrome or histaminic celphalgia) was also seen in Kenyans and Nigerians [59, 60]. In the Nigerian, response to treatment with ergotamine tartrate has been good and most patients have benefited from tranquillisers and sedatives. However, in the Nigerian, tension headache presenting in the usual classical manner is the commonest cause of headache as a primary symptom [61].

Narcolepsy and related disorders have been reported in Nigerian Africans in possibly the same frequency as in Caucasians [60]. Méniere's syndrome and trigeminal neuralgia are relatively uncommon in Africans, probably because of the reduced life expectancy in most developing countries in Africa and the relatively low proportion of elderly people in the population. Hypersensitivity carotid sinus and vasomotor syncope are as common in Africans as elsewhere.

In most African populations it appears that the prevalence of brain tumours is less than in Caucasian populations, and patients are younger than those in Caucasian series. However, primary brain tumours are not uncommon and some large series, each comprising 100 patients or more, have been reported [4, 62, 63]. In most series, meningiomas were commoner than gliomas, or occurred in the same frequency [10, 62]. In one typical series of 134 patients reported from Ibadan, Nigeria [63], the neurogenous tumours, in descending order of frequency—astrocytoma, pineal tumours, medulloblastomas, ependymomas, mixed glioma, retinoblastoma, bilateral acoustic neuroma—constituted 29 per cent of the masses. The percentages constituted by others were as follows: meningiomas, 19 per cent; tumours of the sella turcica, mainly chromophobe adenomas, less commonly craniopharyngioma and eosinophil adenoma, 18 per cent; metastatic neoplasms, 15 per cent; tuberculomas, 10 per cent; and a miscellaneous group including Burkitt's neoplasm, colloid cyst, neurofibrosarcoma, haemangiosarcoma and cyst of the septum pellucidum accounted for the rest. In two series from Senegal and Rhodesia, tuberculomas constituted 14 per cent and 19 per cent of intracranial tumours [62]. Glioblastoma multiforme and the acoustic neuroma are rare in the African. Intracranial tuberculomas are usually supratentorial in location, especially deep in the frontal lobe and less commonly in the temporal, parietal and occipital lobes and rarely in the cerebellum and brainstem [64].

The nervous system is frequently involved in Burkitt's tumour: the meninges and brain in about 60 per cent of cases, the spinal cord and nerve roots in about 20 per cent. Manifestations encountered among Nigerians include those of solitary solid brain tumour, polyneuritis cranialis with bilateral or unilateral proptosis, spinal compression due to epidural deposits, ischaemic infarction of spinal cord, polyradiculopathy and meningeal infiltration with malignant pleocytosis [65, 66]. Not infrequently the involvement of the nervous system is the first manifestation of Burkitt's neoplasm.

In the African, secondary deposits of tumour in the brain are usually from choriocarcinoma of the uterus (hence, females usually predominate in metastatic brain tumours), less commonly from primaries in the breast, kidney, ovarian carcinoma and, very rarely, from hepatoma. Bronchial carcinoma as the primary tumour is relatively uncommon in most Africans except, perhaps, in the Bantus in South Africa [10]. Uterine choriocarcinoma is a highly vascular tumour and the neurological syndromes produced include cord compression, encephalopathy, intracranial space-occupying lesion and, most importantly, acute cerebrovascular accident, commonly in the form of cerebral haemorrhage; for this reason, choriocarcinoma should be excluded as a cause of stroke in an African female in the childbearing period of life [67]. Although primary carcinoma of the liver or hepatoma is very common in Nigerians, it does not usually metastasise to the brain but may present with skeletal metastatic deposits in the skull and spine and, hence, with neurological deficit such as paraplegia [68]. Carcinoma of the thyroid, more common in the female than the male in the African, not infrequently metastasises to the skull [69].

Head Injury and Sequelae

Head injuries in many developing countries in black Africa are becoming increasingly common and are mostly due to automobile accidents, falls from trees (as occasionally encountered among the palm-wine tappers and kola-nut tree farmers of Nigeria), brawls, and occasionally civil strife and wars, such as the Nigerian civil war (1967–70) and the recent Rhodesian fighting. Nigeria is said to have the highest rate in the world of automobile accidents per million vehicle miles [70] and a particular motor road, 140 km in length, between Lagos, the capital of Nigeria, and Ibadan, (the largest Negro city in the world, with a population of 4 million or more) is said to be the most dangerous road in the world. Hundreds of patients with head injuries from automobile accidents are treated every week in Nigerian hospitals. In Rhodesia, 50 per cent of neurosurgical beds are occupied by patients with head injuries. Domestic head injuries are common in children, due to the increasing number of high-rise buildings and the rising percentage of working mothers with children left in care of domestic help.

The postconcussion syndrome, characterised by postural dizziness, lack of concentration, impaired memory and insomnia has been reported among Nigerians and Ghanaians [5, 6]. As seen in over 200 Nigerian patients, persistence of these symptoms in association with clear-cut evidence of anxiety neurosis and unwillingness to return to work, or self-declaration of being unfit to work, is seen in peasants who have never heard of insurance companies, as well as among Nigerian soldiers during the civil war after trivial head injury. Anxiety neurosis was not encountered among soldiers with penetrating missile injuries of the head and other forms of severe head injuries; compensation claims among Nigerian patients were only of the order of 3 per cent [71]. The persistence of neurotic symptoms in most Africans with head injury is in keeping with a presumed organic aetiology and financial gain appeared not to be a major motivating factor. However, in a small proportion, especially those in the upper socioeconomic classes, some form of motivation—subconscious or conscious—may be pre-eminent in the aetiology of accident neurosis.

Congenital Neural Malformations

The available reports concerning major neural congenital malformations in various tropical countries of Africa were reviewed by Odeku (1973) [72] (Table II).

In most reports from Africa, hydrocephalus is the commonest congenital neural malformation. In some cases reported from Nigeria, especially those associated with myelomeningocoele, hydrocephalus was associated with the Arnold-Chiari malformation or the Dandy-Walker-Taggert syndrome [69, 72]. Occasionally, the aetiological association of congenital hydrocephalus as well as microcephaly with toxoplasmosis had been proved [69, 73]. The spectrum of spina bifida is similar to that described in Caucasians, except that: (a) at least in the Nigerians, males predominate over females; (b) in addition to the reported frequency of spina bifida among firstborn children, the 3rd child in Nigerian families appeared to be susceptible to the malformation; and (c) children not born in hospitals were usually brought for

67

TABLE II* Incidence of various major neural malformations in Africans compared with Caucasians and American Negroes

Author and year of publication	Location	Spina bifida	Encephalocoele	Hydrocephalus	Anencephaly	Microcephaly	per 1000
1 Rendle-Short (1967)	Uganda (Kampala)	0.20	0.06	1.00	0.29	0.02	total births
Levy (1968)	Rhodesia	0.48	–	0.81	0.64	–	total births
Lesi (1968)	Nigeria (Lagos)	0.12	0.06	0.36	0.83	0.06	total births
Crupta (1969)	Nigeria (Ibadan)	1.41	0.24	2.12	0.94	0.48	total births
Platt (1970)	Nigeria (Ibadan)	0.84	–	2.65	1.2	–	total births
Odeku (1973)	Nigeria (Ibadan)	0.34	0.11	0.31	–	0.10	hospital population
Khan (1965)	Kenya	1.33	–	1.00	1.33	0.33	total births
2 Record and McKeown (1949)	Gr. Britain (Birmingham)	2.67	0.10	1.77	2.31	–	total births
Laurence et al (1968)	Gr. Britain (S. Wales)	3.86	0.27	0.45	3.54	–	total births
Nelson and Forfar (1969)	Gr. Britain (Edinburgh)	3.20	0.70	0.70	3.60	0.20	total births
3 Alter (1968)	USA (S. Carolina)	0.60	–	1.10	0.20	–	live births

*Modified from Odeku, E L (1973) [72]

1 African Negroes   2 British Caucasians   3 USA Negroes

treatment very late, by which time they had relatively good physique, good legs, normal-sized heads and cysts with epithelial coverings [69] the more severe cases had apparently died at home, a form of natural selection. The majority of spina bifida children have myelomeningocoele, usually in the lumbosacral region (in 95% of cases) [72]. Next in frequency is the meningomyelocoele, followed by syringomyelocoele and lipomeningomyelocoele. Simple meningocoele and cervical myeloschisis are extremely rare [72].

A peculiar lesion seen in Africans and described in detail by Adeloye and Odeku (1971) [74] is the subgaleal or subaponeurotic inclusion cyst. It is commoner in females than in males in a ratio of 2 to 1. The cyst usually overlies the anterior fontanelle in a child that is neurologically normal. The oldest patient in the series by Adeloye and Odeku (1971) [74] was a girl aged 18. The cyst is always situated in the subaponeurotic compartment and is entirely extracranial as demonstrable by air cystogram. Surgical excision had been totally curative in 37 patients [72] and histologically the cyst is a dermoid.

Of the 76 cases of small head syndrome reported in Nigerians [75], 31 were due to craniostenosis involving the coronal or sagittal sutures and less commonly pancraniostenosis, and 45 due to microcephaly; in none of them was a significant background history of rubella during pregnancy obtained. True encephalocoeles, for which the subgaleal inclusion cysts may be mistaken, are common; they occur in equal frequency in males and females, are usually occipital, fronto ethmoidal or parietal, and very rarely arise from the anterior fontanelle [69, 72].

Vascular malformations such as aneurysms, arteriovenous malformations and angiomas occur but are generally uncommon in the Africans [62, 69, 72]. However, unlike South-East Asians, ruptured berry aneurysm is a more common cause of subarachnoid haemorrhage than arteriovenous malformations and angiomas, although all were encountered in Africans [62, 76, 77]. Congenital deaf mutes and primary aphasia [78], congenital defects of the special sense [79], pain asymbolia and congenital auditory imperception in siblings [80], tuberose sclerosis and Sturge-Weber syndrome have been reported in Nigerians [60, 72], and the last two in other Africans [4, 7, 72].

Overall, congenital malformations appear to be comparatively less frequent in Africans compared with Caucasians and the proportion of neural defects to malformations in other systems is lower than in Caucasians [72]. Anencephaly and myelocoele are much less frequent in African Negroes than in Caucasians. As Odeku (1973) opined [72], while the average African mother and fetus may not be exposed to the hazards of 'rotten potatoes' encountered in the British Isles, they share the hazards of rubella, dietary inadequacy, syphilis, toxoplasmosis, and, perhaps, others such as solar radiation. Further neuroepidemiological research is needed to highlight the factors that may be responsible for congenital malformations in Africans, especially in view of the high twinning and other multiple births reported from parts of Africa such as the western areas of Nigeria, where the incidence rates of twins, triplets and quadruplets appears to be 4, 16 and 40 times greater than in Caucasian populations [81]. Too few of the congenital neural malformations encountered in the Nigerian populations occurred in dizygotic and monozygotic twins to enable meaningful inferences to be drawn [72].

The hereditary spinocerebellar degenerations are rare in the African; sporadic cases have been described from Senegal [4], Nigeria [6], Kenya [8], and Rhodesia [9], but they are said not to occur in Ghana [5], and Uganda [7]. On the other hand, 'idiopathic' cerebellar degenerations, as well as nonmetastatic cerebellar degenerations, have been described from most African countries. It is in keeping with the culture of most African countries to deny a family history of any disease, which makes the study of hereditary disorders very difficult [4]; for example, Osuntokun and his associates (1970) [82] reported that in the diabetic clinic, a male patient had 'borrowed' insulin from his brother for three years before he was compelled to come to the 'source of the insulin' following a quarrel: initially he denied any blood relationship with his 'supplier'. A family history as a hallmark of genetically determined predisposition to a disease is unreliable in the African. Apart from a few cases of ataxia telangiectasia described in Nigerians [6], peroneal muscular atrophy in Senegalese and black Rhodesians [9], and neurofibromatosis, which is common in most African countries [4, 6, 10], there is notable absence in the African of genetically determined diseases, especially those involving peripheral nerves with or without involvement of other parts of the nervous system, in the reports of spectrum of neurological disorders.

Cerebral palsy, which was found in 0.2 per cent of the hospital population of Ibadan, Nigeria [6], is common and, except in a few cases due to kernicterus, the cause was unknown but probably related to birth injury. This is similar to experience elsewhere in Africa.

Of the other degenerative diseases of the nervous system in the African, motor neurone disease is as common as in the Caucasian, although there are some unusual features described in Nigeria and Rhodesia [83, 84]. Infantile spinal muscular atrophy (the Werdnig-Hoffman syndrome) had also been described in Nigerians [85]. Motor neurone disease appeared to afflict male Africans more than females in the ratio of 3 to 1, as found in other races. However, patients are rather young at onset of the disease: the mean age of onset in 128 Nigerians was 36 years with 27 per cent, 55 per cent and 78 per cent less than 30, 40 and 50 years of age respectively [84]. The frequency in the hospital population at Ibadan, Nigeria, was 2.6 per 10 000. About 5 per cent of the Nigerian patients had poliomyelitis in childhood and, in another 3 per cent, symptoms began in a limb which had been injured 6 to 36 months previously. The outstanding difference in the natural history of motor neurone disease in the African compared with the Caucasian is the prolonged survival of patients [4, 83, 84]. In Nigerians, of 73 patients who presented with the syndrome of amyotrophic lateral sclerosis, the duration of the disease exceeded 6 years in 54 per cent, 10 years in 29 per cent and 15 years in 8 per cent. Even those with bulbar weakness at onset survived several years, especially if they were young. Plumbism was not a factor in the aetiology of the disease. Speculatively, the prolonged survival of African patients who suffer from motor neurone disease may be linked to chronic poliomyelitis viral infections, as there is some evidence to suggest that motor neurone disease developing several years after poliomyelitis or consequent to lead poisoning has an improved prognosis [86], and poliomyelitis virus probably causes widespread subclinical infection in developing countries. Juvenile motor neurone disease with prolonged survival is also common in some parts of India [87]. On the other hand, the prolonged survival of African patients with motor neurone disease may be racially or genetically determined as in the Guamese Chamorros in whom 50 per cent survive 5 years or more, and many patients survive for as long as 16 years after the onset of their disease [88]. The presence in the African of Alzheimer's disease and Pick's disease, which are common causes of dementia in the Caucasian, has not been substantiated by neuropathological evidence.

Disorders of the Extrapyramidal System

Apart from Parkinsonism, Sydenham's chorea, chorea gravidarum and athetosis, the extrapyramidal syndromes are uncommon in Africa. However, Huntington's chorea, spasmodic torticollis, torsion dystonia, Creutzfeldt-Jakob's disease, non-Wilsonian hepatolenticular degeneration and familial essential tremor have all been encountered [4-8]. Kinnier Wilson's hepatolenticular degeneration is extremely rare in the black races of pure negroid ancestry having been reported only in a West Indian Negro [89] and in a Nigerian child [60]. The major causes of non-rheumatic choreoathetosis are birth injury, postexanthemata syndrome, drugs and cerebrovascular disease, although in 50 per cent of a series of 52 Nigerian patients, no cause was obvious [6]. Parkinson's disease is said to be rare in some parts of Africa, notably among the Bantus in South Africa and in black Rhodesians [9, 10], but this is contrary to the experience of neurologists in Senegal [4], Ghana [5], Nigeria [6], Uganda [7], and Kenya [8]. It has also been reported that Parkinson's disease tends to occur in relatively young age groups in the Africans [6, 8] without any equivocal evidence of a viral origin. In a prospective study of 217 Nigerian Africans [90] who suffered from Parkinsonism, the male to female ratio was 3 to 1, with the peak frequency in the 6th decade. Aetiological factors included idiopathic (paralysis agitans) in 38 per cent, vascular disease in 32 per cent, postencephalitic in 8 per cent, drugs in 6 per cent, toxic (typhoid) state in 5 per cent, liver disease in 4 per cent, and association with other neural degenerations including motor neurone disease, cerebellar degeneration, tropical ataxic neuropathy and dementia in 4 per cent. The mean age of onset in idiopathic, 'arteriosclerotic' and postencephalitic Parkinsonism was 55.6, 55.8, and 20.7 years respectively, suggesting that 'arteriosclerotic' Parkinsonism is probably a misnomer, being the same disease as idiopathic Parkinson's disease (or paralysis agitans). The clinical manifestations are as described in the Caucasian except that in some of the young patients Parkinsonism was sometimes reversible. Osuntokun [91] found prevalence rates for Parkinson's disease of 5, 7 and 9 per 10 000 of the population above the age of 10 years in three village communities in Nigeria. Compared with prevalence rates of 5.8 to 10 per 10 000 for England and Wales [2, 92] and 18.7 per 10 000 for the total population of the USA [1] it can be inferred that, at least in the Nigerian Africans, Parkinson's disease is as common as in the neurological admissions among the Senegalese [4] and 2.3 per cent of neurological diseases seen in a teaching hospital in Ghana [5]. In our experience at Ibadan, Nigeria, adverse effects of L-dopa therapy, such as akathisia and tardive dyskinesia, are rare.

Demyelinating Diseases

Multiple sclerosis is virtually absent in African Negroes, although anecdotal reports of three cases with autopsy verification in the Senegalese [4, 94] and two probable cases each in Nigerians [6] and in Kenyans [8] have been published. Dean (1974) [93] stated that multiple sclerosis had not been seen in 16 million Bantus in South Africa and the experience of Haddock [5] in Ghana, Billinghurst in Uganda [7] and Cosnett [10] in Natal, South Africa, is similar. On the other hand, neuro-myelitis optica, acute bilateral retrobulbar neuritis, acute (presumably demyelinating) transverse myelitis, and postinfectious encephalomyelitis, occur commonly in Africans. The frequency of neuromyelitis optica in the hospital population at Ibadan, Nigeria, was 4 per 10 000 [6].

Spinal Cord Syndromes

The spectrum of spinal cord syndromes as seen in the Nigerians is shown in Table III. Except for certain distinguishing features of the nutritional myelopathy which differ in degree, frequency and putative aetiological factors, the pattern described in most African countries is similar.

Acute paraplegia is usually due to injury or tuberculosis of the spine. Paraplegia of subacute or insidious onset is usually due to tuberculosis of the spine or spinal cord compression from primary and metastatic tumours and arachnoiditis. The neuropathology of spinal cord tumours is similar to that described in Caucasians, except that Burkitt's neoplasm, especially in children, is a common cause of spinal cord compression or ischaemic myelopathy in West and East Africa. Metastatic lesions are usually from primaries in the prostate, liver, breast, thyroid, testis, or secondary to multiple myeloma and Hodgkin's disease, for carcinoma of the lung is rare in Africans, although it is becoming increasingly less uncommon than earlier reports suggested. Of the primary tumours of the spinal cord reported, the main ones in descending order of frequency are neurofibroma, meningioma, schwannoma, ependymoma, astrocytoma, chordoma and ganglioneuroblastoma [4, 6, 62]. An unusual cause of spinal cord compression and disease is chronic arachnoiditis, often of obscure aetiology—only in a few instances can it be causally related to previous or concomitant tuberculous or syphilitic infection—and characterised by localised pia-arachnoidal scarring with cyst formation and extradural deposit of granulation tissue. Rare causes of spinal cord compression include epidural

72

TABLE III   Major Spinal Cord Syndromes as seen in University College Hospital, Ibadan, Nigeria, 1957-1970

	No. of cases	Frequency per 1000 in hospital population
Tuberculosis of the spine with spinal cord compression	406	2.10
Intraspinal canal neoplasms	54	0.24
Other causes of spinal cord compression	76	0.34
Nutritional myelopathy (as part of tropical ataxic neuropathy in Nigerians)	395	1.80
Myelopathy of obscure aetiology	90	0.41
Spinal injuries	80	0.36
Spondylotic myelopathy	65	0.30
Arachnoiditis (chronic)	26	0.12
Syringomyelia	3	–
Platybasia	2	–
Syphilitic myelopathy	8	–
Myelopathy secondary to portacaval shunt	2	–

abscesses, schistosomal granuloma (usually intramedullary) cysticercosis and dermoid cyst.

Spinal injuries are often the result of motor accidents, falls from palm trees, or kola nut trees or trauma to the cervical spine in those who accidentally fall when carrying heavy loads on the head—porter's neck [62, 69].

Cervical spondylosis is seen as a cause of myelopathy, but it is only half as common as in Caucasians [95], and ruptured intervertebral disc is rare in Africans [6, 62].

Foramen magnum abnormalities, syringobulbia and syringomyelia are rarely encountered in Africans.

Subacute combined degeneration from undoubted Addisonian pernicious anaemia is virtually unknown in the African Negro.

There are reports from various parts of Africa of 'nutritional' myelopathy resembling the syndrome first described among Jamaicans by Strachan [96]. In the Senegalese [6], the pyramidal tracts or the posterior columns of the spinal cord or both are predominantly involved, with or without peripheral neuropathic components, with impairment of vision and hearing in about 25 per cent of the patients. Overt evidence of malnutrition may be absent, although in a third of the patients gastrointestinal symptoms are present. The aetiological factors were believed to be 'nutritional' although the precise nature is obscure [6], and there was no investigation of chronic cyanide intoxication in these patients who subsisted mainly on rice and millet, which are rich in cyanogenetic glycoside. Patients with this disease constituted 2.3 per cent of neurological admissions in Dakar, Senegal. 'Nutritional' spinal myelopathy with ataxia but without impairment of vision and hearing had also been described in most parts of West Africa [5, 6],

Kenya, Uganda and Natal [7, 8, 10] and was believed to be due to vitamin and other nutritional deficiencies and/or toxins.

In Nigerians and Tanzanians, strong circumstantial evidence has accrued in the last three decades suggesting that the syndrome of tropical ataxic neuropathy is causally related to chronic cyanide intoxication of dietary origin and perhaps also (in Nigerians) to riboflavin deficiency, and low plasma caeruloplasmin levels [91, 97-100]. In Nigerians, the syndrome of tropical ataxic neuropathy comprises myelopathy with predominant involvement of the posterior columns, bilateral optic atrophy, and perceptive deafness, symmetrical peripheral polyneuropathy, and evidence of more diffuse degenerative lesions in the neuraxis with cerebellar degeneration, Parkinsonism, motor neurone disease, dementia and schizophreniform psychosis. In Nigerians, the disease affected all age groups and the sexes equally but was rare in the first decade of life. Familial cases accounted for 40 per cent of 400 patients studied in one series, but there was no evidence of genetically determined predisposition.

Patients subsisted mainly on a cassava diet. The thiocyanate content of food items mainly eaten by Nigerians is low whereas the cyanide content of food items of cassava derivatives is high. Plasma levels of thiocyanate (a detoxication product of cyanide), cyanide and urinary thiocyanate excretion were high in Nigerian patients. The levels fell when the patients were fed on low cassava hospital diet, and rose again when the patients reverted to cassava meals. Levels of free cyanide in blood were raised. Sulphur-containing aminoacids were absent in plasma in 60 per cent of the patients, and greatly reduced in others. In patients, the levels of serum and tissue (hepatic) cyanocobalamin (another product of cyanide detoxication) were high. Total serum and tissue (hepatic) B_{12} levels were normal. Normal methylmalonic acid excretion before and after valine loading excluded abnormal B_{12} metabolism. The prevalence of goitre of 2 per cent to 5 per cent in the patients was significantly higher than in the population and appeared to be related to cassava diet and high plasma thiocyanate levels.

Neuroepidemiological studies in Nigeria showed correlation of the prevalence of the disease with intensity of cassava cultivation, frequency of cassava meals, and plasma thiocyanate levels. The prevalence of the disease in one high cassava-eating village was nearly 3 per cent and, in males in the 6th decade of life, 8 per cent. Those who handled cassava roots, such as cassava farmers and processors, appeared to have the highest risk of developing the disease. Detailed studies to exclude dietary deficiencies (of thiamine, nicotinic acid, riboflavin, B_{12}, folate, panthothenic acid, pyridoxine, proteincalorie malnutrition) other intoxications, infections and metabolic derangements, showed only low plasma levels of riboflavin and caeruloplasmin and low urinary excretion of riboflavin. The effects of riboflavin deficiency might summate with those of chronic cyanide intoxication: the latter may cause conditioned deficiency of thiamine, and pyridoxine. In each area of tropical Africa where the syndrome or variants of it have been described, similar detailed studies as in the Nigerians would be valuable in unravelling the aetiological factors, which need not be the same or necessarily occur in the same proportions or frequencies in all geographical areas of Africa. As illustrated by the diverse aetiologies of peripheral neuropathies, variants of the nutritional myelopathic-neuropathic syndromes reported from various parts of Africa, the West Indies and India need not be aetiologically related to chronic cyanide intoxication of dietary origin.

In many parts of Africa—Senegal, Ghana, Nigeria, Kenya, Uganda, Rhodesia, Natal [4-10]—there have been reports of patients with isolated spinal cord disease of insidious onset, presenting primarily as spastic paraparesis with normal sphincteric function, normal cerebrospinal fluid, absence of radiological evidence of spondylosis, normal myelographic examination and no clinical and laboratory evidence of dietary deficiencies, intoxications, infections, arachnoiditis and intraspinal granuloma. A diagnosis of myelopathy of obscure origin is usually applied to this group, and aetiological factors and pathogenesis so far are unknown. Some of the cases could be due to demyelination and others resemble familial spastic paraparesis.

Diseases of Peripheral Nerves

In all parts of Africa, diseases of peripheral nerves are common. There are so far no reports of studies to determine true incidence and prevalence rates. However, excluding the nutritional or toxonutritional myelopathic-neuropathic syndromes in which peripheral neuropathy, optic and auditory 'nerve' lesions are common, diseases of the peripheral nerves accounted for 8 per cent of 4519 neurological admissions in Senegal [4], 4.7 per cent in Natal, South Africa [10], and were found in 0.3 per cent of the hospital population at Ibadan, Nigeria [6]. Billinghurst [7] stated that among the Ugandans, peripheral neuropathies were less common than elsewhere in Africa. In the experience of Haddock [5] in Ghana, peripheral neuropathies, especially acute infective polyneuropathy (Guillain-Barré syndrome), were as common in Caucasians.

TABLE IV Frequencies of aetiological factors in peripheral neuropathies in the Africans

Aetiological factors	Range of frequencies (%)
Nutritional deficiencies	25–40
Idiopathic	30–60
Guillain-Barré syndrome	5–10
Leprosy*	5–10
Primary presentation of diabetes mellitus	3–4
Diphtheria	2–3
Alcoholism	4–10
Botulism	1–2
Drug-induced (usually INH, nitrofurantoin)	3–4
Porphyria	2–3
Malignant disease	3–4
Miscellaneous	8–10

* Leprosy as a nosological entity is the commonest cause of neuropathy in all parts of Africa, but it is usually confined to leprosaria and therefore patients are not seen by neurologists, unless they present predominantly as primary neurotic leprosy with little or no dermatological manifestations.

75

Evidence about the relative frequencies of aetiological factors has come so far from data obtained in hospitals. With regard to aetiological factors of peripheral neuropathies which were symmetrical, sensory, motor or sensorimotor with or without autonomic manifestations (but excluding isolated diseases of cranial nerves). Table IV gives an approximate representation of the frequencies as encountered in the Africans.

In nutritional neuropathies, there was usually evidence of malnutrition such as mucocutaneous lesions, malabsorption, supporting laboratory data, including specific changes of serum proteins and vitamin deficiencies, predisposing factors such as poverty, lack of care, diarrhoea, excessive vomiting from pregnancy, disease states, etc., mental illness, anorexia, precipitating conditions such as pregnancy, lactation, febrile illness and alcoholism. True pellagroid neurological syndromes are rarely seen in Africa, even in areas where maize is the staple diet.

The Guillain-Barré syndrome (GBS) appears to be as common in Africans as in Caucasians and the predisposing factors, clinical manifestations and prognosis are similar to those reported in Caucasians [4-8, 101]. In Uganda, GBS was the commonest form of peripheral neuropathy [7].

In Africa, most practising physicians interested in neurology, as well as the few neurologists, would not see on a regular basis patients suffering from diabetes mellitus and therefore would only occasionally see the neuropathic complications of diabetes mellitus when these are the presenting symptoms, or very rarely when the patients are referred by diabetologists. However, peripheral neuropathy is a common complication of diabetes mellitus in Africans and was present in 48 per cent of 830 Nigerian diabetics [83, 102, 103]. Of these, in 21 patients, symmetrical sensory or sensorimotor polyneuropathy was the primary presentation of diabetes mellitus. The pattern and frequencies of peripheral neuropathy in non-alcoholic calcific pancreatic diabetes mellitus, a very common condition in developing countries in Africa and other parts of the tropics where malnutrition is also rife, were the same as in Africans who suffered from maturity-onset and hereditary juvenile diabetes mellitus [7, 102].

Alcoholism is becoming increasingly common in Africa and in many Africans other factors apart from ethanol, such as toxins, including methanol, may be important particularly since many natives consume home-brewed intoxicating drinks.

In view of the high prevalence of tuberculosis in many communities in Africa and the frequent use of INH in the treatment, one would expect a higher frequency of INH-induced neuropathy but recent studies have shown that in most Africans, the proportion of slow acetylators of INH is lower than in Caucasians.

The miscellaneous group of causes of peripheral neuropathy included renal and hepatic failure, myelomatosis, collagen disease, and amyloidosis. Paraneoplastic syndromes including peripheral neuropathies were usually secondary to malignancies of gastrointestinal tract, ovary, breast and myelomatosis. Carcinoma of the lung is relatively rare in Africans.

Conspicuously absent in the African environment are the genetically determined metabolic aberrations and diseases due to enzymic defects or other abnormalities, in which peripheral neuropathy is either the sole or predominant feature or a significant concomitant and component of their pathological manifestations.

76

Hence, peroneal muscular atrophy (of which there are a few case reports from Senegal [4], Uganda [7], Kenya [8], Rhodesia [9]), giant axonal neuropathy, hereditary sensory neuropathies, ataxia telangiectasia (2 cases described in Nigerians [6]), polyglucosan body axonopathy, Fabry's disease, Tangier disease, Bassen-Kornzweig disease, familial dysautonomia, neuraxonal dystrophy, Leigh's disease, agenesis of the corpus callosum with peripheral neuropathy, Déjerine-Sotta's syndrome, Roussy-Levy syndrome, Refsum's disease, adrenoleukodystrophy, metachromatic dystrophy, Krabbe's disease and Pelizaeus-Merzbacher's disease, have been virtually unrecognised in all parts of black Africa.

At present, many of the industrial toxins and environmental factors recognised in the developed countries as causally related to diseases of the nervous system are irrelevant and unimportant aetiologically in the diseases of the peripheral nerves in Africans. There are none or few industries that involve the manufacture or use of polymers, plasticisers, pigment, rayon, organic solvents, batteries (lead), rubber, electronics and antineoplastic drugs, although in the near future these industries are bound to be established and grow in size and number. However, farmers in developing countries of Africa increasingly use herbicides, insecticides, rodenticides (which are usually derivatives of organophosphates), hexachlorophene, hexachloro-benzenes, pyrethrum, thallium and arsenic. There are no reliable statistics on the extent of the hazards, morbidity and mortality constituted by these. In the last two decades, annually periodic self-limiting epidemics of a neurological disease character-ised mainly by extrapyramidal dysfunction, convulsions, coma, and ataxia had been described in parts of Nigeria and were believed to be associated with poisoning from organophosphate insecticides used to control cocoa-pod disease [104], although peripheral neuropathies were not overt or conspicuous features of the clinical manifestations. Developing countries in Africa and elsewhere need to be made more aware than hitherto of the existence of the industrial and environmental neurotoxins which have proved to be causally related to peripheral neuropathies and other neural complications in order to avoid repeating the traumatic experience of the developed countries.

Acute intermittent porphyria encountered in West and East Africa [8, 105] is distinct from acute porphyria variegata of the South African Caucasians. Symptom-atic porphyria cutanea tarda linked with liver disease, alcoholism, and peripheral neuropathy had been described as being common in the Zulus in Natal [10].

It must be emphasised that as a nosological entity leprosy is the commonest cause of neuropathy in the world, afflicting some 15 million people. In fact, leprosy is primarily a neuropathic disease for in *all* cases the peripheral nerves are involved, whereas in a series of 11 000 patients, 4.3 per cent had involvement of the peri-pheral nerves without any cutaneous manifestations [106]. A number of cases of primary neuritic leprosy had also been reported [107-110]. Most patients in developing countries who suffer from leprosy are treated in special centres (lepro-saria) and are rarely seen by neurologists. Hence, in most series of peripheral neuropathies presented by neurologists, the pride of place of leprosy as the most important and common cause of peripheral neuropathy is not likely to be obvious.

True subacute combined degeneration of the spinal cord, and vitamin B_{12} deficiency due to Addisonian pernicious anaemia is virtually unknown in Africans

[4–7], although there had been unconvincing isolated reports of one or two cases from Kenya [8] and Zambia.

The commonest causes of isolated diseases of the cranial nerves in Africans were malignant diseases of the paranasal sinuses, Burkitt's tumour (especially in children in whom the jaw, maxillary and other nodal or parenchymal tumours such as abdominal and ovarian, may not be obvious [66]), haemoglobinopathies (especially homozygous sickle cell disease and heterozygous sickle-cell-haemoglobin-C disease), bacterial and carcinomatous meningitis, neurosarcoidosis, medial sphenoidal ridge meningiomas, pituitary tumours with or without suprasellar extensions, supraclinoid aneurysms of the internal carotid and posterior communicating arteries, diabetes mellitus, and the transient cranial nerve palsies often encountered in African patients with migraine who are heterozygous for haemoglobins A and S [44]. There have been few reports of the painful ophthalmoplegia syndrome (Tolosa-Hunt) from Kenya [9].

Isolated optic atrophy (nonglaucomatous), a not uncommon finding in Africans, was generally due to bilateral retrobulbar neuritis (in a third of patients), choroido-retinitis (probably due to toxoplasmosis), occasionally to pituitary and medial sphenoidal ridge tumours, onchocercal infections, trauma (in 15%), unidentified toxins including methyl alcohol as accidental contaminants of home-made alcoholic brews (4% to 20%), sequelae of meningitis (4%) and maturity-onset diabetes mellitus: in 20% to 50% of cases, no identifiable causes were found [7, 111]. Idiopathic optic atrophy with impaired vision in the tropics has been labelled the tropical amblyopia syndrome [112], in the absence of ocular causes, and might either represent variants of the nutritional myelopathic-neuropathic syndrome [113] or neuromyelitis optica sine myelitis [6].

Sciatica due to ruptured intervertebral disc is rarely encountered in Africans [4–8, 10, 24, 62]. When present, it is usually found in those of the upper socio-economic classes and usually at the level of L4–5 instead of L5–S1 as commonly seen in the Caucasian. Levy and Axton [62] attributed the rarity of ruptured discs to unusually increased mobility of the lumbar spine in the African compared with the Caucasian. Cosnett [10] believed that one reason for the rarity of ruptured discs in the African may be the conditioning effects of lifelong strenuous manual work, physical exertion, or mechanical stresses. I suggest that the rarity of ruptured discs in African peasants might be related to the habit of sleeping on mats spread on the flat hard surface of 'Mother Earth'. Pelvic malignant disease, especially in the female, was found to be a common cause of the symptom complex in the Nigerians.

As earlier emphasised, cervical spondylosis, although encountered in Africans, was only half as frequent as in Caucasians over the age of 50 years, as found in a comparative study [95]. Neuralgic amyotrophy and brachial plexitis as a complication of serotherapy and vaccination are commonly seen. Brachial plexus injuries as a result of motor cycle accidents are also common.

The commonest cause of infranuclear facial paralysis was Bell's palsy (idiopathic facial palsy) in 90 to 95 per cent of patients, with a frequency in the hospital population of 5 per 10 000 and with a good prognosis, irrespective of treatment with corticosteroids [6]. Other causes of isolated infranuclear facial palsy encountered in the African are herpetic infections (the Ramsay-Hunt syndrome), trauma, metastatic growths or deposits, Burkitt's tumour and, occasionally, severe hypertension and diabetes mellitus.

Obstetric neurapraxia occurred commonly, following prolonged labour in short, primiparous women with cephalopelvic disproportion. It is usually unilateral, but occasionally bilateral, and as a rule, but not always, the result of prolonged labour. The prognosis was good except when associated with genitovesicorectal fistulas—evidence of severe obstructed and prolonged labour. Neurological pelvimetric and electrodiagnostic assessments, as well as intravenous pyelographic investigation, indicate that the pathogenesis was essentially a neurapraxis of the lumbosacral cord of the sacral plexus, sometimes accompanied by transient hydroureter and transient palsy of the femoral and obturator nerves, as well as ascending reversible ischaemic dysfunction of the lower lumbosacral segments of the spinal cord [6].

The various entrapment syndromes of the peripheral nerves commonly involving the median nerve at the wrist in the carpal tunnel, the ulnar nerve in the olecranon groove at the elbow, the radial nerve in the arm (as in 'Saturday night' paralysis), the medial plantar nerve, the common peroneal nerve, and the lateral cutaneous nerve of the thigh were encountered: their manifestations were similar to those described in Caucasians although some authors [5] believed they were less common in Africans.

Primary Diseases of the Muscles

Of all neurological diseases, the least documented in Africans are primary disease of muscles. Collomb and colleagues [4] mentioned that among the Senegalese dermatomyositis was occasionally seen in childhood, polymyositis and the Duchenne's type of muscular dystrophy in adults, that the limb-girdle and scapulo-facio-humeral types and dystrophia myotonica had never been recognised, and that myasthenia gravis, though seen, was very rare. Haddock [5], in Ghana, reported a similar experience. Among Ugandans, primary diseases of muscles accounted for 4 per cent of neurological diseases, Duchenne's and limb-girdle types were commonly seen, but scapulo-facio-humeral types of muscular dystrophy and dystrophia myotonica had never been encountered. The above pattern appeared to be the same in Rhodesia, Kenya, and Natal (South Africa), although Cosnett considered that among the Zulus in Natal [10] osteomalacia myopathy was common. It appears that our experience of primary muscle diseases among Nigerians is the most comprehensive in Africans. Table V shows the frequencies of primary muscle diseases as seen in the University College Hospital, Ibadan, Nigeria, over a 20-year period. Our earlier experience has been published [60, 114].

The clinical presentations in Nigerians were in no way different from those described in Caucasians. In spite of the fallacy about the use of hospital statistics, it would appear that frequencies of these diseases are similar to those described in Caucasian hospital populations. It is outstanding that, as with migraine, in polymyositis African females predominate over males in a ratio of 2 to 1. Aetiological factors were malignant neoplasms, multiple myeloma, rheumatoid arthritis, and disseminated lupus erythematosus. In 50 per cent of the patients with polymyositis

79

no other predisposing causes were found. In one Nigerian patient it was believed that polymyositis might have been causally related to guinea-worm (*Dracunculus medinensis*) infection. No patient with muscle disease suffered from cysticercosis.

It is important to mention that, generally, the so-called autoimmune diseases are rare in Nigerians [115] as well as in other Africans.

TABLE V Primary Diseases of the Muscles as seen in the University College, Ibadan, Nigeria, 1957–1977

Diseases	No. of cases	Prevalence per 1000 of hospital population
Muscular dystrophies	76	0.22
Duchenne type	31	
Limb-girdle	28	
Facio-scapulo-humeral	12	
Dystrophia myotonica	5	
Polymyositis / Dermatomyositis	60	0.17
Pyomyositis	372	1.10
Myasthenia gravis	32	0.10
Thyrotoxic myopathy	6	
Hypocalcaemic myopathy	4	
McCardle's disease	1	

The one patient in the Nigerian series who suffered from McCardle's disease was of Lebanese parentage, although he was a naturalised Nigerian. None of the classical metabolic diseases of muscles such as familial periodic paralysis, adynamic episodica hereditaria, Gamstorp's disease, or the more recently described exotic dystrophic/ metabolic diseases of the muscles, have been accurately and unequivocally recognised in Africans, other than two isolated dubious reports from Uganda.

By far the commonest primary disease of muscle in Africans, especially in Nigerians [114, 116, 117], Ugandans, Kenyans and Tanzanians [118–120] is pyomyositis, a suppurative disease of muscles occurring mainly or entirely in the tropics. It has also been described in Indonesia, Surinam, New Guinea and Jamaica [120]. The disease is confined mainly to the indigenous population, hardly ever affecting Caucasians who live in the tropics. In some countries it accounted for 4 per cent of surgical admissions, 800 cases having been reported by Horn and Master in 1968 [118]. It was mostly found in those under 30 years of age, the peak incidence being in the 3rd decade of life. The abscesses may be intra- or inter-muscular, the former being common in young people, and may be multiple. Usually, the lower limbs are involved. Fever, pain, tenderness and leucocytosis were usually present in patients with an intramuscular abscess. The commonest muscles involved were the quadriceps femoris in 60 per cent of the patients, but other muscles such as the trapezius, latissimus dorsi, iliopsoas, biceps, brachialis, sacrospinalis, the glutei, hamstrings, gastrocnemius and soleus were not infrequently involved. *Staphylococcus pyogenes* were usually isolated from the pus (and very rarely, *Escherichia coli:* less than 1%) and rarely from the blood. Treatment with drainage and antibiotics achieved cure in about 95 per cent of patients. The aetiological factors are unknown, but speculation has incriminated trauma complicated by viral and bacterial infections, noxious effects of migrating parasites causing muscle necrosis and superadded infections in patients who are malnourished.

Miscellaneous

Self-limiting vestibular neuronitis as a cause of vertigo had been described in Africans, and was reported in 23 Nigerian patients in a hospital population of nearly 400 000 [6].

The picture of writer's cramp and the predisposing factors as well as frequency are similar to those described in Caucasians [6].

Various workers in Africa [4-10, 121] have reported their experience of hysteria in Africans and their cumulative experience did not support Slater's (1965) [122] dictum that the 'diagnosis of hysteria is a disguise for ignorance and a fertile source of clinical error'.

The neurological complications of protein-calorie malnutrition have been well documented in Africans [4, 123-126]. The pathogenesis of the generalised tremor with akinesia and striatal rigidity which may complicate the active, as well as the recovery, stage of protein-calorie malnutrition is unknown, although recent evidence suggests that functional imbalance and variations in the tissue concentrations of the central putative neurotransmitters may be important in causation. The frequency and prevalence rate of this complication is unknown. The demonstrable reduction in peripheral nerve conduction velocity in protein-calorie malnutrition appeared to be reversible [126] but it is still uncertain whether permanent damage occurs in the cerebellum, in the synaptic interconnections of the neuraxis and, particularly, in the cerebral cortex subsequently impairing or preventing in a child the attainment of its intellectual and psychomotor potential and development [127].

There is still an enormous gap in our knowledge of the frequency, severity, pathogenesis and permanency of the neurological effects of many of the endemic diseases that occur in, or are peculiar to, the developing countries of the tropical world. Examples are helminthiasis and malaria; the latter causes a million deaths among African children every year, afflicts over 200 million, as well as some hundreds in the developed countries because of jet-age travel. Some of the main neurological complications of endemic diseases have been sketchily reviewed by Haddock [5]. We also do not fully understand the socioeconomic, intellectual and technological impact of subclinical malnutrition and under-nutrition which may affect as many as 40 per cent of children in countries such as Ethiopia and those in Central America, and even of adults [128].

Equally puzzling are some published neurological phenomena in the African. For example, there are no satisfactory explanations for the finding that as many as 20 to 25 per cent of apparently normal and healthy Nigerian civil servants and normal Tanzanians had absent knee and ankle jerks [6, 129] that the Babinski sign is often unreliable as a sign of pyramidal tract dysfunction in the African [6, 7, 10], and that the pineal gland is less frequently calcified in the African than it is in the Caucasian.

81

Comments and Conclusions

Neuroepidemiology, though the newest discipline in neuroscience, probably has the greatest value to offer by unravelling the aetiology, risk factors and pathogenesis of neurological diseases. Results of neuroepidemiological research are important in determining the most cost-efficient and appropriate intervention measures for the management and prevention of a disease, to the greatest benefit of communities as well as individuals. Hospital statistics are mainly at best only crude measures and indicators of priorities on which neuroepidemiological investigators should concentrate. Some of the outstanding discoveries in our understanding of disease processes, their control and even eradication, have come from studies of the communities.

In developing countries, the major constraints to effective planning and execution of efficient health care include lack of adequate and reliable data. Such data from well-conducted neuroepidemiological studies would enable meaningful determination of priorities and would provide clues and indications for the best methods for prevention, management and control of the common neurological disorders in the African, especially at the primary care level. Community diagnosis is a prerequisite for the effective implementation of appropriate meaningful and maximally beneficial measures at the primary care level.

To achieve control of the common crippling and devastating neurological diseases (many of which are preventable) in developing countries, there is urgent need for neuroepidemiological research to determine the size of the problem, the risk and predisposing factors, the best intervention measures using technology which is effective to within the financial capability of the community and acceptable to it. It is hoped that in the near future neuroepidemiology will receive the appropriate attention it deserves, especially for support from those who wield the political power and will, the scientists interested in research in neurosciences and the medical personnel in training in medical schools. Results of epidemiological research in neurology in developing countries may also have worldwide significance as demonstrated by the evolution of the concept of slow virus diseases in the aetiology of chronic degenerative diseases of the nervous system in man—which emanated from the neuroepidemiological investigation of Kuru [130].

What has been presented above represents no more, with a few exceptions, than a panoramic view of some aspects of neuroepidemiology in black Africa. Boas wrote, 'Some scientists will study two or three pigeons in a laboratory and then write a book "Pigeons". They should call it "Some pigeons I have known"' [131]. When the results of more neuroepidemiological studies of communities in Africa become available, some of the views expressed in this chapter may need to be modified or revised.

Acknowledgements

This manuscript was planned and written during the 1978/79 academic year. I am grateful to the Association of Commonwealth Universities who offered me the appointment for the 1978/79 academic session as Commonwealth Visiting Professor of Medicine (Neurology) in the University of London, on the nomination of the Senate of the University of London. The academic year was spent at the Royal Postgraduate Medical School, London, and as Honorary Physician in Neurology at the Hammersmith Hospital, London. Professor Keith Peters, Professor and Director of Medicine at the RPMS and Hammersmith Hospital, Dr Malcolm Godfrey, Dean of the RPMS, and my colleagues Dr Chris Pallis and Dr Nigel Legg, Consultant Neurologists to the Hammersmith Hospital, made available to me all facilities I needed. The appointment was funded by the United Kingdom Commonwealth Commission and was administered by the British Council. I record my grateful appreciation to all.

References

1 Kurland, LT (1958) *J. Chron. Dis., 8,* 378
2 Brewis, M, Poskanzer, DC, Rolland, C and Miller, H (1966) *Acta neurol. Scand., 42,* suppl. 24.
3 WHO Study Group (1978) *WHO tech. rep. ser.,* 629, p. 72
4 Collomb, H, Dumas, M, and Girard, PL (1974) In *Tropical Neurology* (ed. JD Spillane). London, OUP, p. 133
5 Haddock, DRW (1974) ibid., p. 143
6 Osuntokun, BO (1974) ibid., p. 161
7 Billinghurst, JR (1974) ibid., p. 191
8 Harries, JR (1974) ibid., p. 207
9 Rachman, I (1974) ibid., p. 237
10 Cosnett, JE (1974) ibid., p. 259
11 Lucas, AO (1964) *Brit. Med. J., 1,* 92
12 Adeloye, A and Odeku, EL (1970) *Afr. J. Med. Sci., 1,* 33
13 Hutton, PW (1956) *E. Afr. Med. J., 33,* 209
14 Bademosi, O and Osuntokun, BO (1976) In *Degenerative Disorders in the African Environment* (ed. FJ Bennett et al) p. 185
15 Osuntokun, BO (1979) In *Advances in Neurology,* vol. 25, (ed. M Goldstein et al) N.Y., Raven Press, p. 161
16 Osuntokun, BO, Adeuja, AOG and Familusi, JB (1971) *Trop. Georgr. Med., 23,* 225
17 Kocen, RS and Parsons, M (1970) *Quart. J. Med., 39,* 17
18 Osuntokun, BO, Osuntokun, O, Adeloye, A and Odeku, EL (1973) *Afr. J. Med. Sci., 4,* 137
19 Adetuyibi, A, Akisanya, JB and Onadeko, BO (1977) *Trans. R. Soc. Trop. Med. Hyg., 70,* 466
20 Boorman, JPT and Draper, CC (1968) *Trans. R. Soc. Trop. Med. Hyg., 62,* 269
21 Causey, POR, Kemp, GE, Madbouly, MH and Lee, VH (1969) *Bull. Soc. Path. exot., 62,* 249
22 Laufer, I (1958) *J. Trop. Med. Hyg., 61,* 4
23 Fendall, NRE and Lake, BM (1958) *J. Trop. Med. Hyg., 61,* 135
24 Trowell, HC (1960) *Non-infective Disease in Africa,* London p. 125
25 Lafaix, C, Rey, M, Diop, M and Alitionou, E (1968) *Bull. Soc. Med. Afr. noire Langue Franc., 13,* 517
26 Osuntokun, BO, Bademosi, O, Ogunremi, K and Wright, SG (1972) *Arch. Neurol., 27,* 7
27 Lambo, TA (1961) In *Pan-African Psychiatric Conference* 12-18 November, 1961 (ed. TA Lambo) Ibadan, Government Printer, p. 91
28 Lambo, TA (1965) *Lancet, ii,* 1119
29 Collomb, H, Ayats, H and Martino, P (1962) *J. Med. France Commun. Nancy, 217,* 1

30 Cosnett, JE (1964) *Neurology (Minneap.)*, *14*, 34
31 Powell, SJ, Proctor, EM, Wilmot, AJ and McLeod, IN (1966) *Am. Trop. Med. Parasit.*, *60*, 152
32 Edington, GM, Nwabuebo, I and Junaid, M (1975) *Trans. roy. Soc. trop. Med. Hyg.*, *69*, 153
33 Osuntokun, BO (1978) *Trop. Georgr. Med.*, *31*, 24
34 Gelfand, M (1974) In *Tropical Neurology* (ed. JD Spillane). London, OUP, p. 247
35 Osuntokun, BO (1977) *Afr. J. Med. Sci.*, *6*, 64
36 Osuntokun, BO, Bademosi, O, Oyediran, ABO, Akinkugbe, OO and Carlisle, RC (1979) *Stroke*, *20*, 205
37 Seraviratne, BTB and Amerantunga, B (1972) *Brit. Med. J.*, *3*, 791
38 Dalal, PM, Sham, PM and Kikani, BJ (1968) *Brit. Med. J.*, *3*, 769
39 Ikeme, AC, Bennett, EJ and Somers, A (1974) *E. Afr. Med. J.*, *51*, 409
40 Williams, AO, Resch, JA and Loewenson, RB (1969) *Neurol. (Minneap.)*, *19*, 205
41 Williams, AO, Loewenson, RB, Lippert, MS and Resch, JA (1975) *Stroke*, *6*, 395
42 Russell, WR (1975) *Lancet*, *ii*, 1283
43 Akinkugbe, OO (1974) In *Cardiovascular Disease in the Tropics* (ed. AG Shaper et al) London, BMA, p. 102
44 Osuntokun, BO and Osuntokun, O (1972) *Brit. Med. J.*, *2*, 621
45 Orley, J. (1970) *Afr. J. Med. Sci.*, *155*, 1
46 Hurst, LA, Reef, HE and Sachs, SB (1961) *S. Afr. Med. J.*, *35*, 750
47 Piraux, A (1963) In *First Pan-African African Psychiatric Conference* (ed. TA Lambo). Ibadan, Govt. Printer
48 Dada, TO (1970) *Trop. Georgr. Med.*, *22*, 312
49 Jilek, WG and Jilek-Aall, LM (1970) *Afr. J. Med. Sci.*, *1*, 305
50 Osuntokun, BO, Odeku, EL and Sinnette, CH (1969) *E. Afr. Med. J.*, *46*, 385
51 Dada, TO, Osuntokun, BO and Odeku, EL (1969) *Dis. Nerv. Syst.*, *30*, 807
52 Levy, F (1970) *Afr. J. Med. Sc.*, *1*, 291
53 Giel, R (1970) *Trop. Georgr. Med.*, *22*, 439
54 Osuntokun, BO and Odeku, EL (1970) *Trop. Geogr. Med.*, *22*, 3
55 Levy, LF, Forbes, JJ and Parirenyatusa, TS (1964) *Cent. Afr. J. Med.*, *10*, 241
56 Bird, AV, Heinz, HJ and Klintworth, G (1962) *Epilepsia*, *3*, 175
57 Mundy-Castle, AC (1970) *Afr. J. Med. Sci.*, *1*, 221
58 Osuntokun, BO, Bademosi, O, Familusi, JB and Okei, F (1974) *Develop. Med. Child Neurol.*, *16*, 659
59 Harries, JR (1974) In *Tropical Neurology* (ed JD Spillane). London, OUP, p. 207
60 Osuntokun, BO (1970) *J. Neurol. Sci.*, *12*, 417
61 Osuntokun, BO (1971) *J. Nig. Med. Assoc.*, *1*, 14
62 Levy, LF and Axton, J (1974) In *Tropical Neurology* (ed JD Spillane). London, OUP, p. 223
63 Odeku, EL, Osuntokun, BO, Adeloye, A and Williams, AO (1972) *Int. Surg.*, *57*, 798
64 Odeku, EL and Adeloye, A (1969) *Trop. Geogr. Med.*, *21*, 293
65 Odeku, EL, Adeloye, A and Osuntokun, BO (1973) *Afr. J. Med. Sci.* *4*, 119
66 Osuntokun, BO (1974) In *Handbook of Neurology* (ed GW Bruyn and PJ Vinken) vol. 39. Amsterdam, N. Holland
67 Adeloye, A, Osuntokun, BO, Hendrickse, JP de V and Odeku, EL (1972) *J. Neurol. Sci.*, *16*, 315
68 Lewis, EA, Osuntokun, BO and Bohrer, SP (1971) *Ghana Med. J.*, *10*, 236
69 Adeloye, A (1977) *Trop. Geogr. Med.*, *29*, 325
70 Schram, R (1969) In *Integrating Rehabilitation in Africa* (ed BO Barry). London, National Fund for Research into Crippling Diseases
71 Bademosi, O and Osuntokun, BO (1977) *Afr. J. Psychiat.*, *1*, 81
72 Odeku, EL (1973) In *Neurology Proceedings of the 10th International Congress of Neurology* (ed A Subirana and JM Burrows). Amsterdam, Excerpta Medica, p 179
73 Klenerman, P (1951) *S. Afr. Med. J.*, *25*, 273
74 Adeloye, A and Odeku, EL (1971) *Arch. Dis. Childh.*, *46*, 95

75 Adeloye, A and Odeku, EL (1972) *W. Afr. Med. J., 21*, 73
76 Odeku, EL (1968) *J. Nat. Med. Assoc., 60*, 1173
77 Adeloye, A, Osuntokun, BO and Odeku, EL (1970) *Trop. Geogr. Med., 22*, 20
78 Sinnette, CH (1970) *Courrier, 20*, 355
79 Gupta, B (1969) *W. Afr. Med. J., 18*, 22
80 Osuntokun, BO, Odeku, EL and Luzzatto, L (1968) *J. Neurol. Neurosurg. Psychiat., 31*, 296
81 Nylander, PPS (1971) *Ann. hum. Genet., 10*, 398
82 Osuntokun, BO, Akinkugbe, FM, Francis, TI, Reddy, S, Osuntokun, O and Taylor, GOL (1971) *W. Afr. Med. J., 20*, 295
83 Wall, DW and Gelfand, M (1972) *Brain, 95*, 517
84 Osuntokun, BO, Adeuja, AOG and Bademosi, O (1974) *Brain, 97*, 385
85 Seraki, O and Osuntokun, BO (1970) *Afr. J. Med. Sci., 1*, 267
86 Mulder, DW, Rosenbaum, RA and Leyton, DD (1972) *Mayo Clinic Proc., 47*, 848
87 Jagannathan, K (1973) In *Tropical Neurology* (ed JD Spillane). London, OUP, p. 127
88 Elizan, TS, Hirano, A, Abrams, BM, Need, RL, van Nuis, C and Kurland, LJ (1966) *Arch. Neurol. (Chicago), 14*, 356
89 Miller, GJ and Persaud, V (1968) *Trop. Geogr. Med., 20*, 225
90 Osuntokun, BO and Bademosi, O (1979) *E. Afr. Med. J.* In press
91 Osuntokun, BO (1972) *Plant Foods for Human Nutrition, 2*, 215
92 Garland, H (1952) *Brit. Med. J., 1*, 153
93 Dean, G (1974) In *Tropical Neurology* (ed JD Spillane). London, OUP, p. 273
94 Collumb, H, Dumas, M, Le Mercier, G and Girard, PL (1970) *Afr. J. Med. Sci., 1*, 253
95 Spillane, JD (1969) *Proc. Roy. Soc. Med., 62*, 403
96 Strachan, H (1888) *Annual of the Universal Medical Sciences* (Sajou's Annual Philadelphia), *1*, 139
97 Osuntokun, BO (1973) In *Chronic Cassava Toxicity*. Ottawa International Development Research Centre Monograph, IDRC-010e, p. 127
98 Osuntokun, BO, Matthews, DM, Hussein, AA, Wise, IJ and Linnell, JC (1974) *Clin. Sci. Mol. Med., 46*, 563
99 Osuntokun, BO, Langman, MJS, Wilson, J, Adeuja, AOG and Aladetoyinba, MA (1974) *J. Neurol. Neurosurg. Psychiat., 37*, 102
100 Makene, WJ and Wilson, J (1972) *J. Neurol. Neurosurg. Psychiat., 35*, 31
101 Osuntokun, BO and Agbeba, K (1973) *J. Neurol. Neurosurg. Psychiat., 36*, 478
102 Osuntokun, BO (1970) *J. Neurol. Sci., 11*, 17
103 Osuntokun, BO (1971) *The Neurology of Diabetes Mellitus in Nigerians:* a study of 830 patients. MD Thesis, University of Ibadan
104 Osuntokun, BO (1972) *Brit. Med. J., 2*, 589
105 Makanjuola, RO, Dsunrokun, BO and Boroffka, A (1973) *Nig. Med. J., 3*, 108
106 Dongre, VV, Granapati, R and Chulawala, RG (1976) *Leprosy in India, 4*, 132
107 Joplin, WH and Morgan-Hughes, JA (1965) *Brit. Med. J., 2*, 799
108 Job, CK, Victor, DBJ and Chacko, CJG (1977) *Int. J. Leprosy, 45*, 255
109 McDougall, AC, Harman, DJ, Waudby, H and Hargreave, JC (1978) *J. Neurol, Neurosurg. Psychiat., 41*, 874
110 McLeod, JG, Hargreave, JC, Gye, JC, Polland, RS, Walsh, JC, Little, JM and Booth, GC (1975) *Brain, 98*, 203
111 Osuntokun, O, Osuntokun, BO and Olurin, O (1972) *W. Afr. Med. J., 21*, 69
112 Degazon, TW (1956) *W. Ind. Med. J., 5*, 223
113 Osuntokun, BO and Osuntokun, O (1971) *Amer. J. Ophthal., 72*, 708
114 Osuntokun, BO (1971) In *Actualites de pathologie neuromusculaire*. Paris, Expansion Scientifique, p. 289
115 Greenwood, MB (1968) *Lancet, ii*, 380
116 Anand, SV and Evans, KJ (1964) *Brit. J. Surg., 51*, 917
117 Ladipo, GOA and Fakunle, YF (1977) *Trop. Geogr. Med., 29*, 223
118 Horn, CV and Master, S (1968) *E. Afr. Med. J., 45*, 463
119 Marcus, RT and Foster, WD (1968) *E. Afr. Med. J., 45*, 167

120 Chaudry, NFAM (1972) *E. Afr. Med. J., 49,* 466
121 Osuntokun, BO and Boroffka, A (1975) *Nig. Med. J., 5,* 6
122 Slater, E (1965) *Brit. Med. J., 1,* 1395
123 Kahn, E (1954) *Arch. Dis. Childh., 29,* 256
124 Kahn, E (1957) *Cent. Afr. J. Med., 3,* 398
125 Kahn, E and Falcke, HC (1956) *J. Pediat., 49,* 37
126 Osuntokun, BO (1971) *Afr. J. Med. Sci., 2,* 109
127 Osuntokun, BO (1972) *Trop. Geogr. Med., 24,* 311
128 Osuntokun, BO (1975) *Bull Schwiz. Akad. Med. Wiss, 31,* 353
129 Haddock, DRW (1963) *E. Afr. Med. J., 40,* 601
130 Gajdusek, DC (1974) In *Tropical Neurology* (ed JD Spillane). London, OUP
131 Lawrence, JB (1978) *Johns Hopkins Magazine, 29,* January 4

Part II Cerebrovascular Disease

Chapter 8

EPIDEMIOLOGY OF CEREBROVASCULAR DISEASE: SOME UNANSWERED QUESTIONS

Roy M Acheson and D R R Williams

Introduction

Cerebrovascular disease (stroke) is one of the commonest causes of death in many industrialised countries, including those of the British Isles and North America: thus, stroke constitutes a considerable public health problem, yet many aspects of its aetiology are an enigma.

The term 'stroke' includes several clinical entities: subarachnoid and cerebral haemorrhage (the haemorrhagic strokes), and cerebral thrombosis and cerebral embolism (the non-haemorrhagic strokes). The pathogenesis of each of these is distinct and has been well described. In subarachnoid haemorrhage, extravasation of blood (commonly from a ruptured 'berry' aneurysm) occurs outside the substance of the brain and, in this respect, the disease differs from all other forms of stroke in which, of course, the lesion is within the brain itself. As Kurtzke [1] has indicated, there are also epidemiological reasons for considering subarachnoid haemorrhage separately from other types of stroke; this will be discussed further below.

The rubrics assigned to cerebrovascular diseases in the 6th, 7th and 8th revisions of the *International Classification of Diseases* (ICD) are described in Table I.

TABLE I Comparison of codes for cerebrovascular disease (CVD) under the 6th, 7th and 8th revisions of the ICD

	6th and 7th revisions	8th revision
Subarachnoid haemorrhage	330	430
Cerebral haemorrhage	331	431
Cerebral thrombosis and embolism	332	
Precerebral occlusion		432
Cerebral thrombosis		433
Cerebral embolism		434
Cerebral vascular spasm	333	
Transient cerebral ischaemia		435
Other vascular disease of the CNS	334	
Acute but ill-defined CVD		436
Generalised ischaemia CVD		437
Other and ill-defined CVD		438

In view of their distinct pathogeneses, it is useful to consider subcategories of stroke separately in the analysis of mortality data, and this is done, where appropriate and possible, in this account. On the other hand, these diseases share certain predisposing factors, the most notable of which is hypertension, which, together with the clinical similarities in chronic cases means that the group, for certain purposes, should be considered as a whole, a procedure that has the extra advantage of avoiding inaccuracies in differentiating one subcategory from another.

Two aspects of the epidemiology of stroke will be considered here: first, trends in death rates in the United States and in England and Wales since 1950 will be compared; and, secondly, associations between stroke mortality, in England, Wales and Scotland, and certain possible (mainly dietary) risk factors will be examined. These two aspects are not distinct. Secular trends in levels of exposure to risk factors are among the more probable explanations for observed changes in mortality rates, hence such changes may be clues in the search for explanations of aetiology and the development of control.

Stroke Mortality in the United States and England and Wales 1950-1974

Secular Trends

Figure 1 shows death rates in England and Wales, and in United States whites, for all categories of stroke combined, cerebral haemorrhage, cerebral thrombosis and embolism, subarachnoid haemorrhage, other ill-defined cerebrovascular disease.

The death rates for these countries have been directly standardised to the US 1940 population; values for England and Wales are given for each year, and those for the US for alternate years from 1950 to 1974 except for 1960 when figures for the subcategories were not available in published tables [2]. Figures for subarachnoid haemorrhage in the USA are not readily available to us after 1966; the overall fall there in total rates for the sexes combined is 32 per cent. Trends in stroke mortality in England and Wales from 1950 to 1973, which show a fall of between 15 per cent and 20 per cent over this period, have been discussed elsewhere [3].

These standardised death rates, when viewed in conjunction with the age- and sex-specific rates (Fig. 2) reveal and decline in total stroke mortality in both populations and in all age groups between 35 and 74, particularly in women.

Of the principal categories, deaths from cerebral haemorrhage show the most dramatic decline in frequency in the United States (Fig. 1), and this change is evident throughout the age range and in both sexes (Fig. 3). The England and Wales population shows essentially similar though less dramatic changes (Figures 1 and 3). The acceleration in the decline in death rates seen in both populations at the introduction of the 8th revision of ICD in 1967 is in part due to the transference of death to ill-defined categories of stroke.

Death rates from cerebral infarction, in both the United States and England and Wales (Fig. 4), have shown a net decline in all age groups (except the over 75s) after a transitory rise during the 1950s; since the introduction of the 8th revision of the ICD, thrombosis and embolism have been coded separately, but the contribution of the latter has been of minor importance.

Subarachnoid haemorrhage is the only subcategory to show an increase in death rates, present in most age groups both in the United States (Fig. 5) until 1966,

89

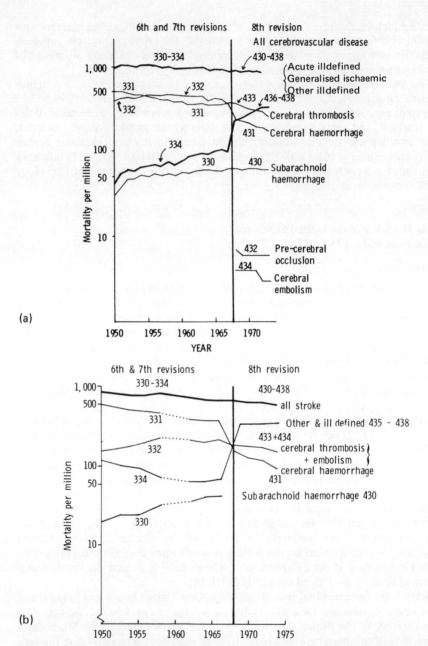

Figure 1 Secular trends for mortality from cerebrovascular disease (a) England and Wales, (b) United States whites, sexes combined. Rates for both countries adjusted by the direct method to the US population in 1940. Thick vertical line denotes 1967 when 8th revision of *International Classification of Diseases* (ICD) was introduced

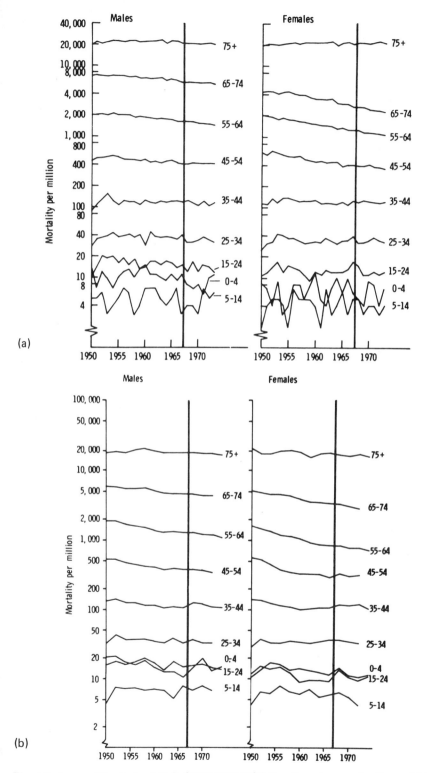

Figure 2 Age-specific secular trends (sexes separately) for all cerebrovascular disease (a) England and Wales, (b) United States. Thick vertical line denotes 8th revision of ICD

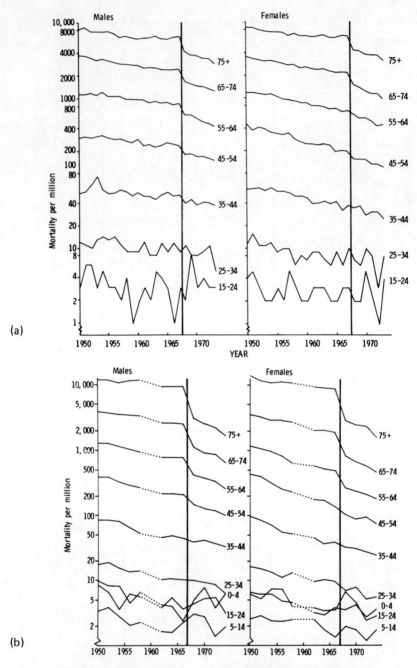

Figure 3 Similar analysis to that shown in Figure 2 for cerebral haemorrhage

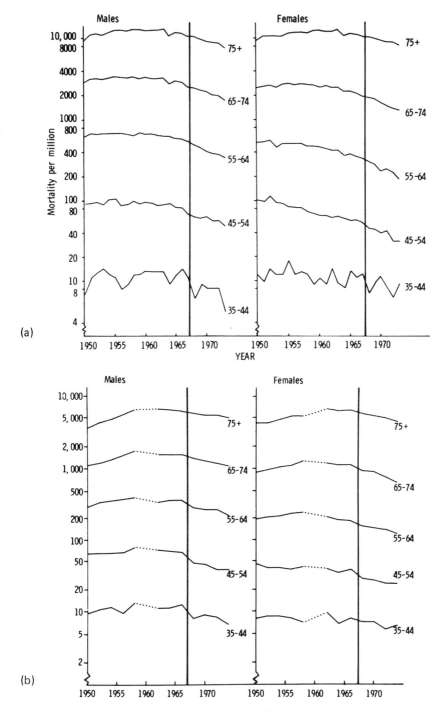

Figure 4 Similar analysis to that shown in Figure 3 for cerebral ischaemia

Figure 5 (a) Similar analysis to that shown in Figure 3 for subarachnoid haemorrhage: (b) age-specific mortality rates (sexes separately) for subarachnoid haemorrhage compared with those for all other forms of cerebrovascular disease.
Note that: (1) while mortality from other strokes increases logarithmically with age, mortality from subarachnoid haemorrhage shows little or no increase with age after 45 years; (2) while other strokes have a higher mortality rate in men than in women at all ages, the reverse is true for subarachnoid haemorrhage after age 40; in the youngest age groups, mortality from subarachnoid haemorrhage is higher than in all other strokes combined

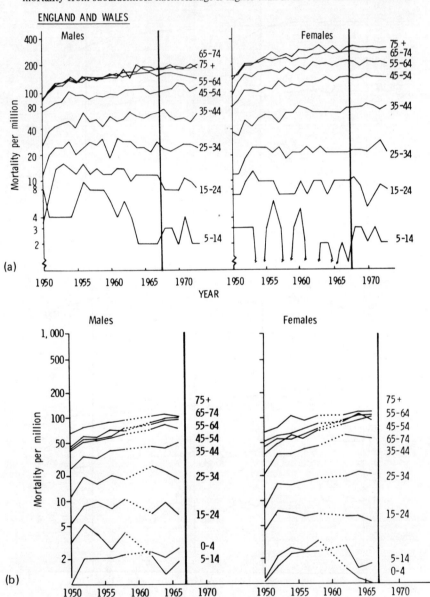

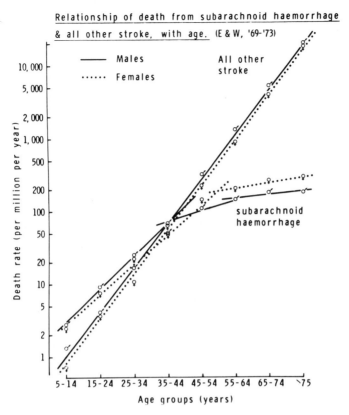

Relationship of death from subarachnoid haemorrhage & all other stroke, with age. (E & W, '69-'73)

Males
Females

All other stroke

subarachnoid haemorrhage

Death rate (per million per year)

Age groups (years)

(c)

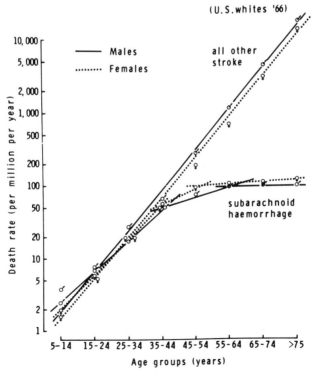

(U.S. whites '66)

Males
Females

all other stroke

subarachnoid haemorrhage

Death rate (per million per year)

Age groups (years)

(d)

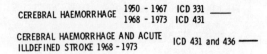

CEREBRAL HAEMORRHAGE 1950 - 1967   ICD 331 ———
                      1968 - 1973   ICD 431

CEREBRAL HAEMORRHAGE AND ACUTE
ILLDEFINED STROKE 1968 - 1973   ICD 431 and 436 ━━━

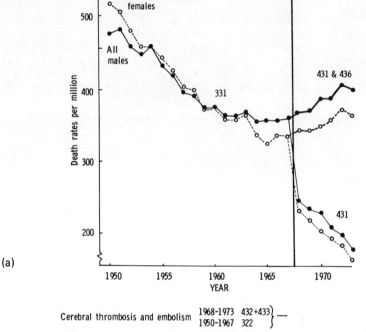

(a)

Cerebral thrombosis and embolism 1968-1973 432+433 ⎫ —
                                   1950-1967 322   ⎭

Cerebral thrombosis 1968-1973   433 only —

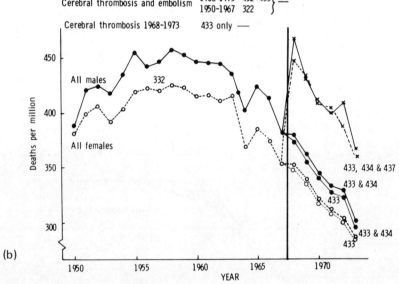

(b)

Figure 6 Age adjusted secular trends (sexes separately) for (a) cerebral haemorrhage, (b) cerebral ischaemia plotted against an arithmetical scale to show the effect on the trends of each, of coding acute ill-defined stroke (ICD 436) and chronic ill-defined stroke (ICD 437) as separate rubrics. It can be seen that after 1967 (thick vertical line) the combined rate for 431 and 436 rises for 5 years; in contrast, after a sharp increase at the time of recording, the combined rates for 433, 434 and 437 fall

and in England and Wales until 1973 (Fig. 5). Why this trend should be contrary to that of other forms of cerebrovascular disease poses an unanswered question.

Consideration of the age-specific death rates for this condition reveals a second epidemiological difference between subarachnoid haemorrhage and other forms of stroke—there is little increase in death rate with increasing age after about 45 years, particularly in British males (Fig. 5). The relationship of death rates (plotted on a logarithmic scale) to age for subarachnoid haemorrhage and for all other forms of stroke combined are also shown in the figure. The difference between the linear relationship in all other forms of stroke and the sharp change in gradient after the age of 45 in subarachnoid haemorrhage is clear, suggesting that, for the latter, there is progressive depletion of susceptible individuals after middle age while, for the former, there is an exponential accumulation of risk with increasing age throughout life. These differences have not, in our view, been adequately explained in pathophysiological terms. Other unexplained characteristics of sub-arachnoid haemorrhage are: first, that in recent years, unlike cerebral thrombosis and haemorrhage, the mortality rate in women is higher than that in men (*see* Figure 5); and secondly, despite this, survival is longer in women [4].

Explanations For Secular Trends

Several factors, alone or in combination, could have been responsible for these secular trends and these are summarised in Table II. Those in the United States have been the subject of recent comment [5], and possible explanations have been discussed.

Change in Diagnostic Habits? The first hypothesis shown in Table II should always be considered when secular trends in death rates are discussed. It has been argued that transference of deaths away from cerebrovascular disease to acute ischaemic heart disease or to hypertensive disease (with greater awareness of the role of raised blood pressure as the underlying cause of stroke), could have taken place. First in the United States, but more recently in England and Wales, death rates from each of these two groups of disease have shown a net fall so that, although diagnostic practice may have changed and may still be changing, in the long run a genuine reduction in mortality from degenerative cardiovascular disease has occurred, rather than a rearrangement of deaths between the categories; never-theless, one cannot conclude from this alone that transference of deaths away from the stroke categories never occurred. There is no longer any simple or satisfactory way of testing this hypothesis further.

Transference of deaths away from cerebral haemorrhage and thrombosis into the ill-defined categories has certainly happened since the 8th revision of the ICD was introduced, as Figures 1 and 6 clearly show. In England and Wales some of the reported fall in cerebral haemorrhage is due to this, but it cannot be true of cerebral thrombosis (Fig. 6). Transference is a possible explanation for some of the rise in subarachnoid haemorrhage, but because of its relative unimportance numerically this cannot have had much of a part to play in the reported trends for cerebral haemorrhage or cerebral thrombosis.

Improved Survival? The second possibility proposed in Table II, that of improved survival after stroke, is unlikely to have been entirely responsible, at least if recent information from the United States [6] can be generalised to other populations. This work has described a decline in the incidence of first strokes between 1945 and 1974 in Rochester, Minnesota, a relatively small but intensively studied population.

TABLE II Possible reasons for secular decline in stroke death rates in England and Wales and in the United States

Reasons	Notes
1. Change in death certification habits of doctors (e.g. transference of deaths to ischaemic heart disease and/or hypertension).	
2. Improved case fatality rate of stroke and/or reduced recurrence rate.	Decline in death rate but incidence rate of first strokes constant.
3. Improved treatment of hypertension.	Decreased incidence of stroke but constant (or increased) incidence of hypertension.
4. Decrease in exposure to risk factors involved in pathogenesis of hypertension (and, therefore, stroke).	Decreased incidence of stroke and decreased incidence of hypertension.
5. Decrease in exposure to risk factors involved in pathogenesis of stroke (independent of hypertension).	Decreased incidence of stroke but constant (or increased) incidence of hypertension.

Treatment of Hypertension? It has been argued that it is unlikely that improved medical treatment of hypertension, with subsequent avoidance of sequelae, has been a major influence in the decline in stroke mortality in the United States [5], and it is true that there has been a steady fall in stroke death rates since about 1914 [7] when Texas decided to collaborate with other States and the analysis of health statistics on a national basis became possible. Effective treatment for hypertension was not available until about 1950 and it was many years later before it became widely used. Similar conclusions have been drawn from an Australian population [8]. Thus, although they cannot have contributed to the original decline, these antihypertensive drugs might well have played a role in recent years; direct testing is again impossible from routine sources of information because of the paucity of data on the incidence (or prevalence) of hypertension in the population in the US until very recently. A further difficulty is that estimates of the consumption of antihypertensive medication must always be based upon information, not only about prescribing habits, but also about compliance of hypertensive patients with their doctors' instructions and, since little information about the latter is available, distribution of drugs can only be regarded as a surrogate of unknown validity.

Environmental Factors? Environmental factors could be related to stroke directly, indirectly through hypertension or by both these routes as displayed in Figure 7,

98

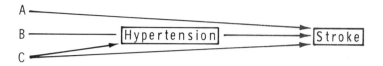

A = directly contributory to stroke;

B = indirectly contributory to stroke via hypertension;

C = both directly & indirectly contributory to stroke.

Figure 7 A simple model which takes account of the strong causal association between hypertension and all forms of cerebrovascular disease, and indicates the various ways in which risk factors might operate

and secular changes in exposure, either to those which are contributory to the development of cerebrovascular disease or may be protective against it, should be considered. We shall present some crude British data relating to nutritional variables and consumption of tobacco.

Stroke Mortality in Relation to Specific Risk Factors in England and Wales

Variations in stroke mortality *between* countries may well, at least in part, be created by differences in the certifying habits of medical practitioners in different cultures. Kurtzke [1] has reviewed the work of authors who consider this to be the major cause of these differences. Consistent differences in mortality rates between different regions of the *same* area, especially one as small as the United Kingdom, however, are more difficult to explain on this basis. Standardised mortality rates for all forms of stroke are higher in the north and west than in the south and east [3] and rates in women are even higher in Scotland [9]. It is difficult to explain them solely on the basis of hypertension, obesity and elevated haemoglobin, even though these are established risk factors. Consistent geographical differences have also been described, among other countries for Ireland [13], Japan [10], Denmark [1] and the United States [14-16] where the same difficulty obtains.

In Britain and elsewhere there are reasons for considering that a very substantial portion of the variability in death rates is environmentally determined. The secular trends in stroke mortality support this contention, if they are not simply artefacts of certifying or recording, and we believe that these are genuine changes, although their extent is unknown.

Social Class. For the purposes of studying health statistics social class in Britain is assigned on the basis of occupation [17]. At the time of the last census, mortality for every category of stroke was shown to be higher in social class V (unskilled manual) than in social class I (professional) and the intermediate social classes showing a gradation between the two [18]. Social class is, clearly, a complex attribute embracing such variables as hazardous exposure at work, dietary differences, variations in the uptake of medical care, family size and organisation, attitudes to health, and many other variables. But as Acheson and Sanderson [3] have shown, although the South East of Britain is much more prosperous than the rest of the country, the geographical differences in stroke mortality in Britain are separate and cumulative to the different admixtures of the social classes in different regions; the national social class gradient obtains within the regions, and SMRs for social classes IV and V in the South East are substantially lower than those for social classes I and II for the North West (Fig. 8).

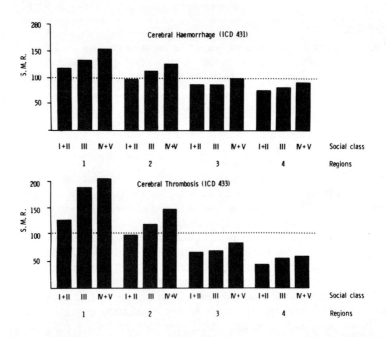

Figure 8 Standardised mortality ratios by social class for grouped regional hospital wards in England and Wales in 1970-1972 for cerebral haemorrhage and cerebral thrombosis in males aged 15-64 years. Note that throughout, although there is a consistent tendency for mortality to be higher in classes IV and V than I and II, with III intermediate, the geographical variation is greater so that mortality in classes I and II in the North and West is greater than that in classes IV and VI in the South East

This striking pattern which has only recently been recognised has not yet been explained. On an island where medical education and practice, and statistical procedures, are all centrally controlled it seems quite unlikely to be a procedural artefact.

Seasonal Differences in Stroke Mortality. Observations in several countries, including the USA [19, 20], Japan [20], and France [21], suggest that mortality from the cerebrovascular diseases is consistently higher in the summer. Responsible factors probably include a lower incidence of the fatal respiratory sequelae of stroke in the warmer weather and the seasonal variation in blood pressure. Takahashi and his associates [22] measured blood pressure in Japanese villagers and not only found significantly higher levels in winter than in summer but also recorded differences in winter levels between villagers living in unheated houses and those who possessed a stove [23, 24]. The order of magnitude of the seasonal variation is, however, slight compared to the geographical differences described above.

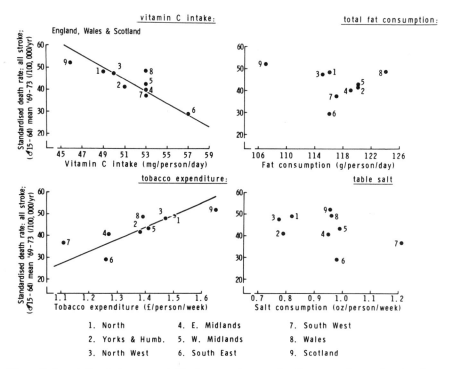

Figure 9 Association between mortality from cerebrovascular disease, on the one hand, and on the other, indices of consumption of four hypothetically related factors in the general population of the nine statistical regions of the UK (see text for discussion)

101

Salt Intake. There is considerable circumstantial and experimental evidence to implicate high salt consumption in the pathogenesis of hypertension [25, 26], and, thereby of course, cerebrovascular disease.

In Japan, where the consumption of salt is high, ranging from 25 g to 30 g per person per day, stroke mortality by prefecture is closely correlated with the consumption of salt and with that of salty foods, such as miso paste and soy sauce [10]. The highest death rates and the highest consumption are in the north of the main island, Honshu [10].

Salt intake in England and Wales is about half that in Japan with a more limited range in intakes between different parts of the country. Thus, the absence of any correlation between salt ingestion and stroke mortality in Figure 9, where population data collected in the National Food Survey [27] are plotted against age adjusted stroke mortality standardised directly to the relevant 1971 census data in the same population, should not be interpreted as indicating that there is no causal relationship between the two elsewhere. Moreover, the most pertinent comparisons would be with total sodium intake, which is not estimated in the NFS; it is difficult to calculate with any accuracy on the basis of usual survey techniques because, depending upon manufacture, methods of preservation and cooking, foods differ considerably in their sodium content.

Dietary Fat. The consumption of a diet high in fat, particularly saturated fat, is widely regarded as being a causative factor in the development of atheroma, and thus, it has been argued, in the production of degenerative cardiovascular disease in general, but prospective studies of stroke incidence have only shown a weak association of the condition with serum lipids [11, 12]. It is beyond the scope of this chapter to assess the complex and often conflicting literature on the subject but the weak correlation shown in Figure 9 is consistent with other epidemiological data.

Vitamin C Intake. The National Food Survey [27] has shown vitamin C to have considerable and consistent gradients by geography (highest consumption in the South East of Britain, lowest in Scotland and the North of England), and Figure 9 shows a strong and statistically significant negative correlation between total stroke mortality in males and vitamin C consumption for Scotland, Wales and the standard regions of England in the years 1969-73. Consumption of this nutrient also varies by income (highest consumption in the higher income groups) and these gradients could vary within geographical area in a manner similar to those that have been observed for stroke mortality in England and Wales (*see* Figure 8).

The consumption of vitamin C in Britain is highest in the third quarter of the year (July-September) and lowest in the fourth and first (October-March) when locally grown new potatoes, fresh green vegetables and soft fruits are not available [28] and so also correlates with seasonal difference in stroke mortality.

Taylor [29] discussed how impaired collagen synthesis and repair arising from relative deficiency of vitamin C may, through increased vascular fragility, be related to the occurrence of haemorrhagic stroke; it may also be associated with reduced fibrinolytic activity [30], and could perhaps play a role in the genesis of non-haemorrhagic strokes as well.

Tobacco Consumption. Apart from a recent report of an association between smoking and subarachnoid haemorrhage [31], there is still little evidence to implicate the use of tobacco in the aetiology of cerebrovascular disease. The most probable explanation of the strong association shown in Figure 9 must therefore be that *per capita* expenditure on tobacco and stroke mortality are both related to other, as yet unidentified, factors.

Summary

In summary, therefore, we draw attention to the following six questions. In our opinion if these could be satisfactorily answered, understanding of the aetiology of cerebrovascular disease would be considerably advanced.

1. The overall mortality rates for cerebrovascular disease in the United States, and to a lesser extent in England and Wales, have been falling for several decades. Why?
2. This trend applies to two of the major subcategories (cerebral thrombosis and cerebral haemorrhage); but not to the third (subarachnoid haemorrhage). Why?
3. What is the explanation for some of the other unusual characteristics of the epidemiology of subarachnoid haemorrhage such as age-specific mortality patterns and sex differences in incidence, mortality and survival?
4. What are the explanations for the geographical variations in England and Wales, and elsewhere?
5. What is the explanation for the social class gradients in England and Wales?
6. Is the strong but crude negative association between stroke mortality and consumption of vitamin C likely to throw further light on the problem?

Acknowledgements

We are grateful to Dr A M Adelstein of the Office of Population Censuses and Surveys for providing unpublished data on stroke mortality in England and Wales and for his permission to include them in this paper.

References

1 Kurtzke, JF (1969) *Epidemiology of Cerebrovascular Disease.* Springer-Verlag, Berlin
2 *United States Department of Health, Education and Welfare. Mortality Statistics for the United States,* vol. II (1950–74)
3 Acheson, RM and Sanderson, CFB (1978) *Population Trends, 12,* 13
4 Acheson, RM and Fairbairn, AS (1970) *Brit. Med. J., 2,* 621
5 Levy, RI (1979) *New Eng. J. of Med., 300,* 490
6 Garraway, WM, Whisnant, JP, Furlan, AJ, Phillips, LH, Kurland, LT and O'Fallon, WM (1979) *New Eng. J. of Med., 300,* 450
7 Acheson, RM (1966) Public Health Monograph, No. 76, US Government Printing Office, Washington

8   Lovell, RRM and Prineas, RJ (1971) *Med. J. of Australia, 2,* 557
9   Fulton, M, Adams, W, Lutz, W and Oliver, MF (1978) *Brit. Heart J., 40,* 563
10   Takahashi, E (1978) In *Ecologic Human Biology in Japan.* Medical Information Services Inc.
11   Kannel, WB (1971) *Stroke, 2,* 295
12   Whyte, HM (1976) *Aust. N.Z. J. Med., 6,* 387
13   Acheson, RM (1960) *Brit. J. Prev. Soc. Med., 14,* 139
14   Wylie, CM (1970) *Stroke, 1,* 184
15   Acheson, RM, Nefzger, MD and Heyman, A (1973) *J. Chron. Dis., 26,* 405
16   Stolley, PD, Kuller, LH, Nefzger, MD, Tonascia, S, Lilienfeld, AM, Miller, GD and Diamond, EL (1977) *Stroke, 8,* 551
17   Office of Population Censuses and Surveys (1970) *Classification of occupations.* HMSO, London
18   Office of Population Censuses and Surveys (1978) *Occupational mortality 1970-1972* (decennial supplement). HMSO, London
19   Wylie, CM (1962) *J. Chron. Dis., 15,* 85
20   Florey, C du V, Senter, MG and Acheson, RM (1969) *Amer. J. Epidem., 89,* 15
21   Aubenque, M, Damiani, P and Massé, H (1979) *Cahiers soc. démogr. med., 19,* 17
22   Takahashi, E, Sasaki, N, Takeda, J and Ito, H (1955) *Hirosahi Med. J., 6,* 181
23   Takahashi, E, Sasaki, N, Takeda, J and Ito, H (1956) *Hirosahi Med. J., 7,* 388
24   Takahashi, E, Sasaki, N, Takeda, J and Ito, H (1957) *Human Biol., 29,* 139
25   Freis, ED (1976) *Circulation, 53,* 589
26   Dahl, LK (1972) *Amer. J. Clin. Nutr., 25,* 231
27   *Household Food Consumption and Expenditure (1969-73).* HMSO, London
28   *Household Food Consumption and Expenditure (1964),* Appendix E, p. 123. HMSO, London
29   Taylor, G (1976) *Lancet, i,* 247
30   Bordia, A, Paliwal, DK, Jain, K and Kothari, LK (1978) *Atherosclerosis, 30,* 351
31   Bell, BA and Symon, L (1979) *Brit. Med. J., 1,* 577

Chapter 9

STROKE REGISTRATION: EXPERIENCES FROM A WHO MULTICENTRE STUDY

Jørgen Marquardsen on behalf of the WHO Collaborative Group for the Community Control of Stroke (see Participants on page 110)

Under the auspices of WHO, a multicentre study of cerebrovascular disease was started in 1971. The aims of the study were to collect comprehensive and reliable data on stroke morbidity and mortality in various parts of the world, to measure the disability caused by stroke, and to estimate the social and economic burden on the community. The ultimate goal was to establish a basis for the planning and implementation of preventive and therapeutic procedures at the community level. The task of acquiring relevant information was undertaken by stroke registers, operating in selected communities, using standardised methods of case-finding and data-recording.

A total of 17 centres from 12 countries participated in the study. The WHO headquarters in Geneva acted as co-ordinating centre and was responsible for the processing of the data. In some of the participating centres the stroke register was part of a regional medical programme for the control of cardiovascular disease, including also registers for hypertension or ischaemic heart disease.

A comprehensive report on the results of the collaborative stroke study is about to be published [1]. The present paper gives a short account of the design of the study and of some of the findings, the emphasis being placed on a comparison of the data collected in European and Japanese centres.

Methods

Study Areas and Populations

Of the participating centres, seven were in Europe (Sweden, Finland, Denmark, Ireland, USSR, Yugoslavia), one in Israel, one in Africa (Nigeria), five in Japan and three in other parts of Asia (Mongolia, India and Sri Lanka). Characteristics of the study areas and populations have been published previously [2]. The size of the populations under study ranged from 803 000 to 36 100, the total amounting to more than three million. The study areas varied considerably with respect to such factors as climate, socioeconomic conditions, standards of medical care, ethnic structure and age distribution of the population, and prevailing cultural patterns.

Criteria of Selection

Registration was based on the following definition of stroke: 'Rapidly developed clinical signs of focal (or global) disturbance of cerebral function, lasting more than 24 hours or leading to death, with no apparent cause other than vascular'. The term 'global' disturbance applies particularly to cases of subarachnoid haemorrhage without focal neurological signs. This purely clinical definition of stroke was chosen because it can be used by doctors, or even paramedical workers, without access to advanced diagnostic facilities.

In a small proportion of initially registered patients the brain lesion was later found to be non-vascular; such cases were excluded from the final data.

Case Finding

In each study area the stroke register, usually operating in a local hospital, was responsible for the registration of new cases. The activity of the register was based on reports from hospital departments, general practitioners, nursing institutions, and health authorities in the area. All sources of information, including death certificates issued in the area, were checked at regular intervals.

Whenever possible, suspected stroke cases were seen by a member of the register staff. For all patients who were eligible for inclusion in the study, relevant information was entered in an 'initial record form'.

Follow-up

At fixed intervals (three weeks, three months, and one year after the stroke) the surviving patients were contacted and a 'Follow-up record form' filled in with a number of clinical and social data. Information about recurrent strokes and/or deaths within a year was also recorded, together with relevant autopsy findings.

Type Diagnosis of Stroke

Although the study was concerned mainly with unspecified stroke, an attempt was made to register also the presumed anatomical type of the stroke. After the initial examination each patient was therefore assigned to one of the diagnostic subgroups 430–434 or 436 (ICD, 8th revision). However, the safety with which such a classification could be made varied widely. For example, the proportion of patients seen by a neurologist ranged from 12 to 85 per cent. Cerebral angiography was performed in less than 10 per cent of the registered patients. None of the centres had access to CT scanning. In fact, even in a large metropolitan hospital (Frederiksberg, Copenhagen) an analysis showed that a type diagnosis confirmed by angiography and/or spinal fluid examination was obtained during life in only 17 per cent of the stroke patients. In the vast majority of the registered cases the diagnosis of the stroke type therefore had to depend on more or less reliable clinical criteria. It is thus clear that local diagnostic habits in the participating centres might seriously bias the assessment of the relative incidences of haemorrhagic and ischaemic strokes.

In order to estimate the influence of observer variation on the diagnosis of stroke, the validity and consistency of diagnoses were tested with 60 randomly selected case reports assessed by European, Japanese and other centres [3]. The diagnosis of stroke versus non-stroke was nearly always correct, whereas the distinction between different types of stroke showed considerable inter- and intra-observer bias, the type diagnoses being inconsistent in about 25 per cent of the test cases. The most reliable type diagnosis was that of subarachnoid haemorrhage.

In rapidly fatal stroke cases the ultimate diagnosis depends to a large extent on the results of autopsy. It is therefore of interest to note that autopsy rates were generally high in Europe—being over 60 per cent in Copenhagen and Moscow—whereas in the Japanese centres, except Fukuoka, autopsy was performed in less than 10 per cent of the fatal cases.

Results

In the study period, May 1971 to December 1974, the participating centres registered a total of 9064 suspected stroke cases, of which 310 were eventually excluded from the analysis. The age distribution of the patients varied widely, reflecting differences in the structure of the background population; for example, the proportion of the registered patients who were under 65 years of age ranged from 29 per cent (Israel) to no less than 78 per cent (Nigeria), the average proportion for the total series being 53 per cent for males, 37 per cent for females.

Incidence

Table I shows the sex- and age-specific incidence rates for first strokes observed in six European and four Japanese centres. The rates are seen to rise steeply with age; in each age group the rate being higher for males than for females. Of the European centres, Espoo, Finland, had particularly high rates; otherwise the variations were only moderate. In nearly all the Japanese centres, on the other hand, rates were as high as in Espoo; extraordinarily high figures were observed in one Japanese community (Akita).

TABLE I Average annual incidence rates for first strokes per 1000 population, in selected communities, 1971–74

Study area	Country	Males				Females			
		45-54	55-64	65-74	all ages	45-54	55-64	65-74	all ages
Gothenburg	Sweden	0.76	2.41	–	–	0.44	1.34	–	–
Frederiksberg	Denmark	0.60	2.83	5.31	1.70	0.34	1.25	3.36	1.93
Dublin	Ireland	0.96	3.70	7.53	1.15	0.54	2.10	6.09	1.22
Espoo	Finland	1.77	4.37	11.98	1.21	1.26	2.30	8.84	1.27
North Karelia	–	1.88	3.61	7.20	1.31	0.86	2.62	6.46	1.35
Zagreb	Yugoslavia	1.04	3.22	3.31	1.31	0.75	1.20	2.61	1.12
Akita	Japan	4.73	9.08	19.30	2.57	2.12	4.74	17.02	1.89
Saku	–	–	4.22	7.85	1.67	–	1.96	5.09	1.31
Fukuoka	–	1.07	5.06	12.02	0.97	0.65	0.93	6.80	0.51
Osaka	–	0.47	3.42	11.53	0.88	0.56	2.80	5.88	0.79

107

The incidence rates for all strokes (including recurrences) were, on the average, 20 per cent to 30 per cent higher than those for first strokes only.

Types of Stroke

Table II shows that in most centres, nearly two-thirds of the cases were diagnosed either as cerebral infarction or 'type unknown', the frequency of the latter diagnosis depending partly on the availability of diagnostic facilities, partly on the strictness of the clinical diagnostic criteria used in individual centres. Subarachnoid haemorrhage, which can be diagnosed with reasonable reliability, accounted for less than 10 per cent of the strokes, except in the Swedish and Finnish centres,

TABLE II Diagnosis of types of stroke, by centre

	Subarachnoid haemorrhage (%)	Cerebral haemorrhage (%)	Cerebral infarction (%)	Type unknown (%)	Total No. of patients (=100%)
Gothenburg	19.6	19.6	26.1	34.7	784
Copenhagen	2.8	14.7	55.0	27.5	891
Dublin	9.9	7.6	7.0	76.5	539
Espoo	14.5	15.2	61.7	8.6	303
North Karelia	15.0	6.1	64.1	14.8	983
Zagreb	2.5	12.7	54.2	30.6	631
Akita	8.4	31.9	52.4	7.3	382
Saku	10.0	26.0	60.0	4.0	708
Fukuoka	9.0	32.9	50.8	7.4	134
Osaka	7.0	35.4	52.5	5.1	158

where somewhat higher percentages were found. It appears that the percentage of patients diagnosed as intracerebral haemorrhage was twice as high in Japan as in Europe.

It is noteworthy that the diagnosis of carotid arterial occlusion, which usually requires angiography, was made in less than 5 per cent of the European patients, and in none of the Japanese.

Clinical Profile

The typical neurological deficit in the acute phase of the stroke was a hemiplegia, which was recorded in about 75 per cent of the patients. Severe impairment of consciousness (coma or semicoma) was seen far more frequently in Japan (43%) than in Europe (25%). A detailed analysis of the neurological findings was outside the scope of the present study.

The systolic blood pressure, as recorded shortly after the stroke, averaged 176 mm in males, and 179 mm in females. The systolic value was consistently 5-6 mm higher in Japanese than in European patients, whereas the diastolic readings differed only slightly.

Types of Management

About 75 per cent of the European stroke patients were admitted to hospital, whereas in Japan over half the patients were treated at home. In Japan, but not in Europe, admission rates were particularly low for old patients and for females. Neither the severity of the stroke nor the living conditions of the patient had any appreciable influence on hospitalisation. Both in Europe and in Japan nearly 80 per cent of the hospitalised patients were admitted on the day of onset.

Long hospital stays after stroke were more frequent in Japan than in Europe: 87 per cent of the Japanese patients stayed in hospital longer than four weeks, as compared with only 50 per cent of the European patients; at three months, the proportion of survivors still in hospital was 34 per cent in Japan, but only 19 per cent in Europe.

Early start of rehabilitation, i.e. within three weeks of the stroke, was recorded in about two-thirds of the European patients, but in less than half of those in Japan. The proportion of patients who did not receive any rehabilitative treatment at all was about 25 per cent in Europe, 50 per cent in Japan. This category of patients was dominated by very mild and extremely severe cases.

At the one-year follow-up, 25 per cent of the European survivors were staying in an institution (hospital, nursing home, etc) whereas nearly all the Japanese survivors, even if severely disabled, were cared for in their homes.

Survival

Most of the deaths in the acute phase of stroke occurred within the first week. The three-week fatality rate, which is traditionally used as measure of 'immediate mortality', was 32 per cent for the total series, with only moderate variations between centres. There were only small differences between death rates in Western Europe and those in developing countries. One year after the stroke, nearly half the registered patients had died.

Comments

In this study, as in previous ones [4, 5], the incidence of stroke (except subarachnoid haemorrhage) has been found to rise steeply with advancing age, and to be higher for males than for females. Distinct geographical variations were demonstrated: age-specific incidence rates were low in Gothenburg, Copenhagen, and Zagreb, markedly higher in the Finnish and three of the Japanese centres, and extremely high in one Japanese community (Akita). Repeated checkings of the sources of information failed to provide evidence of an underreporting of stroke in the Swedish and Danish centres and, in view of the uniformity of the methods of case-finding, together with the small observer variation demonstrated for the diagnosis stroke versus non-stroke, the geographical differences can reasonably be considered real. A valid explanation cannot be given at present, but may emerge from a detailed analysis of environmental factors in the involved communities.

The apparently high frequency of cerebral haemorrhage in Japan, which was found also in the present study, has puzzled many epidemiologists, some of whom [6] believe that the trend is an artefact reflecting differences in diagnostic habits. Support for this view may be found in the fact that autopsy rates in the Japanese centres, except Fukuoka, were much lower than in Europe, and that the percentages of patients dying within a few days of the stroke were not particularly high in Japan. However, in a small series of autopsied cases from the Japanese centres the clinical diagnosis of the type of stroke was confirmed in about 80 per cent. It should further be considered that a history of hypertension was obtained in over 70 per cent of the Japanese stroke patients, but in fewer than 50 per cent of the European patients, and that, in Japan, over 40 per cent of the registered stroke victims were comatose, or semi-comatose, as against 25 per cent in Europe. It is thus probable, although not definitely proved, that cerebral haemorrhage actually occurs more often in Japan than elsewhere, possibly as a result of a higher prevalence of arterial hypertension.

As to the practical aspects of the findings, the impact of stroke on the communities under study has been clearly demonstrated. Provided the data obtained in the participating European centres are applicable to Europe as a whole, it can be estimated that about one million strokes occur in Europe every year, accounting for at least 30 million hospital days and an unknown number of bed days in nursing institutions. Such figures give a rough idea of the social and financial implications of cerebrovascular disease. For a full discussion of the subject the reader is referred to the original report from the WHO study group [1].

In several of the centres the participants were inspired to undertake supplementary stroke studies, such as detailed analyses of risk factors [7], or controlled trials of drug treatment of stroke patients [8].

A particularly important issue is the role of stroke registration as part of community-based medical programmes against cardiovascular disease. Such programmes were established in several of the study areas and, according to the preliminary experience, the stroke registers proved to be valuable as indicators of the success, or failure, of local community campaigns against hypertension. In North Karelia, Finland, such a campaign was started in 1972, at the same time as the stroke register. Over the subsequent three years, when increasing numbers of hitherto unrecognised hypertensives were identified and treated, the annual incidence rates for stroke in the age group 25-74 years fell from 3.6/1000 to 1.9/1000 for males [9]. These results, although still needing confirmation, indicate the important role of disease registers in regional health programmes.

In conclusion, the WHO multicentre Stroke Project has demonstrated that stroke registration, carried out within the framework of existing health services, is feasible in most parts of the world, and that a stroke register can be a valuable tool both for epidemiological purposes and for the evaluation of community programmes for the control of cardiovascular disease.

Participants

K Aho, Department of Neurology, University of Helsinki, Finland.
OO Akinkugbe, Faculty of Medicine, University of Ibadan, Nigeria.
N Dondog, Department of Cardiovascular Diseases, Medical Research Institute, Ulan Bator, Mongolia.

ML Gander, International Classification of Diseases, World Health Organisation, Geneva, Switzerland.
L Geltner, Asaf Harofe Government Hospital, Tel Aviv University Medical School, Zerifin, Israel.
P Harmsen, Department of Neurology, Sahlgren's Hospital, Gothenburg, Sweden.
S Hatano, Department of Epidemiology, Tokyo Metropolitan Institute of Gerontology, Tokyo, Japan.
K Isomura, Saku Central Hospital, Nagano, Japan
S Kojima, Central Institute of Health, Akita, Japan.
Y Komachi, Centre for Adult Diseases, Osaka, Japan.
K Kondo, Central Health Institute, Japan National Railways, Tokyo, Japan.
TA Makinskij, Institute of Neurology, Academy of Medical Sciences of the USSR, Moscow, USSR.
J Marquardsen, Department of Neurology, Frederiksberg Hospital, Copenhagen, Denmark.
T Omae, Faculty of Medicine, Kyushu University, Fukuoka, Japan.
BO Osuntokun, Faculty of Medicine, University of Ibadan, Nigeria.
Z Poljaković, Centre for Cerebrovascular Diseases, Zagreb, Yugoslavia.
P Puska, North Karelia Project, University of Kuopio, Finland.
A Radic, Medico-Social Research Board, Dublin, Ireland.
K Salmi, North Karelia Central Hospital, Joensuu, Finland.
EV Shmidt, Institute of Neurology, Academy of Medical Sciences of the USSR, Moscow, USSR.
VE Smirnov, Institute of Neurology, Academy of Medical Sciences of the USSR, Moscow, USSR.
K Uemura, Division of Health Statistics, World Health Organisation, Geneva, Switzerland.

References

1 Aho, K, Harmsen, P, Hatano, S, Marquardsen, J, Smirnov, VE and Strasser, T. *Bull. Wld. Health Org.* In press
2 Hatano, S (1976) *Bull. Wld. Hlth. Org., 54,* 541
3 Hatano, S (1977) *Jap. Heart J., 18,* 171
4 Matsumoto, N, Whisnant, JP and Kurland, LT (1973) *Stroke, 4,* 20
5 Zupping, R and Roose, M (1976) *7,* 187
6 Kurtzke, JF (1969) *Epidemiology of Cerebrovascular Disease.* Springer-Verlag, Berlin, Heidelberg, New York
7 Aho, K (1975) *Incidence, Profile and Early Prognosis of Stroke.* Academic Dissertation. Helsinki
8 Geismar, P, Marquardsen, J and Sylvest, J (1976) *Acta neurol. Scand., 54,* 173
9 Puska, P (1977) *Excerpta Med. International Congress Series, No. 427,* p. 5

Chapter 10

APPLICATIONS OF A STROKE REGISTER IN PLANNING

Jean M Weddell

Introduction

Ten years ago concern was growing about the quality of care of stroke patients in the United Kingdom. Cerebrovascular disease was the third commonest cause of death in the total population. The proportion of the elderly in the population was rising, and the numbers of deaths and discharges from hospital of patients with cerebrovascular disease was also on the increase [1]. It was felt that stroke rehabilitation units would make a valuable contribution to the care of stroke patients, but at that time virtually no studies had been carried out to evaluate the work of such units. The Department of Health and Social Security commissioned a series of studies of care given to stroke patients, which included one carried out at the Department of Community Medicine, St Thomas's Hospital Medical School. The principal aim of this study was to set up a register to enumerate the stroke patients in a defined population, to establish incidence and prevalence rates, and to analyse the present use of facilities for home and hospital care. Follow-up studies were planned to estimate problems of medical and social rehabilitation of the patients and the present deficiencies and problems of management. It was also hoped to use the register as the basis for randomised controlled trials of the effects of physiotherapy on a domiciliary basis.

When the study was mounted in December 1970, formal planning of health services was in its infancy. When the study was completed in May 1976 the information needed by planners was beginning to be defined. In many respects, a register provides much of this information. When care is being planned for one group of patients it is necessary to define the nature, size and duration of the problems of these patients, the resources that are available and the resources that are needed. The different options of care need to be defined, and evaluated in terms of clinical outcome and use of resources. A register provides a detailed description of a group of patients, but to be a useful planning tool it needs to relate to a defined population, the major demographic characteristics of which are known. Also, if the register is to have a wide application, the group of patients studied should, as far as possible, be representative of all those with the condition, and not restricted to one small subgroup. If the register is continued for several years it is possible to study changes over time of that particular patient group within the defined total population.

112

Method

The design of the study has been described in greater detail [2, 3] in previous publications.

The patients were registered from 1 June 1971 to 31 May 1972 from a defined total population of 272 000, living in the anticipated catchment area of Frimley Park Hospital, which was being built at the time (Fig. 1). The patients received their primary care from 37 of the 38 general practices in the area. Those who survived were seen immediately after the stroke, three weeks, three months, and four years later. The field work was carried out by three state registered nurses, all of whom lived in the study area and worked part-time on this study. Data were also collected and checked by a part-time medical co-ordinator, who lived in the area, and myself.

Before the study started, all the general practitioners in the study area and the physicians, both in and outside the study area to whom patients might be referred for treatment, were visited and the design of the study and the data to be collected were discussed with them. The six months preceding the year of registration were spent developing the questionnaires and streamlining the organisation and running of the register.

In addition, demographic data from the 1971 census were obtained from the Office of Population Censuses and Surveys (OPCS) that related to the individual wards of the study area. These included the age/sex distribution of the population, household size and the numbers of people in households above and below pensionable age.

Information was collected about the services available in each locality provided by the health service, social services and by the voluntary agencies used by the stroke patients. The cost of each service, and the length of the waiting lists, were noted for each service.

Copies of death certificates of those on the register were obtained from OPCS up to the end of the four-year follow-up. Details of the lengths of hospital admissions and the reasons for admission were obtained from all hospitals in and outside the study area, from the date of registration to the end of the four-year follow-up.

The information collected by questionnaire included demographic details, the date of the stroke, places of care, date and place of death, the main neurological features—level of consciousness, presence or absence of paralysis, defects of speech or swallowing, levels of mobility, the capacity to carry out the activities of daily living, the level of occupation, and the amount, nature and frequency of help given to the patient by other people. The data from the survivors were recorded at the time of the stroke, three weeks, three months and four years after the stroke. Baseline data were also recorded of the patients' abilities immediately before the stroke and the help, if any, that they were given by other people. Wherever possible, the information was given by the patient, if not, by a member of their own household or, failing that, by either nursing or medical staff looking after the patient at the time of the visit.

113

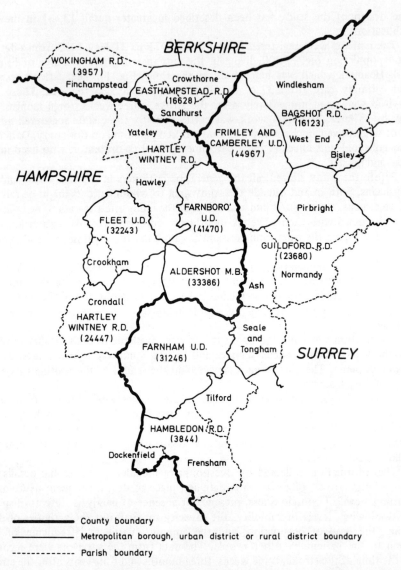

Figure 1 Stroke study area. Figures in parentheses show total population within the study area. (Reproduced from *Planning for Stroke Patients,* Pitman Medical, Tunbridge Wells, by courtesy of HMSO)

In this study a stroke was defined as a focal neurological defect of sudden onset lasting 24 hours or more for which the patient was given medical care. Also included in the register were those who died from a stroke within 24 hours of its onset. Patients of all ages who had suffered a stroke from any underlying cause, including subarachnoid haemorrhage, were placed on the register.

Results

Incidence and Prevalence

The study was designed to register all new patients receiving medical care for a stroke. Between 1 June 1971 and 31 May 1972, 380 patients were registered. From the twelve months' experience which formed the study period we were able to calculate the annual incidence rates of stroke for men and women by age, shown in Table I. The 1971 census ward data were obtained from OPCS for the Farnham and Frimley area.

TABLE I Stroke Study: Annual Incidence Rates per 100 000 of Strokes

Ages	Men	Women
<30	0	0
30–44	14.0	15.0
45–54	76.5	34.0
55–64	298.0	208.0
65–74	942.0	577.0
75–99	1708.5	1914.0
All ages	122.7	156.5

No direct measurement of prevalence rates was possible given the design of this study. However, since the stroke patients were followed for four years, or to death, whichever was the sooner, we were able to make some estimates of the likely length of survival of stroke patients. From these estimates, under certain rather restrictive assumptions, which follow, estimates of the prevalence of stroke survivors have been made. Details of the calculation are given in the Appendix.

The overall annual prevalence rate was estimated to be 548.0 per 100 000: 551.5 for men and 546.1 for women. This is about four times the observed annual incidence rate (139.7 per 100 000). The assumptions behind this calculation are gross and were adopted for ease of calculation rather than realism. They are:

1 The incidence rates are as in Table I for all preceding years back to 1902.
2 The probability of surviving to a certain day after the stroke is as estimated using the study group experience up to 4 years after the stroke. Survival beyond 4 years is based on current adjusted English Life Tables (1969-71). (See Appendix.)

115

3 The age-sex structure of the population is held constant over all preceding years to 1902. The figures used are based on those for the study area at the 1971 census, and the totals for those aged 75 or more have been apportioned to the five-year age groups up to 95+ according to the 1971 figures for England and Wales.

The annual prevalence of stroke survivors was calculated for each year of age from 30 to 99 years for both males and females. This calculation was performed for age 40, for example, by summing

incidence of stroke at age 40
+ incidence of stroke at age 39 X probability of surviving to age 40
+ incidence of stroke at age 38 X probability of surviving to age 40
+ etc., to
+ incidence of stroke at age 30 X probability of surviving to age 40
where, for example
incidence of stroke at age 40 = incidence rate at age 40 X 1/5 (population in age group 40 to 44)

Ignoring the one female child who died of stroke aged under one year, we have taken the probability of stroke in men or women aged under 30 as negligible (i.e. zero). The table of prevalences calculated for different age groups is presented in the Appendix. Adding these together, we found that in a population of 275 000 people (137 000 males and 138 000 females) under the above assumptions, the number of people who have ever had a stroke, counted over a one-year period, is expected to be 756 men and 754 women.

The age-sex adjusted annual prevalence rates for stroke are given in Table II.

TABLE II Stroke Study: Prevalence Rates per 100 000 of Stroke Patients

Ages	Men	Women
<30	0	0
30–44	42.8	46.2
45–54	256.9	159.4
55–64	1031.7	616.2
65–74	3625.7	1874.4
75–99	10 893.3	7821.7
All ages	551.5	546.1

Patients Registered

Out of the 380 placed on the register, 267 were seen by the field workers. Of these, 216 patients were seen within three weeks of the onset of the stroke. The numbers of patients seen at each visit by the field workers are summarised in Table III, with the mean time interval from the onset of the stroke.

116

TABLE III Stroke Study: Total registered 380: Seen alive 267

	Mean time after stroke	No. of patients
Time between Stroke and Visits to all Survivors		
First visit	12 days	267
Second visit	48 days	180
Third visit	104 days	158
Fourth visit	4 years	74
Seen alive by three weeks		
First visit	4 days	216
Second visit	39 days	132
Third visit	100 days	121

Age and Sex Distribution of Patients

The age distribution of the patients at the time of registration, three months and four years after the stroke are given in Figure 2. Of the total patients registered, 77 per cent were aged 65 or over, 14.7 per cent of these were alive at the follow-up four years later, in contrast to 35.6 per cent of those under 65 years.

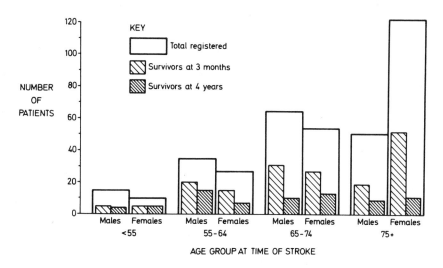

Figure 2 Age distribution of stroke patients at registration, 3 months and 4 years

Disability After Stroke

The analysis of the data on disability immediately following the stroke was restricted to the 216 patients seen within three weeks of the onset of the stroke. Their ability to carry out the activities of daily living were compared at the time

117

of the stroke, three weeks and three months later. The overall changes in the ability to carry out individual activities followed a similar pattern, though continence, both urinary and faecal, was the first to return, closely followed by the patients' abilities to feed themselves. It was not possible to measure the ability of hospital patients to dress themselves as they rarely wore anything but night clothes while in hospital. The ability to get in and out of a bed or chair has been chosen for discussion as this is the activity often used to decide whether or not a patient is able to go home (Table IV). The majority of those completely dependent on others, who had to be lifted in and out of a bed or a chair when first seen, were dead by the time of the second visit three weeks after the stroke, and all but six who were looked after at home initially were in-patients. Of the patients independent of others in respect of the activities of daily living, 14 were still in hospital three months after the stroke. Neither the age of the patients nor social class appeared to contribute to this, but the size of the household and the ages of those in the household did seem to have an important bearing. Patients who lived in small, elderly households were more likely to stay in hospital for social rather than medical reasons, than those who came from younger, larger households.

TABLE IV Stroke Study: Dependency (Transfer) and Place of Care

		First visit		Second visit		Third visit	
		Home	Institution	Home	Institution	Home	Institution
Independent	M	17	8	39	1	37	2
	F	8	6	22	9	35	12
Partially	M	10	16	4	10	4	8
dependent	F	13	28	10	29	9	10
Completely	M	2	38	0	4	0	0
dependent	F	4	65	0	4	0	4
Not known	M	0	0	0	0	0	0
	F	0	1	0	0	0	0
Total		54	162	75	57	85	36
Total survivors		216		132		121	

The abilities of those seen at home four years after the stroke to carry out the activities of daily living were very similar to those seen at home three months after the stroke. But there had been a considerable and steady deterioration in the ability to maintain the same level of function either in full or part-time employment, as a housewife or as a retired person. To assess this the patients were asked if they could do things the same as they could before the stroke, to a limited degree, or not at all. This is an over-simplified, imprecise measure of a person's overall capacity. It is presented here as it may give a crude, but possibly more realistic, measure of the capacity to lead a normal life. These measures apply only to those seen at home at the time of follow-up and are presented in Table V.

TABLE V Stroke Study: Levels of Activity of Patients at Home

Level		3 months		4 years	
		No.	%	No.	%
Men					
As before stroke		16	39.0	10	27.8
Limited		13	31.7	21	58.3
Not at all		12	29.3	5	13.9
	Total	41	100.0	36	100.0
Women					
As before stroke		17	38.6	4	12.9
Limited		25	56.8	19	61.3
Not at all		2	4.6	8	25.8
	Total	44	100.0	31	100.0

Speech Defects

The analysis of speech defects recorded at the first three visits was restricted to the 216 patients seen within three weeks, but at four years all the survivors were included. To make the four sets of data comparable they are presented as percentages (Table VI) and the total number of patients to whom these refer are given for each set.

TABLE VI Stroke Study: Speech Defects in Stroke Survivors

Speech	Percentage distribution			
	1st visit	2nd visit	3rd visit	4th visit
No defect	35.6	86.4	93.4	81.0
Partial defect	33.3	6.0	4.1	13.5
Complete defect	30.1	7.6	2.5	1.4
Not known	0.9	0	0	4.1
Total survivors	216	132	121	74
Dead	0	84	95	193
Mean time seen after stroke	4 days	39 days	100 days	4 years

Speech defects were classified into none, partial, or complete; those with no defect could be fully understood by the field worker, those whose speech could partly be understood were classified as having a partial defect, those who could

119

not be understood at all or who were in coma were classified as having a complete defect.

At the time of the first visit over 60 per cent of the patients had some defect of speech. Three weeks later only 6 per cent had a partial and 7.6 per cent a complete defect. At three months after the stroke there had been little change, though four years after the stroke 13.5 per cent (10 patients) had partial defects of their speech, and 1.4 per cent (one patient) had a complete defect. Two of these had had subsequent strokes.

Hospital Care

Some measure of the hospital care given to the stroke patients is given in Tables VII and VIII. Table VII gives the percentage survivors admitted during the first three and the last nine months of the first year after the stroke, and then annually for the second, third and fourth years after the stroke. The first three months are presented separately as a much higher proportion of patients were admitted during this period, for shorter periods of time. Also, virtually all admissions during this period were for care for the stroke, while between three months and four years in the men over 65 and women over 60, two-thirds of the admissions and transfers were for care of the stroke and a third were for other conditions; 78 per cent of the later admissions in men under 65 were for the stroke. Of the 16 women under 60 who had a stroke, 8 were alive three months later, and between three months and four years had three hospital admissions.

TABLE VII Stroke Study: Hospital Admissions: Percentage Survivors Admitted

Period of time after stroke	Women 60+		Men 65+		Men <65	
	No. alive at start of period	% admitted	No. alive at start of period	% admitted	No. alive at start of period	% admitted
0–3 months	198	73.7	117	64.1	49	77.6
4–12 months	91	45.1	50	28.0	25	20.5
13–24 months	63	36.5	38	28.9	23	13.0
25–36 months	52	34.6	26	50.0	22	22.7
37–48 months	41	41.5	21	42.9	19	10.5
Alive at 4 years	28		19		19	

The mean lengths of stay for all ages (Table VIII) were short in the first three-month period, mainly because so many of these patients died soon after the stroke. The women over 65 were admitted for substantially longer periods than the men, and spent on average five or six months in hospital during each of the last three years of follow-up. In contrast, the older men spent an average of 2.5 to 3.5 months each year in hospital, and the younger men one to two months. This very considerable part played by hospitals in the care of stroke patients has to be taken into consideration against the fact that only six of the 74 survivors were in hospital at the time of the four-year follow-up. Of those alive at four years, 49 had not been admitted to hospital since the three-month follow-up.

120

TABLE VIII Stroke Study: Hospital Admissions—Mean Length of Stay (months)

Period of time after stroke	Women 60+		Men 65+		Men <65	
	No. alive at start of period	Mean length of stay	No. alive at start of period	Mean length of stay	No. alive at start of period	Mean length of stay
0–3 months	198	1.0	117	0.6	49	0.5
4–12 months	91	3.1	50	1.7	25	1.9
13–24 months	63	5.8	38	2.5	23	2.4
25–36 months	52	5.4	26	3.7	22	1.1
37–48 months	41	5.1	21	3.6	19	1.0
Alive at 4 years	28		19		19	

TABLE IX   Stroke Study: Four-year follow-up. Sources of support given to patients out of hospital

	Men		Women		Total
	<65	65+	<60	60+	
Number	19	17	8	23	67
No help	5	–	2	2	9
Source of support					
Own household	12	14	6	13	45
Neighbours	2	–	1	4	7
Extended family	2	4	1	7	14
Health visitor	1	–	2	2	5
District nurse	1	5	–	7	13
Home help	–	3	–	7	10
Domestic help	1	1	1	3	6
Meals-on-wheels	–	1	–	2	3
Chiropody	2	4	1	9	16
Laundry	–	4	–	2	6
Local authority	2	1	2	5	10
Red Cross	2	3	3	7	15
No. of sources of support					
1	6	6	1	5	18
2	7	2	2	4	15
3	1	4	1	4	10
4	–	4	1	3	8
5	–	1	1	1	3
6	–	–	–	4	4
Total	14	17	6	21	58

Community Support

The level of independence of those out of hospital can be gauged to some extent by the amount of help they were given by other people. Table IX summarises this. Nine of those at home were given no help at all. Of those given help by others,

121

65.5 per cent were pensioners. Of those given help 31.0 per cent had one source of support, 26.0 per cent two sources of support and 43.0 per cent three or more sources of support. Most of this help, 77.6 per cent, was given by members of the patient's household. Other much used sources of support were the chiropodist, the Red Cross and other voluntary agencies that provided a great variety of things, such as aids and appliances, transport, lunch clubs, and day centres. The district nurse and home help provided help to 22 per cent and 17 per cent respectively. The small number of people who had meals-on-wheels or were visited by the health visitor is surprising.

Discussion

Use of the Register in Planning

If a register is to provide information relevant to planners it must give a complete, accurate, and useful description of patients from one well-defined group. If the data collected on the register are to be of use then some definition of the main problems of those to be registered has to be attempted before the register is started. In this instance the most important problem was thought to be that of physical disability, and the questionnaires were designed to collect information of various aspects of this.

The information obtained from a register relates specifically to the defined total population in which the patients live. The total population covered by this register now forms the greater part of one health district. It is difficult to assess the comparability of one locality with another, as not only do the measurable variables such as age, sex, household size, level of employment and level of earnings need to be taken into account, but also the organisation of medical care in the locality, which is influenced by the quality of general practice, the quality and nature of the hospital service, the degree of co-operation between the hospitals, general practices and social services and other forms of community care. Another variable difficult to measure, but with an important bearing on the care of stroke patients, is the way each community functions, the degree of awareness each neighbourhood has to the needs of those living there, and the willingness and ability to meet these needs.

Even within the relatively small locality studied here there were considerable differences between the north and the south. The population in the north was young, many lived in new housing estates, the population density was quite high and the provision of services was good. In the south the population was older, living in more isolated but longer-established rural communities, and the provision of services was not so good as these villages were further from the bigger centres of population.

The findings of this study apply specifically to the study area; possibly, in general terms, some of the findings relate to other areas. To that extent the study is of limited value. On the other hand, the method used was simple and worked well in practice and could be applied to any other area in which a total population can be defined that receives its medical care largely within its own area. It would be difficult to apply this method to a large conurbation where many from inside a defined area go long distances outside that area for care, and others are looked after in the area who live outside it.

Incidence and Prevalence

As this register was used to calculate the incidence rate and prevalence rate of strokes it was essential that it should be complete, and include those who died within a few days of the stroke. If the main objective of the register had been confined to a study of physical disability, or the overall care given to stroke patients then the failure to register those who died soon after the stroke would have been relatively unimportant.

The incidence rate calculated from this register, 139.7 per 100 000, is lower than those reported from other studies [4-11] which varied from 144.9 per 100 000 [8] to 764.6 per 100 000 [7]. The considerable difference between reported incidence rates reflects as much the different definitions and study designs used, as the differences associated with race and geographical distribution.

The overall prevalence rate from this study was estimated to be 548 per 100 000. This compares with 440 per 100 000 from a Norwegian study [12]. Harris and his associates [13] in their study of the handicapped and impaired in Great Britain found 130 000 living in private households handicapped from a stroke, a prevalence rate of 266 per 100 000. The age and sex adjusted prevalence rate from Rochester for 1970 was 559 per 100 000 [11]. The number of studies that have produced prevalence rates is small, but the agreement between them is remarkable.

Age Distribution

The age distribution of the cohort of patients studied in this register shows the same dramatic changes over time reported by Marquardsen in his seven-year follow-up study in Frederiksberg [14]. The majority of patients given care in the acute phase of the stroke are elderly; the majority who are still living four years later, most of whom have been given supportive care, are in late middle-age.

Measures of Ability

The limited value of Katz's classification of the ability to carry out the activities of daily living [15] is shown by the 'independent' status in terms of these activities of most of the survivors, which is not borne out by the number of people given help in a variety of ways by other people and also by the fall in their overall level of activity measured by the level of employment and activities at home. The measures of ability to perform the activities of daily living are useful in the acute phase, but 'independence' in these terms can mask a high degree of social dependence in those who survive beyond this time.

The problem of speech defects is considerable immediately after the stroke, but this is largely self-limiting because many of those most severely affected die within three weeks of the stroke. This should give heart to those providing care for these patients, since the problem is of a more manageable size than clinical experience in the acute phase suggests.

The numbers of survivors from this study with physical disability or speech defects were too small to enable randomised controlled clinical trials to be carried out to evaluate physiotherapy or speech therapy. The preliminary findings of one stroke rehabilitation trial [16] have been published. This study compared the

123

effectiveness of different intensities of outpatient rehabilitation following a stroke. One of the main problems faced by the investigators was that only 12 per cent of patients with a confirmed stroke were eligible for the trial. The number of patients referred for physiotherapy by a clinician would be higher than this, but the data from our register do not suggest it would be very much higher after the acute phase. Brocklehurst and his colleagues [17] have compared the use of physiotherapy, occupational therapy, and speech therapy for stroke patients in hospital. They found 79 per cent of those surviving two weeks had physiotherapy, that 22 per cent continued to have this treatment for more than six months. Those who had the most physiotherapy were the most severely affected, with the worst prognosis, and showed little or no response to this treatment. It was suggested that these patients continued to be treated simply because they were in hospital; 26 per cent had occupational therapy and 14 per cent had speech therapy. The smaller proportions of these patients given these treatments were felt to reflect the limited availability of therapists. Far fewer patients stopped having physiotherapy than either occupational therapy or speech therapy because of lack of progress.

The careful assessment of patients to establish their potential for recovery before any type of remedial therapy is started is urged by Brocklehurst and his colleagues [17], together with continuing assessment once treatment has begun.

These authors urge the development of a reliable method of predicting prognosis in patients with a stroke so that physiotherapy may be concentrated on those with the optimum prospect of recovery and continued only while measurable improvement is occurring.

A multicentre randomised controlled trial to assess the effectiveness of speech therapy in stroke survivors is now under way, and this will provide much needed evidence of the place of this treatment in their care.

Hospital Care

The hospital care given to the stroke patients during the four years of the study was almost certainly unique to the study area. At the start of the register one of the topics the general practitioners in the area asked us to study was the difficulty in admitting a patient with a stroke to hospital. The questionnaire was amended to include a record of the number of hospitals the general practitioner had contacted before an admission was arranged, and also how long it took to arrange the admission. From this it was clear that, probably as a result of the study, the stroke patients were much more favoured than they had been in the past, and were admitted relatively quickly, usually to the hospital of the practitioner's first choice. Another feature of the area was that, at the start of the study, five cottage hospitals were open to which the general practitioners in their immediate locality had open access and for which they provided medical cover. This meant that these general practitioners were able to continue to care for their patients after admission, and also that the family were still able to visit their relatives without much difficulty. The existence of these cottage hospitals almost certainly encouraged or enabled admissions which in other localities would not have been contemplated by either general practitioner or relatives. Although the proportion of patients admitted to cottage hospitals was small, the presence of the cottage hospitals coloured the

124

attitudes of families, general practitioners and hospital consultants to the admission of stroke patients.

Another factor that probably influenced the admission and discharge of stroke patients was that during the initial year of the register the first geriatrician was appointed in the area, and a day centre and two geriatric wards were opened in the principal hospital in the area at that time. This appointment not only increased the facilities available for the care of the elderly but also brought additional skills, specific to geriatrics, into the area. This appointment probably affected both discharges and admissions. A much more constructive, positive approach to discharges was soon evident, and more pressure was applied to the community services, both medical and social, to make suitable arrangements to speed the return of a patient to his household. It also engendered more confidence in the family that matters were in the hands of someone fully conversant with all aspects of care of the elderly.

The hospital admissions and the length of these admissions reflect not only the hospital beds available in the study area, but also the organisation of, and attitude to, the delivery of medical care.

Community Support

As well as the largely intermittent, though substantial, amount of hospital care given to the survivors over four years, the majority were given a considerable amount of support when they were at home, particularly by members of their own household. For the household as a whole to live a reasonable life some outside help is often needed. One aspect of the care of stroke patients that was not studied during the life of the register was the difficulty in making arrangements for the care of the patients in their own home after discharge from hospital. That this was a problem became clear during the course of the study, the main reason being the number of people involved working in different organisations—the health service, social services, voluntary agencies, all separately funded and separately accountable. A *Which? Campaign Report* [18] found that there were 54 different forms of financial assistance, and 18 types of supportive services available to disabled people from a total of 17 different kinds of agency.

There is another factor that needs to be considered when community support is being planned for the stroke survivors, and that is the tendency for services such as meals on wheels and home helps to encourage the elderly to withdraw from the community, and the provision of sheltered housing and homes for the elderly tends to isolate them in elderly ghettos [19].

The organisation of care of the patient after discharge from hospital could be greatly improved if one person acted as co-ordinator, and also assessed the needs of the patient and the household if these changed over time.

Conclusion

The register provides a sound base for the comprehensive planning of care for stroke patients, in hospital and in the community, if it relates to a defined total population. Whether the register should be continued indefinitely is open to question. In this study, the register team worked for two years initially, and then the four-year follow-up lasted approximately fourteen months. This discontinuity undoubtedly led to loss of data, but whether the cost of collecting this would have been justified is doubtful. The cost of the first two years' work at 1971 prices has been estimated at £10 000, a small proportion of the budget of a health district but an amount which should show some benefit in terms of improved quality of care. The evaluation of studies such as this is needed as much as the evaluation of specific forms of rehabilitation such as physiotherapy or speech therapy.

Acknowledgements

This study was carried out by the Department of Community Medicine, St Thomas' Hospital Medical School, and I acknowledge the considerable help from Professor Holland and other members of the Department during the study, and members of the Advisory Board, in particular Professor Brian Abel-Smith and Professor A L Cochrane; to Miss Shirley Beresford who was the statistician working on the study throughout and who did all the work on the incidence and prevalence rates and to Chris Wale, the statistical assistant for the greater part of the study; to the field workers, Mrs Bocking, Mrs Hockey and Mrs Large who were responsible for the bulk of the data collection and worked throughout with great cheerfulness and efficiency; to Dr Margaret Anderson who was the local medical co-ordinator during the first part of the study and Mr P Simpson who supervised the four-year follow-up; to the general practitioners, district nurses, physiotherapists and speech therapists in the study area, and the hospital consultants in all the hospitals to which the patients were admitted for their co-operation; to the Department of Health and Social Security, particularly Dr J M G Wilson and Dr J Metters for their interest and support throughout the study; to Mr Leek, the District Records Officer, and his staff for the help they gave during the study, particularly during the extensive search of medical records at the time of the four-year follow-up; to the District Management Team of West Surrey and North-East Hampshire for constructive criticism and encouragement; to the staff of the Office of Population, Censuses and Surveys who provided the death certificates; to Miss Barbara Webster who prepared the figures for the text. My thanks also go to Ms Jenny Griffiths who carried out the work on the hospital admissions data, typed the earlier versions of the paper, and estimated the costs of the first two years of the study. Finally, I would like to thank Mrs Barbara Kneller for preparing the final typescript.

References

1 Department of Health and Social Security and Office of Population, Censuses and Surveys (1972) *Report on Hospital In-patient Enquiry for the year 1970.* Part I. Tables. HMSO, London
2 Weddell, Jean M (1974) Rehabilitation after stroke—a medico-social problem. Skandia International Symposia. *Rehabilitation after Central Nervous System Trauma*, pp. 1–255. Nordiska Bokhandelns Förlag, Stockholm

126

3   Weddell, Jean M and Beresford, Shirley A A *Planning the Care of Stroke Patients:* a four-year descriptive study of home and hospital care. HMSO, London. In press

4   Takahashi, E, Kato, K, Kawakami, Y, Ishiguro, K, Kaneta, S, Kobayashi, S, Ohba, E, Yano, S, Ito, Y, Shiraishi, M, Murakami, N, Sugawara, T, Megure, Y and Suzuki, Y (1961) Epidemiological studies on hypertension and cerebral haemorrhage in north-east Japan. *Tohoku J. Exp. Med., 74* (2), 188

5   Eisenberg, H, Morrison, JT, Sullivan, P and Foote, FM (1964) Cerebrovascular accidents. *J. Amer. Med. Assoc., 189,* 883

6   Kannel, WB, Dawber, TR and McNamara, PM (1965) Vascular diseases of the brain—epidemiologic aspects: The Framingham study. *Amer. J. Publ. Hlth., 55,* 1355

7   Brewis, M, Poskanzer, DC, Rolland, C and Miller, H (1966) Neurological disease in an English city. *Acta Neurol. Scand., 42,* 10

8   Acheson, J, Acheson, HWK and Tellwright, JM (1968) The incidence and pattern of cerebrovascular disease in general practice. *J. Roy. Coll. Gen. Pract., 16,* 428

9   Stensgaard, B (1970) Personal communication. *Apoplexia Cerebri in Bornholm* (English resumé). Unidentified publication

10 Peacock, PB, Riley, CP, Lampton, TD, Raffel, SS and Walker, JS (1972) The Birmingham Stroke Epidemiology and Rehabilitation Study. In *Trends in Epidemiology* (ed GT Stewart). Application to Health Services Research and Training. Charles C Thomas, Springfield, Illinois. Ch. 8, page 231

11 Matsumoto, N, Whisnant, JP, Kurland, LT and Okazaki, H (1973) Natural history of stroke in Rochester, Minnesota, 1955 through 1969: An extension of a previous study 1945-1954. *Stroke: J. Cerebral Circ., 4,* 20

12 Petlund, CF (1970) *Prevalence and Invalidity from Stroke in Aust-Agder County of Norway.* Universitetsforlaget: National Health Association of The Norwegian Council on Heart and Vascular Diseases

13 Harris, AI, Cox, E and Smith, CRW (1971) *Handicapped and impaired in Great Britain. Part I.* Office of Population Censuses and Surveys, Social Survey Division. HMSO, London

14 Marquardsen, J (1969) The natural history of acute cerebrovascular accident—a retrospective study of 769 patients (1940-1952). *Acta Neurol. Scand., 45,* Supplement 38

15 Katz, S, Ford, AB, Moskowitz, RW, Jackson, BA and Jaffe, MW (1963) Studies of illness in the aged: the index of ADL, a standardised measure of biological and psychosocial function. *J. Amer. Med. Assoc., 185,* 914

16 Sheikh, K, Smith, DS, Meade, TW and Brennan, PJ (1978) Methods and problems of a stroke rehabilitation trial. *Brit. J. Occupational Therapy, 41,* 262

17 Brocklehurst, JC, Andrews, K, Richards, B and Laycock, PJ (1978) How much physical therapy for patients with stroke? *Brit. Med. J., 1,* 1307

18 Managing at Home—A *Which? Campaign Report.* (1978) Consumers' Association, 14 Buckingham Street, London WC2N 6DS

19 Lewis, B and Oldfield, C (1977) *The Maintenance of the Elderly Within the Community.* A report on a project sponsored by the Cicely Northcote Trust. Project NT/BL/976

127

Appendix

Stroke Prevalence Calculations

The assumptions and form of the calculations were outlined in the Results.

The probability of a stroke at age x has been taken to be the annual incidence rate of strokes in the appropriate age/sex group.

The probability of survival to day t has been estimated from the study experience up to day 1460 (4 years) using a negative exponential model:

$$\text{Prob (survival to day } t) = ke^{-\alpha t}$$

where the parameter α is defined by

$$\alpha = \frac{\text{number of deaths}}{\text{total man days exposure to risk (of dying)}}$$

and $\quad k = \quad$ 1 for $t \leqslant 30$ and $k = e^{-30\,(\alpha_1 - \alpha)}$ for $t \geqslant 31$

$(\alpha_1$ is the value of α for $t = 30)$.

Eight different models were used according to sex, age (over or under 55) and whether day t was within 30 days of stroke or not. The corresponding values of α and k are given in Table A1.

TABLE A1

Age		Males		Females	
		$<$55 yr	55+ yr	$<$55 yr	55+ yr
day 1 to 30	α	0.039	0.026	0.039	0.028
	k	1.0	1.0	1.0	1.0
day 31 to 1460	α	7.3×10^{-5}	56.1×10^{-5}	7.3×10^{-5}	75.7×10^{-5}
	k	0.962	0.975	0.962	0.973

The survival after 4 years is estimated as follows, using current life tables: if age at stroke is a, the probability of surviving n years is

prob (surviving 4 years) $\times$ prob (surviving from age $a + 4$ to age $a + n$)

$$= ke^{-\alpha \times 1460} \times \frac{1_{a+n}}{1_{a+4}}$$

where 1_a is taken from the current English abridged life table: 1969–1971 (Table A2).

TABLE A2 English abridged life table 1969–1971

Age a	Males	Females
30–	9595	9731
35–	9542	9696
40–	9467	9639
45–	9327	9538
50–	9079	9372
55–	8673	9127
60–	8016	9768
65–	7012	8227
70–	5625	7403
75–	3982	6191
80–	2355	4544
85–	1072	2696
*90–	321	1119
*95–99	55	280

*These were calculated from 1969–1971 mortality and 1971 census figures.

Note: Ages under 30 years have not been included since the incidence rate for stroke at these ages has been taken to be zero.

The population to which the incidence rates and probability of survival was applied is based on the 1971 census population of the study area, and is shown in Table A3.

TABLE A3 Population base for the calculations

Age	Males	Females
under 30	70 150	68 200
30–	10 350	9 900
35–	10 350	8 800
40–	9 200	8 800
45–	8 050	7 700
50–	6 900	6 600
55–	6 400	6 700
60–	5 600	6 300
65–	4 400	5 050
70–	2 600	3 950
75–	1 650	2 950
80–	900	1 850
85–	350	900
90–	80	250
95+	20	50
Total	137 000	138 000

The prevalence calculation was performed for each year of age and each sex from ages 30 to 99, as follows:

129

$$\text{The incidence at age } i = \left\{ \begin{array}{l} \text{annual incidence} \\ \text{rate in appropriate} \\ \text{age/sex group} \end{array} \right\} \times 1/5 \left\{ \begin{array}{l} \text{population} \\ \text{in the 5-year} \\ \text{age/sex group} \end{array} \right\}$$

The probability of survival for $i - j$ years was calculated for each day for the first 4 years, and multiplied by 1/365 of the incidence at age j.

The probability of survival for $i - j$ years was calculated for each year for $i - j > 4$, multiplied by the incidence at age j, multiplied by the probability of surviving 1460 days.

This gave

$$\text{prevalence at age } i = \text{incidence at age } i + \sum_{j=30}^{i-1} \text{incidence at age } j \times \left[\begin{array}{l} \text{probability} \\ \text{of survival} \\ \text{for } i\text{-}j \text{ years} \end{array} \right]$$

Table A4 shows the prevalence of stroke survivors in certain broad age groups which result from a summation of prevalences calculated for the individual ages.

TABLE A4 Prevalences of stroke survivors

Age	Males	Females
<30	0	0
30–44	12.8	12.7
45–54	38.4	22.8
55–64	123.8	80.1
65–74	253.8	168.7
75–99	326.8	469.3
Total all ages	755.6	753.6

Prevalence *rates* can be calculated using Table A4 in conjunction with Table A3.

Chapter 11

STROKE REGISTER IN CARLISLE: a preliminary report

P L Chin, R Angunawela, D Mitchell and J Horne

The burden of care of stroke patients in the United Kingdom falls mainly on Departments of General Medicine and Geriatric Medicine. The clientele of geriatric departments belong to the age group in which the incidence of strokes is greatest, and at any one time 15 per cent of admission beds are occupied by stroke patients and this notwithstanding the fact that geriatric departments are also committed to caring for other no less disabling chronic neurological problems. Haberman and his colleagues (1978) [1] have suggested that there is a declining rate in cerebrovascular disease in the UK. Acheson and Fairbairn, 1970 [2], on the other hand aver that the burden of stroke care on communities appears to be increasing. In the District General Hospital in north-east Cumbria—Cumberland Infirmary—of 450 beds, there has been a trebling of admissions for cerebrovascular disease in the last ten years (Table I). *See* Andrews (1978) [3]; Garraway (1976) [4]. This is partly due to the rising population of over 75s, but it does not fully account for the increased work-load stroke places on the District General Hospital.

TABLE I

Year	Strokes i.e. first diagnosis, admitted to Cumberland Infirmary, Carlisle
1968	99
1969	174
1970	123
1971	176
1972	164
1973	184
1974	201
1975	290
1976	304
1977	274

On the other hand, the major risk factor in stroke illness, namely, hypertension, has been as vigorously attacked in Carlisle as in the rest of the country [5-8]. Hence, we would expect a decline in the death and incidence rate of cerebrovascular accidents, or at least a postponement of the occurrence to the older age groups. Are the presumed increased overall incidence rates reported merely a reflection of the ageing population or just the survival of young hypertensives? It was also evident from preliminary reports from the WHO co-operative study on strokes in different communities that no representative figures from UK were available.

In a search for some answers to such questions we decided to embark upon a prospective one-year Stroke Register. Furthermore, a previous study of central nervous system diseases in Carlisle had been carried out by Brewis and his associates [9] in 1965 for the years between 1955 and 1961 and such information was a valuable base for comparison.

Carlisle, lying in the north of the Lake District National Park, was then said to be a typical English city [9] and perhaps still is, although it is now bypassed by a motorway. It has a reasonably stable population of approximately 100 000 with a slightly greater than national average number of elderly (Fig. 1). With its surrounding rural district the administrative area covers about 112 square miles. There is no major industrial complex but there are small engineering, textile and food factories. The bulk of employment is in agriculture and local and central government work.

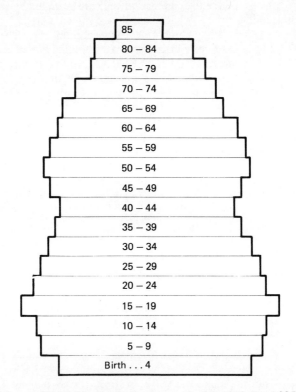

Figure 1 Population distribution by age, Carlisle 1978. Total 99 527

All acute admissions are directed to three main hospitals: the Cumberland Infirmary, the City General Hospital and Garlands Hospital (the main psychiatric hospital). Cumberland Infirmary, with 450 beds, is the District General Hospital and admits over 95 per cent of stroke cases. It has facilities for major specialties required for the care of stroke patients and houses the Assessment Unit for the

Department of Geriatric Medicine. Patients with neurosurgical problems are transferred to the Regional Neuro-Surgical Unit in Newcastle, 60 miles away. A neurologist visits Carlisle fortnightly from Newcastle.

The survey team consisted of 1 consultant physician, 2 medical registrars, 2 parttime clinical assistants, 1 social worker, 1 liaison district nursing officer and a secretary. The Register was patterned on the WHO scheme as described by Marquardsen (1976) [10] but allowed for some minor alterations and additions in data collection as the intention was also to study the part played by certain factors such as hypertension, blood lipids, the content of drinking water, climate and the financial burden of stroke care to the community and hospital. We were also interested in concurrence of acute strokes and myocardial infarction [11]. The definition of stroke used for inclusion in the Register was 'Rapidly developed signs of focal (or global) disturbance of cerebral function of presumed vascular origin leading to death or lasting for more than 24 hours' [10, 12]. This definition included cerebrovascular disease classified according to the International Statistical Classification, 8th Revision, rubrics 430–434 and 436. It excluded cases of transient cerebral ischaemia. The 'work-up', conduct, and difficulties encountered in the keeping of the Register are the subject of another report. We intend following up the small cohort of survivors of the initial episode for several years to study the implications of stroke illness in the family and its impact on life styles. We hope to evaluate the support given by health and social services both in terms of efficiency and cost effectiveness.

Results

The results presented are preliminary observations only and may be subject to revision as some cases reported are still under investigation. This is mainly because the study was concluded only one month ago and the figures presented were compiled only two weeks before the preparation of this chapter.

Altogether, 267 incidents were reported. Excluded from the study were 16 cases, 5 of which were found to have brain tumours (3 primary and 2 metastatic), 2 epilepsy; 1 subdural haematoma; 1 was caused by an overdose, and 7 were certified by general practitioners and other hospital doctors as dying from cerebrovascular accidents, but on examination it was shown that they did not fall within the definition of stroke adopted in this study.

One-hundred and fifty-one (60%) of patients were admitted to hospital. The reasons for admission of these patients were classified as mainly medical (17%), medical/social (63%), mainly social (15%), doubtful necessity (5%). Of those not admitted, a further 9 per cent used either Outpatient consultation or Day Hospital rehabilitation facilities. Thus, 69 per cent of stroke patients reported in Carlisle used hospital facilities of one sort or another—60 per cent as inpatients and 9 per cent as outpatients.

One-hundred and forty-four (58%) died in the first month. Of the 151 patients admitted to hospital 103 (68%) were dead within one month. The average length of stay of the patients who died in hospital was 13 days.

133

The age and sex distribution of reported cases appears in Table II. Over 80 per cent occurred in the over 65s and nearly half were over 75. The preponderance of female sufferers in this age group is probably a function of the proportional increase of aged females in this population. At this age group the male : female ratio is approximately 1 : 2 (0.47). The crude incidence rate by age is shown in Table III.

TABLE II: Age and Sex Distribution of Reported Cases

Age	Male	Female	Total
<44	1	3	4
45–54	4	3	7
55–64	20	5	25
65–74	50	38	88
75–84	35	70	105
85+	3	19	22
	113	138	251

TABLE III

Age	1978 Estimated population	Cases	Incidence per 1000
<44	60 590	4	0.07
45–54	12 242	7	0.56
55–64	11 757	25	2.13
65–74	9 357	88	9.40
75–84	4 729	105	22.20
85+	852	22	25.82
	99 527	251	2.52

TABLE IV Comparing Average Incidence Rate per 1000 in Carlisle (1955–61) with Present Study (1978)

1955–61 Overall 1.42 (excluding subarachnoid haemorrhage)		1978 2.52	
Age	1955–61	Age	1978
0–49	0.11	0–54	0.15
50–59	1.8	55–64	2.12
60–69	4.3	65–74	9.40
70–79	8.3	75–84	22.20
80+	12.1	85+	25.82

The incidence rate by age and sex is shown in Figure 2. The crude overall incidence rate is 2.52 per 1000 and the age adjusted incidence rate (to UK population, 1978) is 2.38. A comparison of the incidence rate with M Brewis's study in the similar locality is shown in Table IV.

134

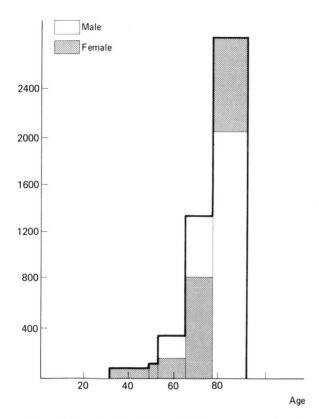

Figure 2 Carlisle Stroke Register 1978. Incidence per 100 000

It should be noted that in Brewis's study the maximum overall crude incidence rate of 1.42 per 1000 excludes subarachnoid haemorrhage cases which were treated separately. If these cases were included the average incidence rate would be 1.57 based on observations made on hospital admission statistics, death certificates and general practitioner records over a 7-year period between 1955 and 1961. It also refers to a smaller population, 69 400, living within the then defined City of Carlisle. The present (1978) estimated population within this old administrative boundary of the City of Carlisle is 71 060. By subtracting the cases occurring outside the old administrative area a comparable incidence rate in 1978 for this particular population would be 2.50. Accepting the inaccuracies inherent in the Brewis retrospective search there appears to have been an increase in the overall incidence rate of 0.91 between the period 1955–61 and 1978–79.

The results of the analysis of other such aspects of the study as diagnostic categories of strokes, medical and social histories and a profile of clinical presentation and prognostic features are not as yet available for presentation.

135

Comments

Over a period of one year new strokes were reported in 251 Carlisle residents. Of these, 151 (60%) were admitted to hospital. Marquardsen reported that 82 per cent of strokes that occurred in Frederiksberg, Denmark were admitted. In South Manchester [3] 64 per cent were admitted to hospital within the first week and in the Farnham Frimley Study 59 per cent [13]. It would appear that there is a rising trend of hospital admissions since the 1962 Report of the College of General Practitioners [14] when 1 in 6 of acute strokes were said to have been admitted to hospital. This is probably due to three factors among others postulated:

1 an increasing absolute number of elderly;
2 changed living conditions of these elderly people;
3 changing attitudes and a growing demand by the public and general practitioners for institutional care for the elderly disabled.

Marquardsen concurs with the last reason given for the increase in hospital admissions in Frederiksberg, Denmark.

Comparing the present incidence rate with that reported by Brewis in the same locale, there appears to have been an increased overall incidence, which is probably accounted for by the ageing population and some inaccuracies arising out of the method of search used by Brewis.

A high mortality of 58 per cent in one month is recorded, most deaths occurring within three weeks. Of those who died in one month, 70 per cent were in hospital. Of those who were admitted to hospital 68 per cent were dead within one month. The average length of stay in hospital of those who were admitted and died in hospital was 13 days. Thus, although there is an increase in the trend of admission to hospital the majority died within one month.

TABLE V UK Studies of Stroke Incidences per 1000 population

	Crude Incidence
Hospital studies	
Brewis (1955–61) Carlisle	1.42
Average (excluding subarachnoid haemorrhage)	
R Acheson (1963–64) Oxford	1.86
Community studies	
J Acheson (1962–65) Stoke-on-Trent [31]	3.94
J Weddell (1971–72) Farnham Frimley	1.35
L Hewer (1972) Bristol Project [32]	1.86
Carlisle (1977–78)	2.52

Mid-point 2.56 (for the four community studies)

The age specific incidence rates found in this study are lower than those observed in some other populations of comparable size and structure [10, 15-17]. Table V shows the distribution of incidence rates in England and Wales from other studies. They are not all strictly comparable because different definitions and methods of registering strokes were used, but it is a reasonable guide to the distribution of stroke incidence in England and Wales.

TABLE VI The Comparisons between Carlisle and Frederiksberg, Denmark
(C = Carlisle F = Frederiksberg)

Males			Females		
Age	F	C	Age	F	C
<54	0.2	0.55	<54	0.1	0.65
55-64	3.7	3.58	55-64	2.1	0.81
65-74	9.6	12.7	65-74	5.6	7.02
75-84	17.8	21.1	75-84	24.4	22.34
85+	26.4	14.7	85+	25.1	29.3

Table VI shows the comparisons between Carlisle and Frederiksberg, Denmark (a study included in the WHO Co-operative Project on Stroke). As both studies were carried out on similar lines, comparison of these two studies is more realistic. There appears to be a higher incidence rate in males between the ages of 55-64 in both studies. No overt explanation is yet available for this observation as the population breakdown in this age group in both areas is similar.

Table VII compares the incidence in Carlisle with other parts of the Western world, age adjusted rate, where available [18].

TABLE VII CVD Average Annual Incidence Rate per 100 000 population

Community Surveys—Total pop., repeat strokes incl.

Source	Locale	Years	No.	Crude incidence rate	Age adj. US pop.
Wallace [33]	Goulbourn	1962-64	(185)	329	
Aho [17]	Espoo, Finland	1972-73	(286)	126	198
Marquardsen [10]	Frederiksberg, Denmark	1971	(287)	287	
Puska [34]	No Karslia, Finland	1972-73	(383)	215	215
Eisenblatter [35]	Berlin-Lichtenberg DDR	1972-73	(377)	202	
					Age adj. UK pop.
Present Survey	Carlisle, England	1978-79	(251)	252	238

137

Risk Factors

Results of analysis of the data collected on risk factors in this study are as yet unavailable. However, two particular aspects are perhaps worth noting. One is the temperature and water story and the other the haemoglobin count of those patients with strokes.

The Water Story

Carlisle, in the northern part of England, has predominantly soft drinking water [19]. There have been several studies into the death rates of cardiovascular disease in relation to hardness or softness of drinking water [20-23]. It appears that death from ischaemic heart disease is slightly greater in soft-water areas. However, on

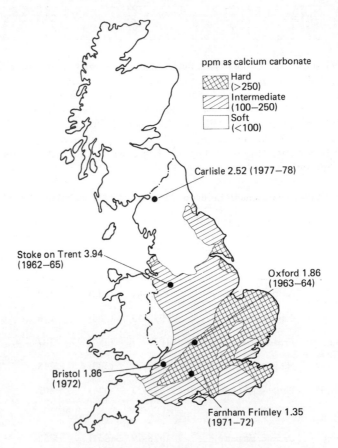

Figure 3 Distribution of hard and soft water areas in the UK

138

epidemiological terms there are certain differences between ischaemic heart disease and cerebrovascular disease [24, 8]. Foder and his colleagues (1972) [25] reported that there is a belt of increased deaths from cerebrovascular disease in the north-eastern seaboard of the United States. Comstock and his associates (1979) [26] were not able to show any association between water hardness and deaths from cerebrovascular disease in Maryland. A glance at the distribution of stroke/incidence rates (from published studies) in this country in relation to areas of hard and soft water so far does not indicate any increased incidence of strokes in soft water areas in England and Wales (Fig. 3). However, the reported incidence rates are not strictly comparable and more information is needed on the incidence rates and water ingredients in several geographical areas before any association between these factors can be established in the UK. A rough map of the UK showing the relationship of standardised mortality ratios from cerebrovascular disease to drinking water hardness is being drawn and will be the subject of a later report.

Weather

Figure 4 shows the month of occurrence of stroke cases in association with mean monthly temperatures in Carlisle over the same period. By plotting the mean monthly temperature against the number of stroke cases in Carlisle it appears that the coldest months are associated with the highest number of strokes. There was no difference between male and female incidences. McDonnell and his colleagues (1970) [27] have suggested that there is a lower incidence rate of strokes in summer. Our study confirms that the onset of stroke follows the pattern of deaths as reported by Bull (1975) [24]. An analysis by month of deaths due to cerebrovascular disease in the last 10 years in Carlisle shows a similar trend. On the other hand, analysis of admissions by month of strokes to the Cumberland Infirmary over the last 10 years shows an opposite tendency (Table VIII). In fact, the highest admission rates occurred in the warmest months. A possible explanation is that fewer stroke patients survive the acute episode in the cold season to require admission to hospital. It also perhaps highlights the problem of interpreting the influence of climatic factors by simply studying hospital admission statistics or attempting to plan hospital resources to cope with seasonal variations of this life-threatening disease based on community incidence surveys only.

TABLE VIII 10 Year Admissions to Cumberland Infirmary by Seasons

December/January/February	628
March/April/May	625
June/July/August	648
September/October/November	595

Blood Counts

Kannel (1972) [28] and his colleagues have shown that stroke patients tended to have a higher haemoglobin count than those who did not develop strokes in Framingham. When allowance was made for associated hypertension a small

139

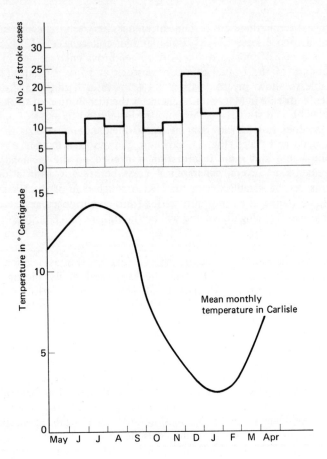

Figure 4 Month of occurrence of stroke cases in association with the mean monthly temperatures in Carlisle

residual independent effect was seen for haemoglobin. In our study the haemoglobin count was taken from stroke patients within 72 hours of the stroke when possible (and this occurred in 75 per cent of the cases reported) and two weeks later. The mean haemoglobin count of those patients with strokes was in the first 48–72 hours 13.2 g/dl, for females; 14.1 g/dl for males compared with a group of controls paired for age and sex of 11.8 g/dl in females and 13.0 g/dl in males. High or higher than normal haemoglobin occurring within a few hours of the stroke can be due to dehydration and haemoconcentration and this was found in some of the patients as the haematocrit was raised. Nevertheless, we found that haemoglobin levels in stroke patients taken two weeks after the initial event tended also to be higher than controls. This confirms the finding of Kannel in 1972 [28]. Perhaps some factors other than haemoconcentration are at play or perhaps a high or

140

higher than normal haemoglobin is a risk factor for stroke [29]? The results of an analysis making allowances for associated hypertension, is being made and will be available in the final report.

Conclusion

An account of the preliminary findings of a Stroke Register compiled in a northern English city with a population of approximately 100 000 is presented. An overall crude incidence rate of 2.52 strokes per 1000 population and an age adjusted rate (to UK population 1978) of 2.38 was found in an area with soft drinking water. Sixty per cent of stroke victims were admitted to hospital and a further 9 per cent used hospital outpatient consultation or rehabilitation facilities. The majority of admissions were due to the lack of social support at home.

Most strokes occurred in the colder months of the year. A one-month mortality of 58 per cent was recorded. The haemoglobin count of both male and female sufferers was relatively higher than a group of controls matched for age and sex. A Stroke Register is a useful tool for delineating the stroke problem in a community, but for the preservation of the sanity of clinicians should be carried out by epidemiologists or trained community physicians.

Acknowledgements

We would like to thank the Cumbria AHA for their financial support, physicians in Cumberland Infirmary, all the general practitioners and community nurses in Carlisle District for so assiduously reporting stroke cases, and Mrs D Norman our co-ordinating secretary for sustaining the enthusiasm of all concerned in the project throughout the year.

References

1 Haberman, S, Capildeo, R and Clifford Rose, F (1978) The Changing Mortality of Cerebrovascular Disease. *Quart. J. of Med.*, New Series XLVII, *185*, 71
2 Acheson, RM and Fairbairn, AS (1970) Burden of cerebrovascular disease in the Oxford area in 1963 and 1964. *Brit. Med. J.*, *2*, 621
3 Andrews, K (1978) *Medical, Social and Psychological Aspects of Stroke.* Final Report Univ. of Manchester, Dept. of General Medicine
4 Garraway, M (1976) The Size of the Problem of Stroke in Scotland. In *Stroke, Proceedings of the 9th Pfizer International Symposium* (ed FJ Gillingham, C Mawdsley, AE Williams). Churchill Livingstone, Edinburgh, London, New York, p. 72
5 Hamilton, M, Thompson, EN and Wishiewski, TKM (1964) The Role of Blood Pressure Control in Preventing Complications of Hypertension. *Lancet, i,* 235
6 Veterans Administration Co-operative Study Group on Antihypertensive Agents (1967) Effect of treatment on morbidity in hypertension. *J. Am. Med. Assoc., 202,* 116
7 Beevers, DG, Fairmain, MJ, Hamilton, M and Harpur, JE (1973a) The influence of antihypertensive treatment on the incidence of cerebrovascular disease. *Postgrad. Med. J., 49,* 905

8 Kannel, WB (1976) Epidemiology of cerebrovascular disease. In *Cerebral Arterial Disease* (ed RW Ross Russell). Churchill Livingstone, Edinburgh, London, New York, p. 288

9 Brewis, M, Poskanzer, DC, Rolland, C and Miller, H (1966) Neurological Disease in an English City. *Acta Neurol. Scand., 42*, Supplementum 24, 1

10 Marquardsen, J (1976) An Epidemiologic Study of Stroke in a Danish Urban Community. In *Stroke—Proceedings of the 9th Pfizer International Symposium* (ed FJ Gillingham, C Mawdsley, AE Williams). Churchill Livingstone, Edinburgh, London, New York, p. 62

11 Chin, P, Kaminski, J and Rout, M (1977) Myocardial Infarction coincident with cerebrovascular accidents in the Elderly. *Age and Ageing, 6,* 29

12 Royal College of Physicians (1974) *Report of the Geriatrics Committee Working Group on Strokes*

13 Weddell, JM (1974) Rehabilitation after Stroke—a medico-social problem. In *The Skandia International Symposium: Rehabilitation after central nervous system trauma,* (ed H Bostrom, T Larsoon, N Ljungstedt). Stockholm: Nordiska Bokhandelns Farlag, p. 71

14 Research Committee of the Council of the College of General Practitioners (1962) *Studies on Medical and Population Subjects, No. 14. Morbidity.* Statistics from General Practice III (Disease in General Practice). London

15 Eisenberg, H, Morrison, JT, Sullivan, P and Foote, FM (1964) Cerebrovascular accidents. *J. Am. Med. Assoc., 198,* 107

16 Eckstrom, PT, Brand, FR, Edlavitch, S and Parrish, HM (1969) Epidemiology of stroke in a rural area. *Publ. Hlth. Rep., 84,* 878

17 Aho, K (1975) Incidence, Profile and Early Prognosis of Stroke in Espoo-Kaunianinen Area, Finland, 1972. *Stroke, 5,* 658

18 Kurtzke, JF (1976) The Distribution of Cerebrovascular Disease. In *Stroke—Proceedings of 9th Pfizer International Symposium,* (ed FJ Gillingham, C Mawdsley, AE Williams). Churchill Livingstone, Edinburgh, London, New York, p. 5

19 Commins, BT (1978) *British Nutrition Foundation Bulletin, 4,* No. 6, 385

20 Crawford, MD, Gardner, MJ and Morris, JN (1968) Mortality and water hardness of local water supplies. *Lancet, i,* 827

21 Gardner, MJ (1976) *Health and the Environment.* (ed J Lenihan and WW Fletcher). Blackie, Glasgow, p. 116

22 Elwood, PC, St Leger, AS and Morton, M (1977) *Brit. J. of Prev. Soc. Med., 31,* 178

23 Schroeder, HA (1960) Relations between mortality from cardiovascular disease and treated water supplies. *J. Am. Med. Assoc., 172,* 1902

24 Bull, GM (1975) A comparative study of myocardial infarction and cerebrovascular accidents. *Geront. Clin., II,* 193

25 Foder, JG, Pfeiffer, LJ and Papezik, VS (1973) Relationship of drinking water quality to cardiovascular mortality in Newfoundland. *Canadian Med. Assoc. J., 108,* 1369

26 Comstock, GW, Cauthen, GM and Helsing, KJ (1979) Stroke-associated deaths in Washington County, Maryland, with Special Reference to Water Hardness. *Stroke, 10,* (2), 199

27 McDonnell, FW, Louis, I and Manohan, K (1970) Seasonal variation of non-embolic cerebral infarction. *J. Chron. Dis., 23,* 29

28 Kannel, WB, Gordon, T, Woft, PA and McNamara, PM (1972) Haemoglobin and the risk of cerebral infarction: The Framingham Study. *Stroke, 3,* 409

29 Thomas, DJ and others (1977) *Lancet, ii,* 941

30 Acheson, RM and Fairbairn, AS (1971) Record linkage in studies of cerebrovascular disease in Oxford, England. *Stroke, 2,* 48

31 Acheson, J, Acheson, HWK and Tellwright, JM (1968) The incidence and pattern of cerebrovascular disease in general practice. *J. Roy. Coll. Gen. Pract., 16,* 428

32 Hewer, RL, Day, RE and McDonald, I (1972) Incidence and cause of non-transient vascular hemiplegia in the community. Royal College of Physicians. Report of the Geriatric Committee Working Group on Strokes

33 Wallace, DC, Clark, MC, Coles, JH, Coombes, BW, Crawford, JNR, Cunynghame, DD, Docker, EB, Hazelton, AR, Ivens, HPH, Lyttle, KP, Lyttle, JO and Woods, RG (1967) A study of the natural history of cerebral vascular disease. *Med. J. Austral., 1,* 90

34 Puska, P, Aho, K and Salmi, K (1974) Incidence of strokes in Finland. *Duodecim, 90,* 965
35 Eisenblatter, D, Zillman, K, Hausding, WD, Todt, B, Ihle, E and Bohm, M (1974) Stroke Registry for Berlin-Lichtenberg. *Deutsche, Gesundh, Wesen, 39,* 2478

Chapter 12

THE DECLINING INCIDENCE OF STROKE*

M Garraway and J P Whisnant

Attempts to follow the changing frequency of major chronic disease are usually limited to the analysis of mortality statistics. These sources are used only because no other data are available and over the past twenty years or so, a number of such studies based on mortality attributed to cerebrovascular disease have been undertaken in several countries [1-7]. These studies have all suggested that the frequency of stroke is declining, but limitations apply to the use of mortality statistics. They may be influenced by changing diagnostic fashion among practitioners completing death certificates [8]. Revisions of coding practice with the introduction of each new edition of *The International Classification of Disease* creates anomalies [9]. Coverage of cerebrovascular disease as the underlying or even secondary cause of death may be incomplete [10]. Low diagnostic accuracy among deaths attributed to cerebrovascular disease is well recognised, one study revealing that 29 per cent of hospital deaths certified as being due to cerebrovascular disease had no evidence of such on autopsy, and a further 12 per cent of deaths having evidence of cerebrovascular disease on autopsy with no mention of such on the death certificate [11]. Unfortunately, autopsies cannot be used as a way of validating death certification attributed to cerebrovascular disease in practice because of the very low proportion of deaths that subsequently undergo autopsy examination [12].

Morbidity studies based on the actual occurrence of stroke give more accurate information, and several such studies have been undertaken [13-17]. But problems of comparability between studies and long-term continuity within studies have prevented these contributions from being heard in the debate on the apparent decline in cerebrovascular disease in recent years. An opportunity to overcome these limitations arose in the population of Rochester, Minnesota, by utilising the Mayo Clinic medical records linkage and indexing system described in detail in Chapter 5. This system has been used recently to examine the incidence of stroke in a defined population during the same period for which other studies have reported a decline in mortality from cerebrovascular disease [18].

The definition of stroke used throughout was the onset of a focal neurological deficit lasting for more than 24 hours and due to a presumed local disturbance in blood supply to the brain. Stroke was considered to include brain infarction due to arterial thrombosis, stenosis or embolism, primary and secondary intracerebral haemorrhages and subarachnoid haemorrhage. The criteria of diagnostic categories used are as follows—

---

* This investigation was supported in part by Research Grant GM 14231, National Institutes of Health, Bethesda, Maryland, USA.

144

Cerebral Infarction. Abrupt or relatively rapid onset of focal neurological deficit persisting for more than 24 hours, with clear cerebrospinal fluid, with or without a recognisable source for embolus.

Intracerebral Haemorrhage. Any combination of rapid progression for focal neurological deficit, headache, altered conscious level, evidence of meningeal irritation and gross blood in the spinal fluid and/or frank focal haemorrhage on computer assisted tomography, includes both primary intracerebral haemorrhage and secondary cases due to leukaemia or arteriovenous malformations.

Subarachnoid Haemorrhage. Abrupt onset of headache with or without altered consciousness, with signs of meningeal irritation, without focal neurological deficit, or with late occurrence of such deficit after other criteria were observed. Includes primary subarachnoid haemorrhage due to presumed aneurysm, and secondary cases due to haematological causes or arteriovenous malformations.

Stroke of Uncertain Type. Incomplete clinical details at the onset of the acute episode, but a history of onset and residual deficit sufficiently well documented to ensure a high likelihood that stroke had occurred.

The following results are based on the 1854 new cases of stroke that occurred during 1.2 million person-years of observation in residents of Rochester, Minnesota during the period January 1, 1945 to December 31, 1974.

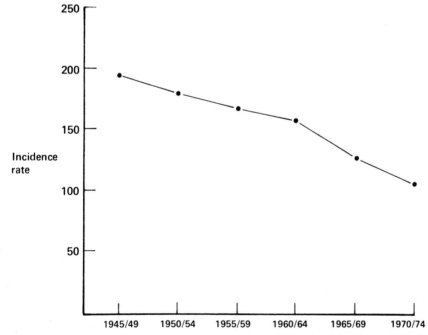

Figure 1 Average annual incidence per 100000 population for stroke, 1945-49 to 1970-74 adjusted for age and sex to the 1950 US white population

Incidence

The overall incidence of stroke has declined consistently when the rates are adjusted for age and sex in six quinquennial periods (Fig. 1). The reduction appears to have occurred in two phases; from 1945-49 to 1955-59, the overall average annual decline in the incidence rate adjusted for age and sex was 3.1 per 100 000. A plateau was then reached between 1955-59 and 1960-64, after which the decline continued at an accelerating rate, the average annual decreases in the rate adjusted for age and sex being 4.8 and 5.2 per 100 000 for the quinquennial periods 1965-69 and 1970-74 respectively. The overall effect of the decline has been to reduce the age and sex adjusted rate from 190 per 100 000 population in 1945-49 to 104 per 100 000 population in 1970-74. Table I demonstrates that the magnitude of the reduction was similar for males and females, but the timing differed. An early decline in the rate for males was followed by a plateau, before another reduction occurred between 1965-69 and 1970-74. The rate in females was a more progressive decline, beginning between the quinquennia 1950-54, and 1955-59.

TABLE I

Sex	1945–49		1950–54		1955–59		1960–64		1965–69		1970–74	
	Rate	No.	Rate	No.	Rate	No.	Rate	No.	Rate	No.	Rate	No.
Male*	214	119	177	115	181	142	186	157	174	175	122	142
Female*	166	136	180	178	139	168	125	179	90	162	87	181
Totals †	190	255	179	293	159	310	154	336	130	337	104	323

* Age-adjusted to 1950 US white population
† Adjusted for age and sex to 1950 US white population

Age Analysis

When the trend is examined in age-specific groups (Fig. 2), it is apparent that the greatest reduction has occurred in the more elderly groups who had the highest rates at the beginning of the period of observation. This has had the effect of narrowing the range of rates between the younger and older age groups in successive quinquennia, particularly during the later period of observation. Thus, in 1960-64, the average annual rates for those aged 55-59 years and 80 years of age and over were 209 and 2932 per 100 000 persons, producing a ratio of one stroke in the younger age group for every fourteen strokes in the older age group. By 1970-74, the average annual rates for the same age groups had declined to 205 and 1287 per 100 000 respectively, producing a ratio of one stroke in the 55-59 year age group for every six strokes in the age group 80 years and over. Rates were higher for men in all age groups up to 75 years of age, but women had the higher age-specific rates above this age.

146

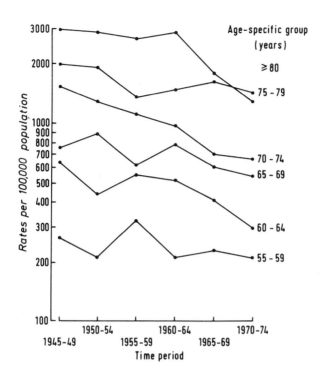

Figure 2 Age analysis of the incidence of stroke according to 5-year periods (Reproduced with permission of the *New England Journal of Medicine*)

Diagnostic Categories of Stroke

Strokes were separated into diagnostic categories using the clinical criteria previously defined. Table II summarises the changing pattern of stroke in consecutive quinquennia. The rates for cerebral infarction show a consistent decrease beginning in 1955-59 such that by 1970-74, the rates were only two-thirds of those seen 15 years before. Rates for intracerebral haemorrhage fluctuate with a sharp fall in the period 1955-59, being followed by a rise in 1960-64 before a more gradual decrease in the two subsequent quinquennia of 1965-69 and 1970-74. The rates for subarachnoid haemorrhage and strokes of uncertain type do not show a clear trend by quinquennial periods. This could be due to the relatively small number of episodes in each quinquennium. Consequently, average annual incidence rates were calculated by amalgamating the quinquennia into three decennial periods 1945-54, 1955-64, and 1965-74. The rates for subarachnoid haemorrhage did not show a fall during these periods, producing average annual incidence rates of 10.6, 11.8, and 10.3 per 100 000 persons respectively. However, strokes of uncertain type did not show an accelerating decline during these periods, with average annual incidence rates of 13.1, 11.3, and 6.8 per 100 000 persons respectively. No change

147

TABLE II

	1945–49	1950–54	1955–59	1960–64	1965–69	1970–74
Cerebral infarction	140 (191)	153 (237)	139 (253)	121 (260)	108 (268)	92 (247)
Intracerebral haemorrhage	18 (24)	19 (29)	8 (15)	13 (29)	12 (29)	10 (26)
Subarachnoid haemorrhage	12 (17)	8 (13)	8 (15)	14 (30)	10 (24)	11 (30)
Stroke of uncertain type	17 (23)	9 (14)	15 (27)	8 (17)	6 (16)	7 (20)

Figures in parentheses are actual number of cases

was noted in either the relative proportion of the different diagnostic categories of stroke or the age at onset during the 30-year period of observation.

The reason for the decline in stroke is not clear. Given the present evidence of risk factors for stroke [19], it is unlikely that trends in recent years of a reduction in the consumption of cigarettes or a decreased dietary intake of saturated fat could have had much bearing on the declining incidence of cerebral infarction in particular. Although the trend in cerebral infarction is of a steady decline during the last 20 years of the study, the rates for intracerebral haemorrhage fluctuated during this period. There is evidence from this population suggesting that anticoagulant therapy after myocardial infarction or transient cerebral ischaemic attacks could have been responsible for the temporary increase in the rate seen in the quinquennium 1960-64, at least for the component of primary intracerebral haemorrhage [20]. The factor most likely to account for the overall decline in incidence is increased surveillance and treatment of hypertension in the community [21]. However, as effective antihypertensive therapy was not even available until the mid-1950s, it is difficult to account for the decline up to the end of that decade. A decrease in blood pressure could have been an important factor during the later, more prominent decline which began from the quinquennium 1960-64. There is some evidence of an increased awareness of the importance of blood pressure surveillance in this community during this period [22]. However, there was a delay of about 10 years between increased recognition of hypertension in this community and a subsequent increase in the use of antihypertensive therapy in patients who had cerebral infarction between 1955 and 1974. Moreover, the proportion of patients with diastolic blood pressures of more than 105 mmHg who were not receiving treatment before the onset of cerebral infarction remained surprisingly high at 53 per cent during the period 1970-74. Thus, the accelerating decline in incidence which began in 1960-64 could well continue in future years, although information on the extent of blood pressure surveillance and subsequent treatment in all persons in the community who did not have a stroke during this period of observation is required to substantiate these observations. One possible result of antihypertensive therapy might have been to create a cohort effect, and evidence of this was sought by undertaking a birth cohort analysis.

148

Birth Cohort Analysis

A birth cohort analysis was undertaken among the specific birth cohorts born during successive five-year periods from 1865 to 1915. The increasing age of these birth cohorts was plotted against the semi-logarithm of the age specific incidence rates for five-year age groups (Fig. 3). While the analysis of birth cohorts confirmed the trend in declining incidence rates in all age groups, among the birth cohorts no differences that could help to explain further the decline in incidence rates were seen. However, it is too early to be certain whether any cohort effect is present in the later birth cohorts of 1900, 1905 and 1910. It will be interesting to see how the trends in these three birth cohorts develop when the next quinquennial period of 1975-79 becomes available for analysis from the Mayo Clinic medical records and linkage system. The absence of a birth cohort effect would not preclude antihypertensive therapy from having the effect that therapeutic trials have suggested it should have. But it would suggest that any reduction in stroke through increased community surveillance and treatment of hypertension may be a more gradual process.

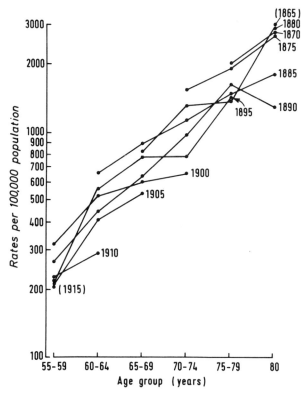

Figure 3 Birth cohort analysis of the incidence of stroke according to age group (Reproduced with permission of the *New England Journal of Medicine*)

149

References

1 Acheson, RM (1960) *Brit. J. Prev. Soc. Med., 14,* 139
2 Wylie, CM (1962) *J. Chronic Dis., 15,* 85
3 Borhani, NO (1965) *Am. J. Public Health, 55,* 673
4 Prineas, RJ (1971) *Med. J. Aust., 2,* 509
5 *Stat. Bull. Metropol. Life Ins. Co., 56,* 2
6 Haberman, S, Capildeo, R and Rose, FC (1978) *Quart. J. Med., 47,* 71
7 Soltero, I (1978) *Stroke, 9,* 549
8 Katsuki, S and Hirota, Y (1966) *Jpn. Heart J., 7,* 26
9 Israel, RA and Klebba, AL (1969) *Am. J. Public Health, 59,* 1651
10 Matsumoto, N, Whisnant, JP, Kurland, LT et al (1973) *Stroke, 4,* 20
11 Heasman, MA and Lipworth, L (1966) *Studies on Medical and Population Subjects, No. 20,* HMSO, London
12 Garraway, WM (1976) In *Stroke Proceedings of the Ninth Pfizer International Symposium.* (ed FJ Gillingham, C Mawdsley, AE Williams). Churchill Livingstone, Edinburgh, page 72
13 Eisenberg, H, Morrison, JT, Sullivan, P et al (1964) *JAMA, 189,* 883
14 Aho, K and Fogelholm, R (1974) *Stroke, 5,* 658
15 Abu-Zeid, HAH, Choi, NW and Nelson, NA (1975) *Can. Med. Assoc. J., 113,* 379
16 Christie, D (1976) *Med. J. Aust., 1,* 565
17 Hansen, BS and Marquardsen, J (1977) *Stroke, 8,* 663
18 Garraway, WM, Whisnant, JP, Furlan, AJ et al (1979) *N. Engl. J. Med., 300,* 449
19 Kannel, WB, Wolf, PA and Dawber, TR (1975) *Millbank Mem. Fund. Q., 53,* 405
20 Furlan, AJ, Whisnant, JP and Elveback, LR (1979) *Ann. Neurol.* In press
21 Walker, WJ (1977) *N. Engl. J. Med., 297,* 163
22 Garraway, WM, Whisnant, JP, Kurland, JT et al (1979) *Stroke.* In press

Chapter 13

RISK FACTORS FOR CEREBROVASCULAR DISEASE

Bruce S Schoenberg

Despite the encouraging reports of decreasing mortality [1-7] and morbidity [8,9] from cerebrovascular disease, stroke remains a significant cause of mortality throughout the world. Figure 1 presents the annual age-adjusted mortality rates for cerebrovascular disease coded as the underlying cause of death. The data shown are for 28 countries from 1967 to 1973. Even for nations with a low reported death rate for cerebrovascular disease, such as Poland and Mexico, stroke is a major force of mortality.

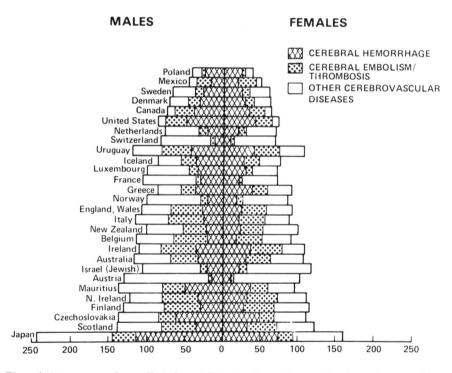

Figure 1 Average annual age-adjusted mortality rates for cerebrovascular disease by sex and by type. Various countries, 1967-73. Adjusted to the US population of 1950 as the standard, using the direct method of age-adjustment. (Reproduced with permission from Schoenberg, BS (1979) *South. Med. J., 72,* 331)

151

It has been estimated that approximately 50 per cent of stroke victims die within 30 days of the acute event [10]. The case fatality ratio is greatest for intracerebral haemorrhage, followed in order by subarachnoid haemorrhage and cerebral infarction [10, 11]. Of those who survive more than 1 month, approximately 10 per cent are left with little discernible disability, 40 per cent have mild residual disability, 40 per cent have sufficient residual impairment to require specialised care, and 10 per cent require institutional care because of profound neurological impairment [10].

At the present time, there is little to suggest that improved medical management of the completed stroke will substantially affect the cerebrovascular disease problem. It would seem that greater benefit could be achieved by dealing with the precursors of stroke, rather than delaying treatment until after the event has occurred. This makes it essential to identify the stroke-prone individual, and to provide treatment before the occurrence of long-lasting neurological dysfunction.

General Considerations in Epidemiological Studies of Risk Factors

The investigation of stroke risk factors is in the province of analytic epidemiology, and research designs can generally be categorised into two groups: case-control and prospective. These two approaches are outlined in Figure 2. The case-control study begins with a group of individuals with stroke (cases) and a comparable group (controls) without stroke. One explores their current status (cross-sectional investigation) or past history (retrospective study) for factors differentially distributed in the stroke group as compared to the control group. For any given risk factor examined, this study design allows one to estimate a parameter known as relative risk. Relative risk is the ratio of the risk of stroke in those with the factor present to the risk of stroke in those without the factor. Such studies can usually be done quickly and without great expense. The advantages and disadvantages of this type of research strategy are described in detail elsewhere [12]. One particular problem of case-control studies is that they cannot provide an estimate of absolute risk (the risk of stroke in those with a given risk factor).

To obtain measures of absolute risk, one must employ a prospective study design (Fig. 2). This begins with a group or cohort with a particular factor (thought to be related to the disease of interest) and a group without the factor. The two groups are observed over a period of time in order to see how many develop the disease under investigation (in this case, stroke). The frequency of stroke in the group with the factor is compared to the stroke frequency in the group without the factor. These studies typically require many years to carry out and are quite expensive. Furthermore, such investigations are generally suitable only for relatively frequent disorders such as stroke. The prototype for illustrating the advantages of the prospective approach in studying stroke is the Framingham, Massachusetts investigation [13-15]. Observations were begun in 1950 on an original cohort of approximately 5000 men and women who were between ages 30 and 62 at the start of the study period. The group was followed with standardised biennial examinations.

152

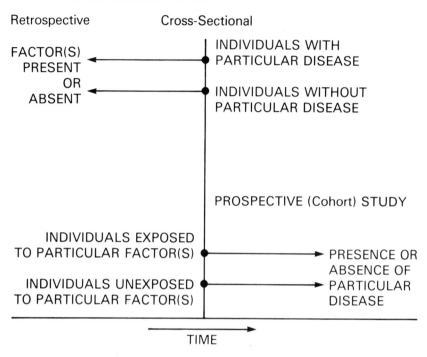

CASE-CONTROL STUDY

Retrospective   Cross-Sectional

FACTOR(S) PRESENT ◄——— INDIVIDUALS WITH PARTICULAR DISEASE

OR

ABSENT ◄——— INDIVIDUALS WITHOUT PARTICULAR DISEASE

PROSPECTIVE (Cohort) STUDY

INDIVIDUALS EXPOSED TO PARTICULAR FACTOR(S) ———► PRESENCE OR

ABSENCE OF

INDIVIDUALS UNEXPOSED TO PARTICULAR FACTOR(S) ———► PARTICULAR DISEASE

TIME

Figure 2 Format for analytic epidemiological studies of stroke risk factors. (Reproduced with permission from Schoenberg, BS (1978) In *Advances in Neurology, Vol. 21: The Inherited Ataxias: Biochemical, Viral, and Pathological Studies*. Raven Press, New York, page 15)

Note that the vertical line along the time axis in Figure 2 is not labelled. The traditional prospective study begins in the present and continues into the future. However, under certain circumstances it may be possible to begin the point of observation at some time in the past and look at disease outcome in the present. This is possible if cohorts of those with and those without a given risk factor were examined and questioned in a standardised manner in the past to determine health and exposure status. The two groups must then be followed in a uniform, standardised manner. Such an investigation is called a nonconcurrent prospective study or a prospective study in retrospect. This approach has the advantage of greatly reducing the time and expense often associated with prospective studies. On the other hand, it is most unusual to find cohorts of individuals who have been examined, questioned, and observed in a standardised manner over a number of years. In reality, we must settle for cohorts who are examined and followed in a more or less uniform manner that does not achieve the level of standardisation available with prospective studies beginning in the present and continuing into the future. This nonconcurrent prospective research design is at present being employed by the author in an evaluation of the role of cardiovascular disease as risk factors, for both completed stroke and transient ischaemic attacks. A cohort of about 2000 residents of Rochester, Minnesota was identified; these individuals met the following criteria in 1960: (a) they were 50 years of age or older, and (b) they underwent a medical evaluation during that year. The group was then followed over 13 years. The cardiovascular status of each individual was defined at the start of observation, and was modified according to the findings of evaluations throughout the 13-year period.

Analytic epidemiological studies of stroke risk factors pose a number of difficulties. The case-control approach is often restricted to studying survivors, and this can result in serious biases since survival following stroke is a function of the type of cerebrovascular disease (cerebral infarction, intracerebral haemorrhage, etc.) and the degree of residual disability [13]. Furthermore, the level of a given risk factor may change following the occurrence of a stroke. Some authors have suggested that for certain risk factors, levels in the remote past may be a better predictor of stroke occurrence than levels of such factors closer to the onset of the acute neurological dysfunction [13]. This means that prospective studies of such risk factors must incorporate lengthy periods of follow-up. If certain risk factors (e.g. transient arrhythmias) are present for only brief periods of time, they may be missed altogether. With such investigations it is also important to specify the type of cerebrovascular disease and the location and extent of vascular lesions in as much detail as possible. For example, a given risk factor may be an important predictor of cerebral infarction due to occlusion of the internal carotid artery near its origin from the common carotid, but the same risk factor may have no predictive value for subarachnoid haemorrhage secondary to rupture of an aneurysm.

It should also be emphasised that in any of these studies, the identification of a risk factor does not indicate a direct, causal relationship. A particular characteristic under consideration may be only indirectly related to a biologically significant factor. Despite this, it may be possible to make a significant impact on the occurrence of disease by dealing with this indirect association; for example, there is a strong relationship between cigarette smoking and bronchogenic carcinoma. Although the exact pathogenic mechanisms for the development of squamous cell carcinoma of the lung have not been clearly elucidated, it is possible to lower the risk of lung cancer through cessation of cigarette smoking.

In evaluating the results of studies reported in later sections of this paper, one must consider whether the risk factor is related to a particular type of stroke, or whether the risk factor is important only for certain demographic subgroups of the population defined on the basis of age, race, sex, geographic location, etc. One must also search for a dose–response relationship between the factor and the disease (i.e. do increased levels of the risk factor correspond to an increased risk of the disease?). Furthermore, is there a threshold level of the risk factor below which there is no increased risk of the disease? Finally, the reduction or removal of the risk factor should correspond to a reduction in the rate of disease occurrence. This last association has important implications not only for primary prevention, but also for providing aetiological clues.

From the results of several analytic epidemiological studies, a profile of the stroke-prone individual is beginning to emerge. Such factors as pre-existing hypertension, heart disease, diabetes, and transient ischaemic attacks have been shown to increase the risk of completed stroke by a factor of between two and 12 times [14, 15]. Results concerning potential risk factors such as cigarette smoking, elevated cholesterol levels, and elevated triglyceride levels have been more equivocal [15]. The present tabulations from Framingham suggest that 10 per cent of the asymptomatic population in which 50 per cent of all strokes will occur can be identified [16].

TABLE I Currently Recognised Risk Factors for Cerebrovascular Disease

Risk factors	Relationship to cerebrovascular disease*
Hypertension	+
Diabetes mellitus	+
Heart disease	+
Transient ischaemic attacks	+
Blood lipids	±
Obesity	±
Cigarette smoking	±
Exogenous oestrogens	+
Others	+

* Code: + Indicates that several studies have documented that the presence of this factor increases the risk of cerebrovascular disease; ± indicates that results are equivocal as to whether the presence of this factor increases the risk of cerebrovascular disease. (Reproduced with permission from Schoenberg, BS (1979) *South. Med. J., 72*, 331)

Table I outlines a number of currently recognised risk factors associated with stroke in adults. Each of these will be considered separately in the remainder of this paper. Risk factors for cerebrovascular disease in children are considered in detail in Chapter 25 [17].

Hypertension

Of the currently identified stroke risk factors, hypertension is the most important. This holds true for cerebral infarction, intracerebral haemorrhage, and subarachnoid haemorrhage [15, 18–20]. Some report a linear relationship between the level of either the systolic or diastolic blood pressure and the risk of stroke; this relation remains true for both sexes and all age groups studied in Framingham, Massachusetts [15, 21]. But other investigators feel the curve relating blood pressure and stroke may be more complex [10]. The Framingham experience indicated that the first casual blood pressure at the initial examination was an adequate predictor of subsequent stroke risk. Repeated blood pressure measurements, averages of pressures on subsequent examinations, calculations of pulse pressure or mean arterial pressure, and the lability of the blood pressure yielded little additional information [21]. The relationship between blood pressure and stroke has also been studied extensively in Japan, and the results are consistent with the findings in the United States [22]. The higher levels of blood pressure among the US black population and their high risk of stroke are observations consistent with the relationship noted above [23]. However, geographic variations in stroke incidence and mortality in the US cannot be explained by geographic variations in blood pressure [24]. Furthermore, the correlation between increased blood pressure and increasing stroke rates does not hold for Japanese-US comparisons. Japanese residing in California have higher blood pressures than Japanese living in Hawaii or Japan, yet the California Japanese have lower stroke death rates and lower stroke prevalence than their counterparts in Hawaii or Japan [25].

The application of blood pressure control programmes would be expected to have an effect in reducing the risk of stroke. This has been demonstrated in both the United States and Japan [26-27]. Therapy was most successful in those with markedly elevated blood pressure [13]. In addition, clinical trials of treating patients with mild [28] and moderate [29] hypertension resulted in fewer initial strokes of all types.

Diabetes Mellitus

The association between diabetes mellitus and ischaemic cerebrovascular disease is well documented. A high percentage of death certificates on which stroke is listed as the underlying cause of death also contain diabetes mellitus as a contributing cause [30]. In addition, diabetic patients followed over many years had an increased risk of dying of stroke than did age-matched controls [31]. The findings of these studies based on stroke mortality are supported by investigations of stroke morbidity. A number of case-control investigations report a higher prevalence of diabetes mellitus among stroke patients when compared to controls [32]. The stroke incidence rate among all diabetics identified among the population of Rochester, Minnesota was compared to the stroke rate among all Rochester residents adjusted by age and sex. Those with diabetes mellitus had 1.7 times the risk of stroke than the general population [33]. Similar results were obtained in the Framingham cohort [15, 34, 35]. When these data are adjusted for the presence of other major stroke risk factors, the relative risk of ischaemic stroke among diabetics is approximately 2 [34]. There was no evidence that treatment of the diabetes (with diet, oral hypoglycaemic agents, or insulin) resulted in a reduction of the stroke risk [36]. Variations in the prevalence of diabetes or geographic variations in blood glucose levels cannot explain national differentials in stroke mortality or morbidity [13]. In one study of three areas in the United States, however, there was a consistent trend between blood glucose levels one hour after ingesting 50 g of oral glucose and the risk of stroke in that area of the country [24]. In this same investigation, blacks were found to have higher blood glucose values than whites. This is consistent with their higher risk of stroke.

156

Heart Disease

The most extensive information on the importance of heart disease as a risk factor for stroke is derived from the Framingham cohort. Over the course of 24 years of observation, 204 ischaemic strokes occurred in this group [46]. A number of electrocardiographic abnormalities are associated with an increased risk of cerebral infarction. Electrocardiographic evidence of left ventricular hypertrophy results in a tenfold increase in the risk of ischaemic stroke. The relative risk of stroke in those with ST-T wave abnormalities or intraventricular block is 4.2 and 2.5, respectively. The presence of coronary heart disease (coronary insufficiency, angina pectoris, and myocardial infarction) heightens the risk of cerebral infarction regardless of sex. This relationship held for all ages included in the Framingham cohort. The relative risk of stroke in those with congestive heart failure was 9. In the Framingham cohort, the risk of stroke in persons with rheumatic heart disease and atrial fibrillation was 25 times the expected rate. Those with atrial fibrillation in the absence of rheumatic heart disease had 8.5 times the risk of stroke compared to individuals of the same age, sex, and blood pressure who did not have atrial fibrillation. The Framingham study revealed that those with rheumatic heart disease without atrial arrhythmia are also at increased risk of stroke. However, the number of such cases was too small to reach statistical significance. Coronary heart disease and congestive heart failure not only increased the risk of stroke, but were also associated with decreased survival following a stroke.

These associations of an increased risk of stroke in the presence of heart disease are also supported by the findings of other studies [10, 37–40]. With regard to previously unsuspected risk factors, a recent case-control investigation documents an association between cerebral ischaemia and the presence of mitral valve prolapse [41]. The results of the nonconcurrent prospective study in Rochester, Minnesota should provide further documentation of these important relationships.

Transient Ischaemic Attacks

A number of early studies based on case series indicated that as many as 30 per cent–50 per cent of hospitalised patients with thrombotic cerebral infarction recall a transient ischaemic attack (TIA) prior to the onset of the completed stroke [42, 43]. When this analysis was restricted to all patients derived from a well-defined population (thereby minimising the problems of selection bias inherent in a case series), the percentage of patients with a previous history of TIA dropped to 10 per cent [44]. Observations concerning the natural history of patients with TIA indicate that between 2 per cent and 35 per cent of such individuals suffer a subsequent cerebral infarction [45–53]. It is difficult to compare these reports because of the varying ages of the patients in each series, the varying periods of follow-up, etc. The prognosis of the TIA patient with regard to subsequent stroke does not seem to be related to the duration or number of TIA's or to the presence of heart disease [53].

Longitudinal observations of the stroke experience of TIA patients derived from

157

the well-defined Rochester, Minnesota population revealed that the risk of completed stroke was a function of time interval following the initial TIA [54]. The probability of remaining stroke-free for TIA patients was compared to the probability of remaining stroke-free for the general population adjusted for the age and sex distribution of those with TIA's (Fig.3). The ratio of observed-to-expected strokes among TIA patients dropped from 16.5 at the end of the first year following the initial TIA to 9.5 at ten years following the first TIA. Over 50 per cent of all strokes occurring in the TIA cohort occurred within one year of the first ischaemic episode.

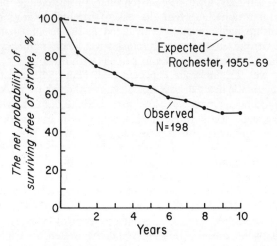

Figure 3 Conditional probability of surviving free of stroke after first transient ischaemic attack, given survival. Expected survivorship is for a population of the given age and sex and is based on the stroke incidence rates of the Rochester, Minnesota study for 1955 through 1969. (Reproduced with permission from Whisnant, JP, Matsuomoto, N and Elveback, LR (1973) *Mayo Clin. Proc., 48,* 194)

Blood Lipids

The relationship between blood lipid levels and the risk of stroke is much less clear-cut. Despite no significant differences in serum cholesterol levels in selected areas of the United States, these same regions have markedly different stroke death rates [24]. No relationship could be found between serum cholesterol levels and stroke risk in a Japanese study as well [55]. Furthermore, although Japanese remaining in Japan have lower cholesterol levels than Japanese living in California or Hawaii, they have higher death rates for stroke [56-58]. Among the Framingham cohort, the risk of cerebral infarction was related to serum cholesterol levels only for men in the youngest age group studied [15]. No relationship was found in women. In several other community studies of stroke risk factors, no clear or consistent relations were found between serum cholesterol and the rate of subsequent stroke [10]. If the relationship only holds for younger individuals, as suggested by the

158

Framingham data, this could explain the lack of consistent findings in the other studies which dealt with older populations. Furthermore, it has been suggested that since cholesterol levels are highly correlated with coronary disease, those with hypercholesterolaemia may die of a myocardial infarction before developing clinically apparent cerebrovascular disease [13].

Obesity

The relationship between obesity and cerebrovascular disease is equivocal. There is no consistent international pattern between the presence of obesity and stroke mortality [59]. In a study of college students at two universities, those who subsequently died of stroke (at a mean age of 49) had a lower ponderal index at the time they were in college than age-matched surviving controls. However, these tabulations were not adjusted for the subsequent development of hypertension or diabetes mellitus prior to the stroke [60]. Gain in weight from age 20 was related to an increased stroke risk in the Evans County, Georgia population, but the weight gain was also correlated with increases in blood pressure [61]. Obesity was found to be related to the risk of cerebral infarction in the Framingham cohort for both men and women. The excess risk reached statistical significance only for women, however [15]. In Framingham, obese hypertensives had higher stroke rates than nonobese hypertensives [62].

Cigarette Smoking

Like blood lipids and obesity, there is no consistent relationship reported for cigarette smoking and cerebrovascular disease. Variations in cigarette smoking could not explain geographic differences in stroke mortality and morbidity in the United States [24]. A large study of stroke in the population of Washington County, Maryland found no relationship with cigarette smoking [63]. With regard to positive results, former college students who smoked while in college had a higher subsequent stroke mortality than their nonsmoking counterparts [60]. In the Framingham cohort, nonsmoking men in the youngest age group had a lower incidence of cerebral infarction than smokers of the same age. There was no correlation between the risk of cerebral infarction and cigarette smoking over all age groups, and even in the youngest group of men, there was no consistent dose-response relationship with the number of cigarettes smoked [15]. There were too few heavy cigarette smokers and too few cerebral infarctions among the Framingham women to allow one to draw any reliable conclusions. In an investigation of a cohort in Chicago, there was a strong positive correlation between stroke and cigarette smoking for those who were free of illness at the beginning of the study. For those with pre-existing illness, there was a strong negative association between cigarette smoking and stroke [10].

159

Exogenous oestrogens

Case-control studies have demonstrated that the use of oral contraceptives increases the incidence of stroke [64, 65]. It has been postulated that the increase may be due to increased thrombogenesis, increased blood pressure, and increased blood glucose associated with the use of exogenous oestrogens [13]. However, despite this increased relative risk, a study of stroke incidence among all female residents of Rochester, Minnesota (from ages 15 to 49) in the years just before and just after the introduction of oral contraceptives failed to demonstrate any change in the stroke rate [66]. A case-control study of oestrogen use and stroke risk among post-menopausal women found no significant overall association. However, there was a significant excess of oestrogen users among 70–79-year-old women who had suffered a nonembolic cerebral infarction [67]. This was thought to be due to increased blood pressure associated with oestrogen use. Exogenous oestrogens also heighten stroke risk in men, prostatic cancer patients receiving high doses of stilboestrol having an increased risk of stroke [68–69].

Other Factors

The presence of a host of other factors such as sickle-cell anaemia, collagen vascular disease, polycythaemia, high haemoglobin concentrations, prosthetic heart valves, syphilitic vascular disease, etc. increase the likelihood of stroke [57, 70]. Although these factors probably account for only a small percentage of all cases of cerebrovascular disease, they are important clinically in that they represent potentially treatable precursors of completed stroke.

Summary

The most important currently identified risk factors for completed stroke in the adult are hypertension, diabetes mellitus, heart disease, and transient ischaemic attacks. Despite the array of potential risk factors that have been studied and identified, we cannot at present provide an adequate explanation for a large proportion of the strokes that occur. The paradoxical distributions of certain of these risk factors (for example, in US–Japanese comparisons) further emphasise that other currently unknown risk factors remain to be discovered, and that currently recognised factors are poorly understood. This area of research must be actively pursued if we are to realise the goal of stroke prevention.

References

1 Acheson, RM (1960) *Brit. J. Prev. Soc. Med., 14,* 139
2 Wylie, CM (1962) *J. Chron. Dis., 15,* 85
3 Borhani, NO (1965) *Am. J. Public Health, 55,* 673
4 Prineas, RJ (1971) *Med. J. Aust., 2,* 509

5   Anonymous (1975) *Stat. Bull. Metropol. Life Ins. Co., 56,* 2
6   Haberman, S, Capildeo, R and Rose, FC (1978) *Quart. J. Med., 47,* 71
7   Massey, EW, Schoenberg, DG and Schoenberg, BS (1979). Submitted for publication
8   Wolf, PA, Dawber, TR, Thomas, HE Jr et al (1978) *Stroke, 9,* 97
9   Garraway, WM, Whisnant, JP, Furlan, AJ et al (1979) *N. Engl. J. Med., 300,* 449
10 Stallones, RA, Dyken, ML, Fang, HCH et al (1976) In *Fundamentals of Stroke Care* (ed AL Sahs and EC Hartman). US Govt Printing Office, Washington, DC., page 5
11 Wylie, CM (1976) In *Fundamentals of Stroke Care* (ed AL Sahs and EC Hartman). US Govt Printing Office, Washington, DC, page 381
12 Schoenberg, BS (1978) In *Advances in Neurology, Vol. 19: Neurological Epidemiology (Principles and Clinical Applications)* (ed BS Schoenberg). Raven Press, New York, page 43
13 Kuller, LH (1978) In *Advances in Neurology, Vol. 19: Neurological Epidemiology (Principles and Clinical Applications)* (ed BS Schoenberg). Raven Press, New York, page 281
14 Wolf, PA, Dawber, TR and Kannel, WB (1978) In *Advances in Neurology, Vol. 19: Neurological Epidemiology (Principles and Clinical Applications)* (ed BS Schoenberg). Raven Press, New York, page 567
15 Wolf, PA, Kannel, WB and Dawber, TR (1978) In *Advances in Neurology, Vol. 19: Neurological Epidemiology (Principles and Clinical Applications)* (ed BS Schoenberg). Raven Press, New York, page 107
16 Wolf, PA, Dawber, TR, Kannel, WB et al (1973) *Neurology, 23,* 418
17 Schoenberg, BS and Schoenberg, DG Chapter 30 of this volume Rose). Pitman Medical Publishing Co Ltd, Tunbridge Wells
18 Kannel, WB (1966) In *Cerebral Vascular Diseases* (ed RG Siekert and JP Whisnant). Grune & Stratton, New York, page 53
19 Kannel, WB, Wolf, PA, Verter, J et al (1970) *J.A.M.A., 214,* 301
20 Wolf, PA (1975) In *Cerebral Vascular Diseases* (ed JP Whisnant and BA Sandok). Grune and Stratton, New York, page 105
21 Kannel, WB, Dawber, TR, Sorlie, P et al (1976) *Stroke, 7,* 327
22 Komachi, T, Iida, M and Shimamoto, T (1971) *Jpn. Circ. J., 35,* 189
23 U.S. National Center for Health Statistics (1964) Series 11, No. 5, US Dept of Health, Education, and Welfare, Washington, DC, page 1
24 Stolley, PD, Kuller, LH, Nefzger, MD et al (1977) *Stroke, 8,* 551
25 Marmot, MG, Syme, SL, Kagan, A et al (1975) *Am. J. Epidemiol., 102,* 514
26 Veterans Administration Cooperative Study Group on Antihypertensive Agents (1972) *Circulation, 45,* 991
27 Komachi, Y, Iida, M, Shimamoto, T et al (1971) *Ann. Rep. Center for Adult Disease (Osaka), 11,* 1
28 Veterans Administration Cooperative Study Group on Antihypertensive Agents (1970) *J.A.M.A., 202,* 1028
29 Veterans Administration Cooperative Study Group on Antihypertensive Agents (1967) *J.A.M.A., 202,* 1028
30 Kuller, L and Seltser, R (1967) *Am. J. Epidemiol., 86,* 442
31 Kessler, II (1971) *Am. J. Med., 51,* 715
32 Gertler, MM, Leetma, HE, Rusk, HA et al (1969) *N.Y. State J. Med., 69,* 2664
33 Palumbo, PJ, Elveback, LR and Whisnant, JP (1978) In *Advances in Neurology Vol. 19: Neurological Epidemiology (Principles and Clinical Applications)* (ed BS Schoenberg). Raven Press, New York, page 593
34 Kannel, WB and McGee, DL (1979) *J.A.M.A., 241,* 2035
35 Gordon, T and Kannel, WB (1972) *J.A.M.A., 221,* 661
36 Golden, MG, Knatterud, GL and Prout, TE (1971) *J.A.M.A., 218,* 1400
37 Peacock, PB, Riley, CP, Lampton, TD et al (1972) In *Trends in Epidemiology: Application to Health Service Research and Training,* Chapter 8 (ed GT Stewart). Charles C Thomas, Publisher, Springfield, Illinois
38 Friedman, GD, Loveland, DB and Ehrlich, SP (1968) *Circulation, 38,* 533

39 Harrison, DC, Fitzgerald, JW and Winkle, RA (1976) *N. Engl. J. Med., 294*, 373
40 Fairfax, AJ, Lambert, CD and Leatham, A (1976) *N. Engl. J. Med., 295*, 190
41 Barnett, HJM, Bougher, DR and Cooper PF (1978) *Ann. Neurol., 4*, 163
42 David, NJ and Heyman, A (1960) *J. Chron. Dis., 11*, 394
43 Fisher, CM (1958) In *Cerebral Vascular Diseases. Transactions of the Second Princeton Conference* (ed CH Millikan). Grune and Stratton, New York, page 81
44 Whisnant, JP, Matsumoto, N and Elveback, LR (1973) *Mayo Clin. Proc., 48*, 194
45 Baker, RN, Schwartz, WS and Rose, AS (1966) *Neurology, 16*, 841
46 Ziegler, DK and Hassanein, RS (1973) *Stroke, 4*, 666
47 Baker, RN, Broward, JA, Fang, HC et al (1962) *Neurology, 12*, 823
48 Fields, WS, Maslenikov, V, Meyer, JS et al (1970) *J.A.M.A., 211*, 1993
49 Pearce, JM, Gubbay, SS and Walton, JN (1965) *Lancet, i*, 6
50 Marshall, J (1964) *Quart. J. Med., 33*, 309
51 Ostfeld, AM, Shekelle, RB and Klawans, HL (1973) *Stroke, 4*, 980
52 Karp, HR, Heyman, A, Heyden, S et al (1973) *J.A.M.A., 225*, 125
53 Heyman, A, Leviton, A, Millikan, CH et al (1976) In *Fundamentals of Stroke Care* (ed AL Sahs and EC Hartman). US Govt Printing Office, Washington, DC, page 33
54 Whisnant, JP (1974) *Stroke, 5*, 68
55 Omae, T, Takeshita, M and Hirota, Y (1976) In *Cerebrovascular Diseases* (ed P Scheinberg). Raven Press, New York, page 261
56 Schoenberg, BS (1976) In *Cerebrovascular Diseases* (ed P Scheinberg). Raven Press, New York, page 284
57 Schoenberg, BS (1979) *South. Med. J., 72*, 331
58 Nichaman, MZ, Hamilton, HB, Dagan, A et al (1975) *Am. J. Epidemiol., 102*, 491
59 Blackburn, H, Taylor, HL and Keys, A (1970) In *Coronary Heart Disease in Seven Countries* (ed A Keys). American Heart Association, New York, page 154
60 Paffenbarger, RS and Williams, JL (1967) *Am. J. Public Health, 57*, 1290
61 Heyden, S, Hames, CG, Bartel, A et al (1971) *Arch. Intern. Med., 128*, 956
62 Gordon, T and Kannel, WB (1976) *Clin. Endocrinol. Metab., 5*, 367
63 Nomura, A., Comstock, GW, Kuller, L et al (1974) *Stroke, 5*, 483
64 Collaborative Group for the Study of Stroke in Young Women (1973) *N. Engl. J. Med., 288*, 871
65 Vessey, MP and Doll, R (1969) *Brit. Med. J., 2*, 651
66 Schoenberg, BS, Whisnant, JP, Taylor, WF et al (1970) *Neurology, 20*, 181
67 Pfeffer, RI and Van Den Noort, S (1976) *Am. J. Epidemiol., 103*, 445
68 Veterans Administration Co-operative Urological Research Group (1967) *Surg. Gynecol. Obstet., 124*, 1011
69 Byar, DP (1973) *Cancer, 32*, 1126
70 Whisnant, JP, Anderson, EM, Aronson, SM et al (1976) In *Fundamentals of Stroke Care*. US Govt Printing Office, Washington, DC, page 14

Chapter 14

ASSESSING THE EFFECTIVENESS OF REHABILITATION FOLLOWING STROKE

T W Meade and D S Smith

Introduction

Remedial therapy in the patient disabled by a stroke is now considered usual practice. This kind of treatment is particularly labour-intensive and, unless domiciliary care is available, it may involve the patient in a considerable amount of travel between home and hospital. It is by no means obvious, however, that attempts to rehabilitate the stroke patient are effective. How can the uncertainty be resolved? How much time should therapists devote to stroke patients, and should the patients be put to the trouble of undergoing treatment? Proponents of different rehabilitation regimes claim that theirs are effective provided they are applied to the 'right' patients. But the encouraging results claimed may be due as much to spontaneous improvement as to treatment. Comparisons based on different centres using different methods are difficult or impossible to interpret. Patients attending one centre may very well differ in several respects from those attending another. Contrasts in outcome may then be due to contrasts in the characteristics of the group being compared, rather than to treatment.

Randomised controlled trials

The best solution to these difficulties is the randomised controlled trial. Each patient is allocated to one or other of the treatment regimes at random. This process establishes two (or more) groups of patients which are, as groups, and under ideal circumstances, identical. They will be identical not only in terms of features that can be identified and measured, such as age or height, but will also be identical in terms of unidentifiable features. In these circumstances, subsequent differences in outcome can really be due only to treatment.

It is not possible to evaluate every facet of health care by randomised trials, but stroke rehabilitation is a suitable topic. If rehabilitation is effective, a worthwhile outcome will be achieved, but this may depend on a large investment of effort and resources by the patient and by the rehabilitation team. There is, thus, a clinical cost-benefit question to be answered in the interests of the individual patient. There are also cost-benefit questions to be answered in the interests of the best use of health service facilities.

163

The Northwick Park stroke trial

The Northwick Park trial is a randomised controlled comparison of different intensities of out-patient rehabilitation following stroke. There are ethical difficulties in the way of an in-patient rehabilitation trial, for this would involve withholding or reducing early treatment. Doctors and therapists understandably find this difficult to accept. Once the patient has left hospital, however, the situation is different. He or she may benefit from further rehabilitation. On the other hand, frequent travel between home and hospital is likely to be tiring, and the consequences could even cancel out the advantages of treatment. The crucial question, however, is whether rehabilitation is effective anyway.

The Northwick Park trial described elsewhere by Sheikh and his colleagues [1] compares two active regimes with one involving little or no rehabilitation. One active regime (Group I) consists of very intensive treatment given during four whole days each week. The other (Group II) consists of a 'conventional' level of treatment occupying three half days a week. Patients allocated to the third regime (Group III) receive no routine rehabilitation. They are regularly visited at home by a health visitor, who can refer them to hospital if necessary.

Recruitment to the trial took place between 1972 and 1978. Patients entered in 1978 will be followed up for the last time in 1979. Results on the clinical and social value of rehabilitation are therefore not yet available. However, some of the trial's problems can be usefully discussed. They are likely to be relevant to similar trials in the future.

Standards for Rehabilitation Trials

A randomised controlled trial of rehabilitation should be designed and carried out like a double-blind drug trial, as far as possible. Remedial therapy and similar trials certainly raise difficulties not encountered in most drug trials, but there is no reason why the best of the latter should not be the model. Good drug trials are the source of most of our experience.

Reasons for randomisation and some ethical considerations have already been referred to. Other substantial questions that have arisen in the Northwick Park trial concern how it is managed, recruiting adequate numbers, recording 'dosage' of treatment, methods of measuring outcome, the need for 'blind' assessments and the policy to be adopted on divulging the main results.

Management of the Trial

The day-to-day conduct of a remedial therapy trial should be in the hands of the clinicians and therapists with responsibility for the routine service. A consultant and therapists might be willing to hand over their patients to a special team for a trial that they did not want to be involved in themselves. This arrangement might have some advantages in terms of strict adherence to the trial's schedule, but would be removed from day-to-day realities. There might then be difficulties about the acceptability of the results. An epidemiologist or statistician should be responsible for the overall design of the study, for seeing that this is adhered to and for analysing the results.

164

Numbers Required

Recruiting adequate numbers into a randomised controlled trial is often difficult. Estimates of numbers of patients likely to be available are nearly always much too optimistic. Inadequate allowance is usually made for reasons of exclusion. The first step should be, though it is often not taken, to specify some basic statistical criteria. The first is the improvement in outcome that is to be detected, e.g. a 30 per cent increase in those actively treated who achieve a particular result, compared with those in the control group. The larger the percentage, the smaller the numbers will have to be. The second is to have some idea about the rate at which those in the control group will achieve the particular result, i.e. the 'natural' event rate. Again, the larger the rate, the smaller the required numbers. Finally, the level of statistical significance for a positive result should be decided, together with the probability (power) of being able to detect a positive result.

The Northwick Park trial aimed to recruit 200 patients, but has fallen somewhat short of this. The reasons are summarised in Table I. Of all the patients admitted to Northwick Park Hospital with a confirmed stroke between 1972 and 1978, 34 per cent died within two months or so. Many patients, about 30 per cent, were too old or frail, or had other serious illnesses, and would not normally be considered for rehabilitation anyway. Nearly a fifth (19.3%) made an early and complete recovery. Out-patient rehabilitation was obviously not indicated. Thus, only about 12 per cent of the patients were eligible for the trial. Eligibility had to be assessed in terms of eligibility for *intensive* rehabilitation, in case the patient drew this regime. With this one reservation, however, it seems likely that those who were suitable for the trial were fairly representative of patients who would be considered for rehabilitation in district general hospital practice. Eligibility for rehabilitation in residential centres might be higher than in a hospital out-patient setting.

TABLE I Proportions of Patients Considered for Northwick Park Stroke Trial

	%
Death within two months of stroke	34.0
Too old, other serious illness, etc.	30.5
Full recovery within two months of stroke	19.3
Other exclusions	4.5
Included in trial	11.7

These proportions are based on the first five years of the trial. Final (6 year) figures may differ slightly.

Interest in particular sub-groups of patients who may respond better than others also affects the overall numbers required; for example, rehabilitation might be more effective in young patients than in old, or where visual disturbance has not occurred. These are valid scientific questions of a specific nature. On the other hand, the doctor's or therapist's approach is to do the best he or she can for each individual patient, whatever the circumstances; neither will want to be too rigidly bound by *dicta* as to whether or not the patient is likely to do well. For them, a more general answer to the value of rehabilitation may be needed. Under ideal conditions, this general answer would be based on the results of a number of trials on very specific questions. There are obvious research limitations to this approach. The pooled experience of different sub-groups of patients in a single trial, regardless of treatment regime, may indicate which are likely to do best.

The limited numbers available to the Northwick Park trial meant that entry was spread over six years. The objective was to compare intensities of rehabilitation, not different types. Thus, even marked changes in rehabilitation practice between 1972 and 1978 would not necessarily have affected the chief aim of the trial. In the event, such changes seem to have been limited. But a six-year entry period is unsatisfactory. Staff change, and it may be difficult to maintain standard procedures for this long. In any future trials, multicentre co-operation will be essential. Weddell (1974), [2] has also shown that the number of stroke patients likely to benefit from rehabilitation is rather small.

Measuring Dosage

As in drug trials, so in remedial therapy it is necessary to state an intended dosage of treatment, and to record how far the actual dosage departs from this. In this respect, a stroke rehabilitation trial is at an advantage. Hospital rehabilitation, unlike pill-taking at home, is supervised. So quite accurate estimates of treatment given are possible. In the Northwick Park trial, two factors have caused some departures from the intended schedules for Groups I and II. Some Group I patients found the full course too tiring. This bears out the relevance of the clinical cost–benefit balance already referred to. The other problem has been with ambulance transport. This has been described by Beer and his associates [3]. Despite these difficulties, however, Group I patients have on average received twice as much physiotherapy and occupational therapy as those in Group II.

Measuring Outcome

Stroke rehabilitation studies are mainly concerned with 'soft' end-points related to quality of life and functional ability. These are notoriously difficult to measure compared with 'hard' events such as death. The profusion and diversity of suggested indices for general health bears this out. The Northwick Park trial uses change in a modified Activities of Daily Living (ADL) index as its chief measure of outcome. The index can be used to derive a total score, or scores for its individual components can be used. Sheikh and co-workers [4] have shown that the ADL is repeatable, subject to little within-person variability over a short period of time, and valid to the extent that this point can be established. The trial also measures various aspects of limb and total body function.

Active treatment in the Northwick Park trial consists of physiotherapy, occupational therapy and speech therapy (where necessary). It also involves much non-specific contact between patients and therapists, ambulance staff, receptionists and others. Differences in outcome, if any, can therefore only be attributed to differences in the three regimes as a whole. Other trials would be necessary to identify the individual components of the effective regime(s).

166

Blind Assessments

Remedial therapy trials cannot be double or even single blind. Both the therapist and the patient are bound to know what treatment is given and received. Views on the value of rehabilitation are often held with extreme degrees of conviction. Opportunities for biased assessments of outcome are plentiful. These assessments should therefore be made by someone not involved in treatment, and preferably in complete ignorance about it. This may not be easy, but should certainly be attempted.

Policy on Results

Even in double-blind trials, it is increasingly the practice not to make interim disclosures about the main results. If early indications are known to favour one treatment, new biases might be introduced, affecting the actual delivery of treatment or assessments, or both. It is asking a great deal of therapists to remain in ignorance about something that might eventually affect the approach to rehabilitation quite fundamentally. But it has proved possible to run the Northwick Park trial on this basis in spite of its long duration.

Conclusion

Experience at Northwick Park suggests that the effectiveness of rehabilitation after stroke can be studied without unacceptable breaches of the basic rules of clinical trials. The small numbers of patients recruited, and the reasons for this, are in themselves valuable practical findings. That only a small proportion of patients were eligible may imply that the need for rehabilitation is less than has been generally thought. But stroke is a common disease. There will still be many patients who are eligible and stand to benefit from rehabilitation, if it is effective.

References

1   Sheikh, K, Smith, DS, Meade, TW and Brennan, P (1978) *Brit. J. Occup. Ther., 41,* 262
2   Weddell, Jean M (1974) In *Rehabilitation after Central Nervous System Trauma.* Skandia International Symposia, Nordiska Bokhandelns, Förlag, Stockholm, page 71
3   Beer, TC, Goldenberg, Eva, Smith, DS and Mason, AS (1974) *Brit. med. J., 1,* 226
4   Sheikh, K, Smith, DS, Meade, TW, Brennan, P and Kinsella, G (1979) *Int. Rehab. Med., 1,* 51

Part III   Multiple Sclerosis

Chapter 15

MULTIPLE SCLEROSIS: AN OVERVIEW*

John F Kurtzke

Introduction

For over a century, multiple sclerosis (MS) has intrigued workers in all the neural sciences, with perhaps more publications resulting than for any other neurological disease. However, we face today a situation little different from that of Charcot: MS is still really a disease of unknown cause, inadequate treatment, and unpredictable outcome.

To attack all these areas of ignorance, a number of investigators had turned to epidemiology. In the period since World War II especially, there have been an increasing quantity and quality of works designed to define the natural history of MS. Although we have today some useful information on survival, on risk factors, and on prognostic features, this chapter concentrates on the geographic distribution of MS and what it seems to tell us. In this regard, we will pay special attention to the studies of migration in MS, because they provide us with our best clues as to aetiology, *and* because they pose the greatest problems in performance and interpretation.

It is well to recall that in virtually all series of MS cases, whether defined for the laboratory or for an epidemiological inquiry, we are dealing with a clinical diagnosis without recourse to a pathognomonic diagnostic test or to pathological verification. A number of schemes for diagnostic criteria have been put forth; none with universal acceptance. In almost all of these, though, there are several grades relating to the degree of confidence in the correctness of the label. If we limit attention to the classes considered 'best', and discard 'possible MS' and 'uncertain MS', we do in fact have defined groups that are quite similar one to another in time and space. Thus, the assessments to follow are based upon series of cases variously labelled 'definite', 'clinically definite', and 'probable' MS.

Geographic Distribution of MS

The geographic distribution of MS has been best delineated from prevalence surveys of defined communities. Their number at present is approaching 200. Almost all of these have been performed since World War II. In 1975 I tried to collect all such studies extant as well as to rate them as to quality [1].

*Supported by the Veterans Administration and the National Multiple Sclerosis Society

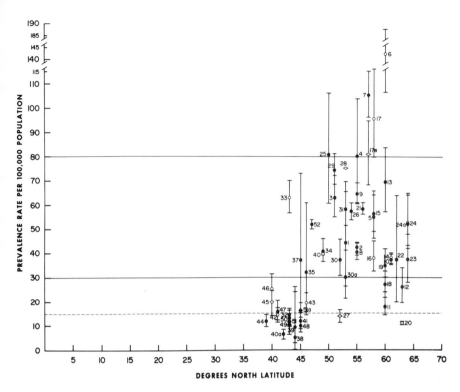

Figure 1 Prevalence rates per 100000 population for probable MS in Western Europe, correlated with geographic latitude. *Numbers* identify the survey in Kurtzke (1975). *Solid circles* represent Class A studies, *open circles* Class B, *diamonds* Class C, and *squares* Class E. *Vertical bars* define 95 per cent confidence intervals on the rates. (From Kurtzke (1975) [1])

In Figure 1 are studies then available for Western Europe, with the prevalence rates per 100 000 population for 'probable MS' correlated with the latitude of the locus of the study. The numbers refer to the specific surveys as previously described [1]. The solid circles are what I have considered Class A studies, as representing proper surveys with well-defined and comparable methodology and diagnostic standards. Those I rated Class B (open circles) are good surveys but there are reason(s) why they are not fully comparable to those of Class A. Surveys denoted by diamonds are Class C; these have obvious defects which make them unreliable. Open boxes are Class E surveys, which represent an *estimate* of the prevalence from the ratios of MS to amyotrophic lateral sclerosis (ALS) cases in series from hospital. Taking this ratio and a likely prevalence for ALS of 5 per 100 000, we can calculate estimated prevalence rates for MS applicable to the region in question. This has been quite useful where there are no proper prevalence surveys. The vertical bars define the 95 per cent confidence intervals for each rate. What this means is that, if the cited rate arose from a random sample of its parent

171

universe, the 'true' rate for this universe would be found to lie within this interval 19 times out of 20. It might be better then were the bar to be taken to represent the likely prevalence for the community rather than the locus of the symbol. At least, one should not pay too much attention to the precise digits.

It seems that MS in Western Europe is distributed according to latitude within two clusters: a high frequency zone with prevalence of some 30–80 (or more) per 100 000 population extending from about 43° to 65° north latitude; and a medium frequency zone with prevalence of some 5–25 per 100 000, and mostly 10–15, from about 38° to 46°.

Numbers 8 and 9 in the figure refer to two national surveys of Northern Ireland. In the Republic of Ireland, the prevalence rate for probable MS with 1982 patients as of 1971 was 67 per 100 000 population [2]. The provisional rate of 106 provided for northeastern Scotland (No. 7) as of 1970 has been confirmed: For 'probable' and 'early probable and latent' MS the rate is 105 with 464 patients [3]. The Shetland-Orkney rate of 143 for 1962 denoted by No. 6 in Figure 1 has been updated by Poskanzer and his associates [4]. As of 1 December 1974, the 73 cases of probable MS gave a prevalence rate of 203 per 100 000.

Number 30 in Figure 1 represents Lower Saxony with a rate of 37 for 1970. The same authors now provide a prevalence of 63 per 100 000 as of 31 December 1975 for 161 'definite plus apparent' ('eindeutig bzw. wahrscheinlich') MS; excluded were 'questionable' cases [5]. With 52 'MS-cases' a prevalence of 25 per 100 000 was calculated for the southeastern Swiss canton(s) of Wallis: 38 in Oberwallis and 19 in Unterwallis as of 31 December 1972 [6].

In Figure 1, Nos 41–51a refer to Italy, with Sardinia. A series of eight later studies from Italy have been summarised by Caputo and his co-workers [7]. All rates are still between 5 and 25 per 100 000. On Sicily, a prevalence of 5 per 100 000 was calculated for Messina in 1975. Specifics as to methodology for this last are lacking; it was apparently part of a presentation on MS throughout Italy by Tavolato and Borri at the 1975 Italian Congress of Neurology in Genoa. Tavolato [7a] has recently stated: 'I'm sure that Messina's prevalence (of 5) is too low. . . . On the other hand, Dean's prevalence rate is really too high. . . . It is still my opinion that the prevalence in Sicily, with some possible local variations, is between 10 and 20/100 000'.

Similar prevalence data for Eastern Europe are drawn in Figure 2. Note the relative paucity of good quality studies. There still seems to be a disposition of rates into the same two frequency zones: high from about 45° to 65° and medium from 32° to perhaps 50° or so, but latitude alone does not serve fully to separate the two. As to later information, we do have available a good study for Bucharest, Romania. The prevalence for probable MS was 41 per 100 000 with 798 patients as of 5 January 1977 [8]. Bucharest lies in southern Romania at 44°N. In the northwestern part of its western neighbour, Yugoslavia, the Rijeka region is at 45°N, and this area provided a prevalence of 32 per 100 000 with 95 probable MS on 31 December 1969 [9]. In Czechoslovakia the prevalence of MS as of 1970 among attendants at a national rehabilitation spa in Bohemia was calculated at 19 per 100 000 with 2760 patients 1970–76. The authors estimated this to represent 'almost one third of patients with MS in Czechoslovakia' [10].

172

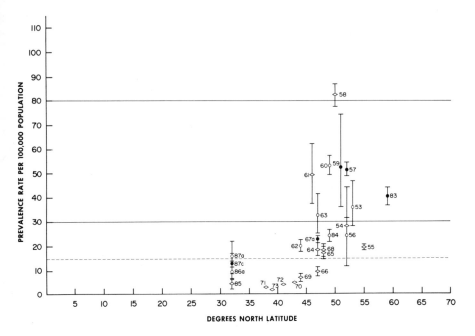

Figure 2 Prevalence rates per 100000 population for probable MS in Eastern Europe and Israel, as in Figure 1 (From Kurtzke (1975) [1])

Data were presented previously to indicate clustering of MS in Switzerland and Scandinavia, and the statement was made that the disorder in the latter region comprises a 'Fennoscandian focus' extending from the waist and southeastern plains of Norway across the southern part of Sweden to southwestern Finland, and thence back to Sweden near Umeå [11]. This focus is taken to define the northern boundaries of high MS in Europe.

The geographic distribution of MS in Europe may thus be considered to follow the pattern of Figure 3. The high-frequency region of northern Europe is rather sharply separated, both north and south, from a medium frequency area. The more recent studies suggest that not only that part of the Balkans to the south of the dotted line but also its extension from the head of the Adriatic Sea to the Black Sea may all be part of the high risk zone. This is based on the recent Romanian and Yugoslavian works.

Prevalence surveys from the Americas are denoted in Figure 4. Here we see all three risk zones: high frequency from 37°-52°, medium frequency from 30°-33° and low frequency (prevalence less than 5 per 100,000) from 12°-19° and from 63°-67° north latitude. The coterminous United States and southern Canada are represented by all the surveys from Number 88 to 119a, except for Numbers 106 (Greenland), 109 (Jamaica), 113 (Alaska), 117 (Netherland Antilles), and 118 (Mexico City). The Alaskan rate of 0 refers to natives of that state. The prevalence

173

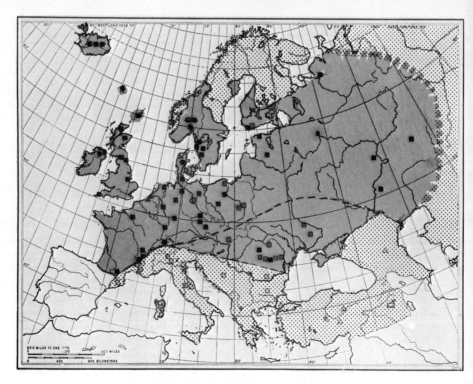

Figure 3 MS prevalence zones of Europe with survey sites spotted on the map. *Heavy shading* represents high frequency MS (prevalence 30 or more per 100000); *dotted shading* medium frequency MS (prevalence 5 to 25); no European area is low (prevalence 0–4). *Solid squares* are high frequency rates, *open squares* medium frequency, and *triangles* likely but not surely medium frequency. *Dashed line* may be the proper dividing line between high and medium, but later data suggest a more southerly line from the northern Adriatic to the Black Sea. Surveys are listed regardless of quality (From Kurtzke (1977) [11])

rates for the northern United States and southern Canada then are quite similar to the high frequency rates of Western Europe. Note that there are no data referable to South America. Krauss [12] presented a map with prevalence rates from four or five regions (Chile, Argentina, Brazil) in South America indicated, but provided no information as to their source.

However, Christiansen has published prevalence estimates for several regions of that continent, based on the ratio of MS to ALS cases seen at major clinics in the same intervals [13]. Together with the data he later provided [14] and an estimated prevalence of 5 per 100 000 for ALS, it would seem that South America from 36° south latitude as far north as perhaps 12° south might fall within the medium prevalence zone for MS (Table I). (I hope Christiansen will publish his findings in full, including identification of foreign-born patients.) He had also reported that in Brazil the disease might be of low prevalence, since only 136 cases were known to have been seen by neurologists of that country of over 70 million population in the five years to 1974 [14].

174

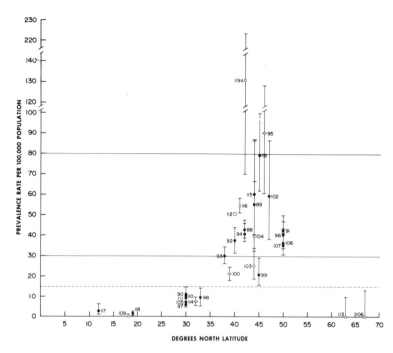

Figure 4 Prevalence rates per 100000 population for probable MS in the Americas, as in Figure 1 (From Kurtzke (1975) [1])

TABLE I Estimated* prevalence rates per 100 000 population for multiple sclerosis in South America: data of Christiansen (1975, 1977) [13, 14]

	Locus	Interval	MS cases	Prev. rate	Latitude
(a)	Buenos Aires, Argentina	1965–74	81	21	36.00°S
(b)	Buenos Aires, Argentina	1965–74	30	15	36.00°S
	Tucumán, Argentina	1955–74	65	18	27.00°S
	Mendoza, Argentina	–	–	18	32.54°S
	Montevideo, Uruguay	1964–73	86	18	34.50°S
	Lima, Peru	1945–73	50	5	12.00°S

*Estimated by ratio of MS/ALS cases seen at neurological clinics, with ALS prevalence taken as 5 per 100 000 population.

In the United States, the modest number of prevalence surveys of Figure 4 leave much of the country undefined as to the distribution of MS. Visscher and his colleagues recorded a prevalence of 69 per 100 000 for probable MS among 399 native-born whites of King and Pierce Counties, Washington, and 22 for 356 of Los Angeles County, California, as of April 1970 [15]. These rates confirm the high-north and medium-south partition of the country, but still leave wide gaps in our knowledge. However, by taking advantage of our recent history, we can provide a rather detailed delineation of the disease throughout the United States.

175

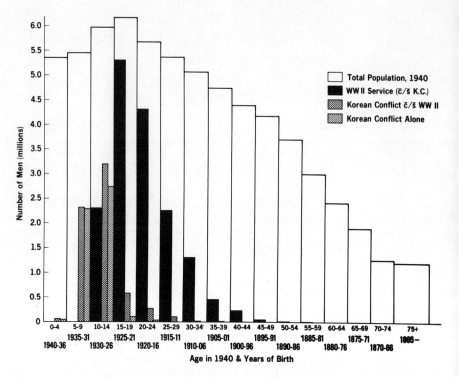

Figure 5 United States males by age in 1940, total population and those destined to serve in the military in World War II and/or Korean Conflict (From Kurtzke (1978a) [16])

In the World War II period, some 16.5 million Americans served in the armed forces. In the Korean Conflict there were 6.8 million, including 1.5 million who had also served in World War II. When the servicemen are plotted by age against the US male population of 1940, we see that the vast majority of young males were destined to serve in those wars (Fig. 5) [16].

For diseases or injuries that were either incurred in or aggravated by military service, the US Congress has decreed that they are to be declared 'service-connected disabilities'. For MS, the laws have been amended to include manifestations not only during service but also within seven years of discharge from service. This rating is totally independent of social or economic status, or of severity of illness. Thus, for World War II males, we have available an approximately ten-year incidence series of nationwide composition. Further, if we match such individuals with their military peers according to age, branch of service, date of entry and survival of the wars, we have an unbiased, pre-illness case-control series of unprecedented size.

This is precisely what we have done [17]. In Table II is our series of 5305 cases and matched controls from both the wars according to sex and race. In Figure 6 are the case-control ratios for white males of World War II according to residence

176

TABLE II Multiple sclerosis. Case-control ratios by race and sex for veterans of World War II and/or Korean Conflict 'service-connected' for MS. Data of Kurtzke et al (1979a) [17]

Race and Sex	Ratio	Case/control
White male	1.04	4923/4741
White female	1.86	182/98
White total	1.05	5105/4839
Black male	0.45	177/390
Black female	1.33	4/3
Black total	0.46	181/393
Other male	0.23	17/73
Other female	–	2/–
Other total	0.26	19/73
All male	0.98	5117/5204
All female	1.86	188/101
All total	1.00	5305/5305

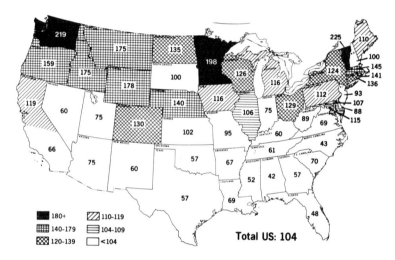

Figure 6 Case-control ratio percentages for MS according to state of residence at entry into active duty (EAD): white males of World War II (Data of Kurtzke et al (1979a) [17])

at service entry. Figure 7 provides the same data for these cases vs. the 1940 distribution of white males in the United States. This is virtually identical with that for the MS/C ratios. In Figure 8 are the *controls* for the MS cases, also against the 1940 US population. In formal testing, this last distribution is homogeneous. We can thus state that this MS series is indeed representative of MS among males in this country. As to the validity of the diagnosis, fully 96 per cent of a random sample of 80 cases upon review met all criteria of the Schumacher Committee [18] for definite MS.

177

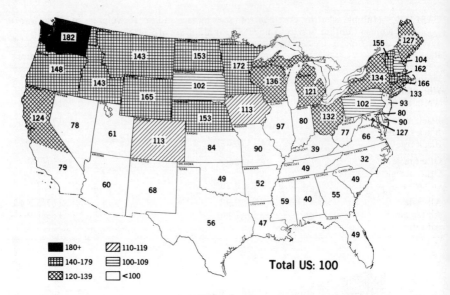

Figure 7 Ten-year incidence rates or risk ratios for MS in white males with service in World War II by state of residence at EAD, versus US white males age 15 to 34 in 1940 by state of residence, expressed as percentages of national (mean) rate of 21.118 per 100000 population (From Kurtzke (1978a) [16])

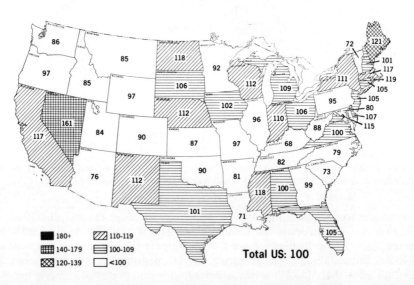

Figure 8 Distribution of white male matched controls for World War II MS cases by state of residence at EAD, versus US white males age 15 to 34 in 1940 by state of residence, expressed as percentages of the national (mean) rate of 20.333 per 100000 population (From Kurtzke (1978a) [16])

178

Returning to the international prevalence studies, we see that Australia–New Zealand comprise principally a high frequency zone for 44°–34° south latitude, and a medium frequency region for 33°–15° south (Fig. 9). The recorded rates, though, which are considered high, are toward the lower end of this range [1].

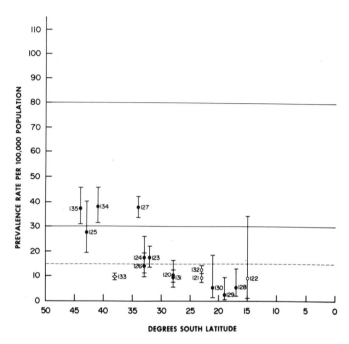

Figure 9 Prevalence rates per 100000 population for probable MS in Australia–New Zealand, as in Figure 1 (From Kurtzke (1975) [1])

Rates from Asia and the Pacific in the northern hemisphere are all low, except that Hawaii (Nos 145, 146) is likely to be in the medium zone (Fig. 10). These study sites extend from 8° to 47° north latitude. Hospital series comparing MS and ALS frequencies as of 1973 indicate a low rate for MS in Bombay, Jakarta, Seoul, Taipei, Chenghua, and Bangkok [19]. Asahikawa at 43° north in Japan had a prevalence of 2.5 per 100 000 for MS (including Devic's disease) in 1975 [20]. There is then no site in Asia thus far demonstrated to have more than a low frequency for MS.

In the southern hemisphere, with surveys from 30° to 6° south, all rates from Asia and Africa are also low, except for English-speaking native-born whites (No 156) of South Africa (Fig. 11). Their rate of 11 contrasts with that of 3 for the Afrikaans-speaking native-born whites, a difference still without an answer. It should be noted, though, that over the entirety of this vast continent there are data otherwise available only for Ethiopia, Natal and Senegal. In particular, there

179

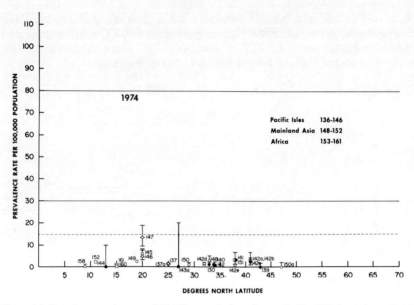

Figure 10 Prevalence rates per 100000 population for probable MS in Asia and Africa (northern hemisphere), as in Figure 1 (From Kurtzke (1975) [1])

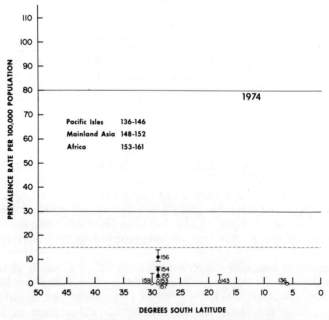

Figure 11 Prevalence rates per 100000 population for probable MS in Asia and Africa (southern hemisphere), as in Figure 1 (From Kurtzke (1975) [1])

is no information on the Mediterranean littoral. Ben Hamida was able to collect 73 cases of 'typical and probable' MS from his neurological centre in Tunis, Tunisia, in a three-year period [21]. All but one of these were Tunisian natives, and he sees about one new case of MS each week [22]. With some 700 000 or so residents of greater Tunis, this could *suggest* a prevalence near 10 per 100 000, well within the medium risk range. Clearly, many interpretations of the distribution of MS would be altered if this were a fact, which holds whether this rate reflects a recent event or is of long standing. However, Ben Hamida could provide no denominator data; even the number of ALS cases seen was unknown at this time [22].

In summation, we may thus consider the world-wide distribution of MS as comprising three zones of frequency or risk. The high risk zone, with prevalence rates over 30 per 100 000 population, includes northern Europe, northern US and southern Canada, New Zealand, and southern Australia. These regions are bounded by areas of medium frequency, with prevalence rates between 5 and 25 per 100 000. Asia, Latin America, and almost all of Africa are of low frequency with prevalence rates less than 5 per 100 000 (Fig. 12). Much of Africa and all of South America remain unknown, though, from formal prevalence studies.

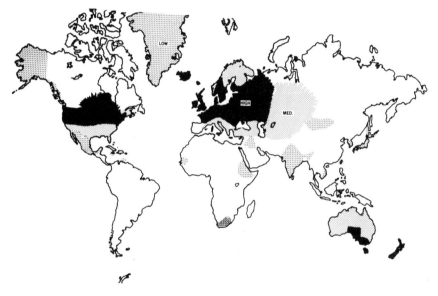

Figure 12 World-wide distribution of MS according to high (*solid*), medium (*dotted*), and low (*diagonal dashed*) risk areas. The high risk area of Europe may reach the head of the Adriatic Sea in the Balkans

Race

One aspect of the general distribution worth noting is that all the high risk and the medium risk areas have predominantly white populations. Thus, MS can be considered the white man's burden. Further evidence to this point is provided by our

181

TABLE III Multiple Sclerosis: Case Control Ratios by Tier of Residence at Entry into Active Duty (EAD) for the Major Sex and Race Groups, Entire Series. From Kurtzke et al (1979a) [17]

| Sex and Race | Tier of Residence at EAD | | | |
	North	Middle	South	Total*
MS/C ratio				
White male	1.41	1.02	0.58	1.04
White female	2.77	1.71	0.80	1.86
Black male	0.61	0.59	0.31	0.45
Total series**	1.41	1.00	0.53	1.00
Normalised MS/C ratio				
White male	1.36	0.98	0.56	1.00
White female	1.49	0.92	0.43	1.00
Black male	1.36	1.31	0.69	1.00
Total series***	1.41	0.99	0.53	1.00
MS/C				
White male	2195/1544	2059/2022	668/1161	4922/4737
White female	97/35	65/38	20/25	182/98
Black male	28/46	88/150	61/194	177/390
Total series**	2323/1647	2213/2219	762/1425	5298/5291*

*Excludes 1 male case and 11 male controls inducted in foreign countries.

**Includes Black females and Other (non-white, non-black) persons.

***White male, White female, Black male only.

veteran series (Table III). Regardless of residence in the US, white females have nearly twice the risk of MS as white males, while blacks or Negroes have only half the risk. The group consisting of the 'Other' races suggests a paucity as well in American Indians and in Orientals (Table IV). Detels and his colleagues in California have presented good evidence for a low prevalence among Japanese-Americans [23]. The apparent deficit we found among Spanish-Americans would seem more a reflection of geography than race. This is borne out when comparisons by each race are made among the foreign-born cases in the veteran series (Table V).

Migration

Having defined areas of the world where MS is common or rare, the fate of migrants among these regions is vital to our interpretations of the distribution and, thus, to the definition of this disease. Table VI summarises material on prevalence rates (all ages) among immigrants to and from different MS risk areas. The rates are those regardless of age at immigration and of time of clinical onset of MS in reference to migration.

In broad terms, the immigrants tend to retain the MS risk of their birth-place.

TABLE IV Multiple Sclerosis Case/Control Ratios for 'Other' Males by Birthplace and Race, Entire Series. From Kurtzke et al (1979a) [17]

Birthplace and race	Ratio	Total	N**	S**
		Case/Control		
Coterminous United States	0.48	11/23*	6/12	5/11
Amerindian	0.38	3/8	3/6	0/2
Mexican - Spanish American	0.60	6/10	1/1	5/9
Japanese	0.50	2/4	2/4	0/0
Mexico, Latin America, Total	0.29	6/21		
Mexican - Spanish American	0.00	0/5		
Puerto Rican	0.38	6/16		
Hawaii, Total	0.00	0/15		
Japanese	0.00	0/10		
Other	0.00	0/5		
Asia, Total	0.00	0/14		
Chinese	0.00	0/4		
Filipino	0.00	0/9		
Other	0.00	0/1		
Total	0.23	17/73		

*Includes 1 Filipino control.

**N = Northern and middle tier of birth, S = Southern. For white males the MS/C ratios are 1.2 N and 0.6 S.

TABLE V MS Case/Control Ratios According to Race and Birthplace in Selected Regions, Data from First Match, both Wars. From Kurtzke et al (1979a) [17]

Region	Ratio	Total	White	Black	Other
		Case/Control			
Mexico, Central America	0.14	2/14	1/9	1/-	-/5
Puerto Rico	0.42	14/33	6/14	2/3	6/16
Hawaii	0.06	1/16	1/1	-/-	-/15
Japan, Korea	-	4/-	4/-	-/-	-/-
China	0.00	-/4	-/-	-/-	-/4
Philippines, SE Asia	0.00	-/12	-/2	-/-	-/10

'Risk' is defined according to the same three frequency zones previously discussed. The evidence for risk retention is better for immigrants from high risk areas to low than is the reverse, where there are in fact almost no data.

Two points are worth noting. First, in no survey is the rate for immigrants born in high frequency areas *higher* than that expected of their home lands. This is important when we come to interpretations. Secondly, the migrants to Australia—all but one group from high risk countries—*appear* to have appreciably lower rates than expected for their birth place. This though is explicable by Australian immigration laws dealing with the disabled. Few of these MS migrants would be likely to

183

TABLE VI Prevalence Rates per 100 000 Population for Probable Multiple Sclerosis among Native-born and Immigrants. From Kurtzke (1977) [11]

Immigration site according to its MS risk	Native born	Prevalence rates among		
		Immigrants from risk areas		
		High	Medium	Low
High				
(1) South Australia	38	37	4	...
Medium				
(2) Perth, W. Australia	40 [b]	87 [b]	...	...
(3) Perth, W. Australia	14	22	...	...
(4) W. Australia	10	31	...	...
(5) Queensland	9	15	...	...
(6) Israel [a]	9 [c]	----- 19[c] -----		6 [c]
(7) Israel	4	33	8	3
Low				
(8) South Africa	6	48	15	...
(9) Neth. Antilles	3	59	...	...
(10) Hawaii [a]	5	----- 35 -----		...

[a] may include 'possible' MS.

[b] age-specific rate, 40–49 years.

[c] age-adjusted to 1960 US population.

have had clinical onset, or at least diagnosis, before immigration. In the South African study to be discussed below, about half the European immigrants were symptomatic before their move. Were this to apply to Australia, then the immigrant rates there could perhaps be doubled.

The Israeli data should be considered from the age adjusted rates, since their several populations have strikingly different age compositions. The European immigrants too include many survivors of the concentration camps of World War II, who are a very select group. It *may* be that the Afro-Asian immigrants (low risk) to Israel (medium risk) have an increased frequency of MS over that presumed for their birthplace, but it is really too early to be sure.

Other data on low to high areas are sparse. Dassel [24] recorded three instances of MS among immigrants from Indonesia to Holland. Their onsets were at age 17, 23 and 25 years, and took place respectively 7, 9 and 8 years after their arrival in the Netherlands. They are probably whites of Dutch origin, but neither this nor the population at risk was provided. Regardless, three cases out of what is likely to be a small migrant group looks impressive. Unfortunately, this group could not be traced any further.

Three instances of exacerbating–remitting MS have been found among a series of some 3400 children who were born in Vietnam of Vietnamese mothers and French fathers, and who came to France under the age of 20. At interview in 1975, 80 per cent were age 20–39. The three MS patients each had clinical onset about 15 years after immigration, which for them was under the age of ten. The cumulative risk of MS, which was also their prevalence rate, was 89 per 100 000, with a 95 per cent confidence interval of 18–260. The age-specific prevalence rate was 169 per 100 000 age 20–29 (confidence interval 35–494). Both measures are similar to such rates for Denmark, but the confidence intervals are very wide. Even so, the lower limits are clearly higher for these half-Orientals than for Vietnamese in Vietnam. Whether their disease is really as frequent as expected for natives of France is unknowable at the present [25]. Further evidence on migration arises from consideration of the age of migration.

Age of Migration

If one grants there is to some degree a retention of birthplace risk in MS for migrants from high to low frequency areas, the next question would be whether this is dependent on age. If this risk is acquired at or near birth (or is innate), then birth-place alone and time of birth would be the critical point, and for low-to-high migrants there should be no increase in the risk of MS.

In the United States, death rates for MS are distributed so that the states to the north of 37° north latitude have twice the rates of those to the south. One should see the mirror image of this distribution for those who exchange risk areas (between north and south) between birth and death, if birth is the critical time. In fact, though, one sees almost an *obliteration* of the north–south difference when such migrants are considered (Table VII). In the US the ratios of Table VII are also the actual death rates. Regardless of direction, those who change risk areas no longer differ significantly, north vs. south, as to their MS death rates. However, the death rate for US southern-born MS who had died in the north (0.68) was significantly higher than that for the southern-born who died in the south (0.46). Thus it would also appear that moving north does increase the risk of MS [11].

TABLE VII   Migration in multiple sclerosis. Ratios* of death rates for residence at birth and death in high and low MS risk areas of Norway and United States. From Kurtzke (1977) [11]

	Place of birth			
Place of death	US (1959–61)		Norway (1951–65)	
	High	Low	High	Low
High	1.00*	0.68	1.00*	0.57
Low	0.87	0.46	0.59	0.44

*High/High = 1.00.

Detels and his colleagues [26] have studied migrants to the west coast of the US (Table VIII). Northern migrants to (southern) Los Angeles have significantly lower MS prevalence rates than similar migrants to (northern) King-Pierce Counties. There is no significant increase in the rates for southern migrants to the north, but their numbers are too small for confidence.

185

TABLE VIII Age and sex adjusted prevalence rates per 100 000 population among white residents age 20+ who migrated from northern or southern US before onset of MS, with 95% confidence intervals on the rates*

Birthplace	Residence	
	Los Angeles, CA	King-Pierce, WA
Northern US	30 (27.5–32.7)**	55 (47.7–63.1)
Southern US	15 (12.2–18.3)	19 (11.1–30.4)

*data of Detels et al [26]
**95% confidence intervals

The case-control series of US veterans mentioned previously gives further evidence to this point. In Table III above we noted distributions by residence at entry into service allocated within three horizontal tiers for the coterminous United States: a northern tier of states above 41–42° north latitude; a middle tier; and a southern tier below 37° including California from Fresno south. Migrants would be those born in one tier who entered service from another.

Because of the differing risk for blacks and the selection bias among women found in the military, we shall limit attention to white males. Table IX defines the case-control ratios, with their numbers, for white males of World War II according to residence at birth vs. entry into service.

TABLE IX   MS/control ratios for white males of World War II* by tier of residence at birth and at entry into active duty (EAD): US only. From Kurtzke et al (1979b) [27]

Birth tier	EAD tier			Birth total
	North	Middle	South	
MS/C ratio				
North	1.41	1.26	0.70	1.38
Middle	1.30	1.04	0.72	1.04
South	0.73	0.62	0.56	0.57
EAD Total	1.39	1.04	0.58	1.04
Case/Control				
North	1611/1140	112/89	32/46	1755/1275
Middle	125/96	1544/1482	68/94	1737/1672
South	16/22	42/68	439/788	497/878
EAD Total	1752/1258	1698/1639	539/928	3989/3825

*Includes those who also served in Korean Conflict.

The ratios decline from north to south. This is true for birthplace and for residence at service entry. Those for whom these residences are the same provide the ratios along the major diagonal: 1.41 north, 1.04 middle, and 0.56 south.

186

Movements *off* the diagonal provide the ratios for the migrants. Those born north and entering service from the middle tier have a ratio of 1.26; if they enter from the south their ratio is 0.70, only half that of the nonmigrants. Birth in the middle tier is marked by an increase in the MS/C ratio for northern entrants to 1.30 and a decrease to 0.72 for the southern ones. Migration after birth in the south seems to raise the ratios to 0.62 (middle) and 0.73 (north). The migrant risk ratios are intermediate between those characteristic of their birthplace and their residence at entry.

TABLE X   MS/C ratios (with 95% confidence limits for migrants) by tier of residence at birth and at entry into active duty (EAD): (a) white males of World War II, (b) white males of World War II or Korean Conflict. Data of Kurtzke et al (1979b) [27]

Birth tier	EAD tier		
	North	Middle	South
(a) WM-WW II			
North	1.41	1.26	0.70
	–	(0.95–1.68)	(0.43–1.11)
Middle	1.30	1.04	0.72
	(0.99–1.72)	–	(0.52–1.00)
South	0.73	0.62	0.56
	(0.36–1.45)	(0.41–0.92)	–
(b) WM-both wars			
North	1.45	1.19	0.76
	–	(0.91–1.56)	(0.49–1.18)
Middle	1.34	1.02	0.72
	(1.04–1.72)	–	(0.53–0.96)
South	0.67	0.63	0.56
	(0.36–1.22)	(0.43–0.92)	–

Confidence intervals on these ratios indicate that these differences are likely to be real—at least for the northern and middle tiers of birth (Table X). In the middle tier, moving north clearly increases the risk of MS and moving south decreases it. Therefore the risk of MS *is* altered by changing residence between birth and entry into service, and thus well before clinical onset. This is further evidence that MS is an acquired, exogenous, environmental disease, and that it is acquired well before the onset of clinical symptoms. The environmental factor would appear to be either more common or more effective in those geographic areas where the disease itself is more common. These data therefore support what Acheson [28] called the 'simple' hypothesis, and Nathanson and Miller [29] the 'prevalence' hypothesis as to the cause of MS.

Residence at birth has about the same gradient of risk as does residence at service entry, and therefore about age 24 for World War II veterans. There is also no clear difference in risk for the migrants from high to low regions versus low to high. We do not know the specific ages of migration, but if we assume that they took place at an even rate between birth and service entry for all migrants, then we are

187

still left with two hypotheses as to the likely age of acquisition of MS. *If* the disease is acquired over a short interval, then the point midway between birth and 24 would seem the most reasonable to account for our findings. This would therefore indicate age 10 to 15, which would be in accord with other data on migrants. However, the findings are equally compatible with the idea that prolonged or repeated exposure to the presumed pathogen is required for its acquisition, and that what we are seeing here is a dose-response curve to duration of exposure during the earlier years of life.

From ages of maximal clustering of MS in Denmark and several other features, it was 'tentatively concluded that (for natives of high-risk areas) the actual onset of MS appears to take place on the average between the ages of 10 and 15 years, and that there is probably a "latent" or "incubation" period of some 20 years before the onset of clinical symptomatology' [30]. More specific was the survey of European immigrants to South Africa [31]. For such immigrants, the MS prevalence rate, adjusted to a population of all ages, is provided in Table XI according to age at immigration [32]. For immigration under age 15 there is the same medium prevalence rate as for the native-born English-speaking South Africans [33]. But for all older age groups, the prevalence is about what one would expect from their high risk homelands. This change is sharp, as seen from Figure 13, where each MS immigrant is represented by his own horizontal bar. The height of the bar on the *Y* axis reflects his age at immigration, and the length of the bar denotes the number of years between immigration and clinical onset. The diagonal is the average age of clinical onset for the entire group. It is clear that there were very few immigrants who developed MS if they arrived under age 15, as opposed to the large number who arrived beyond age 15. In this series then, age 15 was critical for the acquisition of MS among those who came from high risk areas.

TABLE XI MS prevalence rates, all ages, per 100 000 immigrants in 1960 according to age at immigration (AAI) for northern European immigrants to Republic of South Africa. (Modified from Kurtzke et al 1970 [32]

AAI	UK	all
0–14	12.8	12.9
15–19	66.1	81.1
20–24	31.8	31.3
25–29	59.4	58.4
(20–29)	(45.7)	(44.9)
30–39	58.2	52.4
40–49	57.7	62.4
50+	70.5	80.8
N	65	114

Two other high-to-low migrant surveys also suggest, though with small numbers, that age 15 divides those who retain the risk of their birthplace from those (younger) who acquire a lower risk. These pertain to immigrants to Israel [35] and to Hawaii [36]. More recently Alter and his associates have suggested that Afro-

188

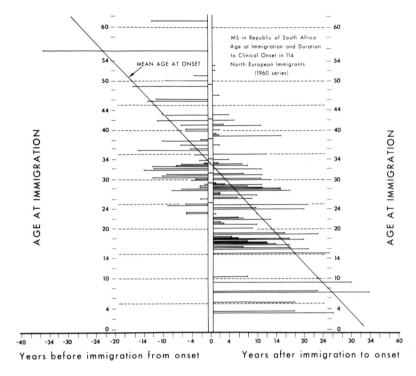

Figure 13 Age at immigration (Y axis) and years from immigration to clinical onset (X axis) for each of 114 northern European immigrants to South Africa ascertained as MS in 1960 prevalence survey (From Kurtzke (1972) [34])

Asian immigrants arriving in Israel below the age of 5 years have age-specific incidence rates similar to such immigrants from Europe, whereas those arriving beyond age 5 tend to differ: European rates *appear* higher [37]. However, here too the number of cases, especially for those under age 15 at immigration, would appear too small for meaningful interpretation.

Geoffrey Dean and colleagues have concluded that: 'Emigrating to England from low risk parts of the world did not seem to increase the risk of developing MS' [38]. This was based on a comparison of hospital admission rates for MS in greater London according to land of birth, with expected numbers provided by the London population by birthplace. They later pointed out that motor neurone disease ascertained in similar fashion did not differentiate those immigrants [39]. Chapter 21 reports further stages in this work, but the conclusions have been criticised [40].

Problems of Migration Studies

'The question of risk of MS in migrant populations gets very involved, being dependent not only on a sufficiency of people who change their residence from one

189

risk area to another but also on their ages at immigration, their length of stay in the new land, *and* their ages at prevalence day. . . . Another problem further to confound the issue is the apparent racial predilection of MS, regardless of geography . . .' [40].

The true population at risk according to age at survey *and* age at migration *and* age at clinical onset can be very difficult to define, and the choice of denominator—or the type of rate required (incidence, prevalence, death, cumulative risk)—can get very involved. The desired population denominator is generally not available from routine sources. In the South African study [31] we attempted to reconstruct the population at risk at prevalence day from annual counts of immigrants by age, adjusted for expected survival. Age in 1960 for estimated survivors seemed to differ from the actual census count, and this was not well corrected by deleting the survival adjustment (Figure 14). However, similar calculations for age at immigration provided an excellent fit with either method when compared with a population sample surveyed (MRA) for radio listening habits (Figure 15). We believe the 1960 age differences, as well as the absolute over-count for 1960 UK immigrants, resulted from the inclusion in our estimates of Republic of Ireland immigrants before 1921, and the early outmigration of considerable numbers of immigrants; the latter is a situation impossible to quantitate but known to have occurred. Our population data in Table XI were, however, adjusted to the actual 1960 counts.

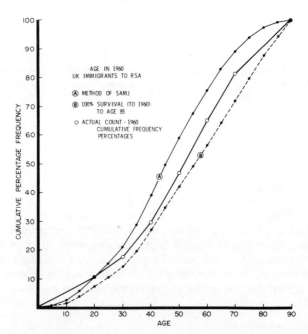

Figure 14 Cumulative percentage frequency for estimated numbers by age in 1960 for UK immigrants to South Africa, compared with actual census count. Two estimates are provided: one adjusted for survival, as used in Table XI; the other with 100% survival from birth to age 85

190

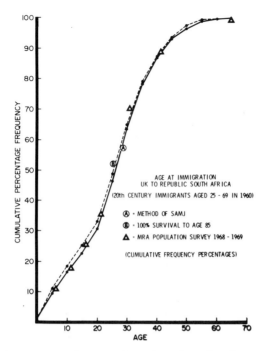

Figure 15 Cumulative percentage frequency for estimated numbers by age at immigration for UK immigrants to South Africa age 25–69 in 1960, contrasted with population sample (MRA) actual counts. The two estimates provided are as in Figure 14

In our Vietnamese study [25] we had the complete study population at hand, and could readily calculate the several age and duration factors (Table XII). The problem was that our sample was small and any similar total enumeration would also be small. For the prevalence estimates of Detels' group in California and Washington, they had to carry out a special survey of 'a probability sample of residents in both areas' [26]. Our veteran series [16, 17, 27] provided us with both numerator (cases) and denominator (controls), and the latter were shown to be fully representative of the population at risk. But this gives us data for only two specific ages, and obviously is of little value for general use.

It was for these reasons that I attempted to provide, for one area at least, estimates as to the risk of MS by age, sex and interval [41]. Table XIII gives a summary of the period risk for MS in Denmark by age at entry for both sexes combined. The cumulative lifetime risk from birth is 201 per 100 000, or one chance in 500. At age 20, the risk of MS beginning within the next five years is 34 per 100 000; after 20 years this figure is 142, and after 30 years 181. Conversely, at age 10 the five-year risk is only 2 per 100 000 and the 20-year risk 92. By 30 years, it reaches 159. For entrants age 50, the lifetime risk of 13 per

191

TABLE XII   Age Distribution of Half-Vietnamese Immigrants to France*

Age at Immigration	Age in 1975											
	0-4	5-9	10-14	15-19	20-24	25-29	30-34	35-39	40-44	45-49	50-54	Total
0-4	1	3	21	64	160	24	9	3	1	1	1	288
5-9		8	39	88	413	513	66	44	–	–	–	1171
10-14			15	114	151	318	321	107	102	–	–	1128
15-19				17	141	44	110	262	112	23	–	709
20-24					–	13	6	14	28	6	1	68
25-29						–	2	2	2	1	1	8
30-34							–	1	1	–	–	2
35-39								–	3	1	1	5
Total	1	11	75	283	865	912	514	433	249	32	4	3379

*Data of Kurtzke and Bui (1977) [25].

TABLE XIII   Period cumulative risk of multiple sclerosis in Denmark. Approximate number of new cases expected by period per 100 000 population of given age at entry, both sexes combined*

Age at entry	Period						
	5 yr	10 yr	15 yr	20 yr	25 yr	30 yr	lifetime
0	0	2	4	20	52	89	201
5	2	4	21	54	94	128	211
10	2	19	53	92	126	159	210
15	17	51	90	125	158	181	209
20	34	74	109	142	165 ·	181	193
25	40	75	108	131	148	157	160
30	35	69	92	108	118	120	120
35	34	58	74	83	86	86	86
40	24	41	50	53	53	53	53
45	17	27	30	30	30	30	30
50	10	13	13	13	13	13	13
55	3	3	3	3	3	3	3
60	0	0	0	0	0	0	0

*Data of Kurtzke (1978b) [41].

100 000 is attained within ten years. Differences such as these make 'man years of exposure' regardless of age at entry difficult to interpret.

If we assume that the duration of MS is constant regardless of geography, then the ratios of prevalence rates in different areas are equivalent to the ratios of incidence rates. Then, too, such ratios can also be applied to these risk estimates. For example, if 100 000 Japanese migrate to Denmark at age 10, they would be expected to provide 4 MS cases after 20 years if they retained the low risk of their birthplace, but 92 cases if they acquired the high risk of Denmark.

Perhaps more meaningful would be a statement as to the number of cases, all ages, to be expected to occur within given intervals among a disease-free sample of the general population. Remember this refers to those whose prior lifetime has been spent in the same high-risk area. No account is taken of the presumed 'incubation' period between disease-acquisition and symptom-onset. Also, no account is taken of the usual interval between onset of symptoms and date of diagnosis.

Table XIV gives the number of cases of MS expected to develop over time when the Danish risk estimates are applied to the 1960 US population, all ages. In five years there will be only 14 per 100 000 or some 12 per cent of the total anticipated. After 20 years we will have accumulated only *half* the total cases expected. It is this kind of information that must be borne in mind when trying to interpret data for MS among migrants.

TABLE XIV MS: Number of cases per 100 000 population expected to develop in given intervals among a disease-free cohort of a high-risk populace*

Interval (years)	Cases per 100 000
5	14.1
10	28.8
15	44.4
20	61.3
25	77.9
30	92.2
life	121.2

*Risk estimates for Denmark applied to 1960 US population distribution.

Summary

Geographically, MS is distributed into three zones of high, medium and low frequency. High frequency areas, with prevalence rates over 30 per 100 000 population, comprise Europe between 65° and 45° north latitude, southern Canada and northern United States, New Zealand and southern Australia. These regions are bounded by areas of medium frequency with prevalence rates of 5-25 and mostly 10-15 per 100 000, which then comprise southern Europe, southern US, and most of Australia. Known areas of Asia and Africa (save for one white group in South Africa) are all low, with prevalence rates under 5 per 100 000 population.

All high and medium risk areas are among predominantly white populations: MS is the white man's burden. In America, blacks and Orientals have much lower rates of MS than do whites, but still demonstrate the geographic gradients found for whites.

Migration studies indicate that, on the whole, migrants retain much of the risk of their birthplace. However, this risk is clearly *not* defined at birth: MS death rates for migrants born in one risk area and dying in another are intermediate. Prevalence studies for migrants from high to low risk areas indicate the age of adolescence to be critical for risk retention: those migrating beyond age 15 retain the MS risk of their birthplace; those migrating under 15 acquire the lower risk of their new residence. Several low-to-high studies show that those migrating in child-hood are adolescence do in fact increase their risk of MS. Best data to this point arise from a nationwide series of MS cases with pre-illness controls from the US military-veteran population. For white male veterans of World War II service, case-control ratios are clearly decreased by moving from north to south between birth and entry into military service, and clearly increased by similar moves in the opposite direction.

The migrant data, plus the geographic distributions, serve to define MS as an acquired, exogenous (environmental) disease, whose acquisition in ordinary circumstances takes place years before clinical onset. The data fit best the 'simple' or 'prevalence' hypothesis: that the cause of MS will be found where the clinical disease is common.

Further migrant studies are required to support (or refute) this interpretation. However, all migrant studies are beset with major difficulties in ascertaining the denominator, the true population at risk, since this is a threefold function of age at migration, duration of residence, and age at prevalence day, each aspect of which will have a major influence in defining expected numbers of cases. To obviate those difficulties in some measure, period risk estimates have been calculated for MS in Denmark. They indicate that, after five years a disease-free population, all ages, would be likely to provide only some 12 per cent of the MS cases expected over its life time, and only half the expected total would be found even after 20 years follow-up.

References

1   Kurtzke, JF (1975) *Acta Neurol. Scand., 51,* 110, 137
2   Dean, G (1975) *The Medico-Social Research Board Annual Report,* page 55
3   Shepherd, DI and Downie, AW (1978) *Brit. Med. J., 2,* 314
4   Poskanzer, DC, Walker, AM, Yonkondy, J and Sheridan, JL (1976) *Neurology, 26 (Part 2),* 14
5   Wikström, J., Ritter, G, Poser, S, Firnhaber, W and Bauer, HJ (1977) *Nervenarzt, 48,* 494
6   Bärtschi-Rochaix, W (1977) *Multiple Sklerose im Wallis. Eine epidemiologische Studie.* Huber, Bern
7   Caputo, D, Palestra, A and Zibetti, A (1978) *Archivio per le Scienze Mediche, 135,* 1
7a Tavalato, B (1979) personal communication, March 14
8   Verdeş, F, Petrescu, A and Cernescu, C (1978) *Acta Neurol. Scand., 58,* 109
9   Septić, J, Ledić, P, Antončić, N and Milohanovič, S (1977) presented at 11th World Congress of Neurology, Amsterdam
10 Lenský, P (1978) *Čas. Lék. ces., 117,* 36
11 Kurtzke, JF (1977) *J. Neurol, 215,* 1
12 Krauss, N (1977) *Fortschr. Med., 95,* 539
13 Christiansen, JC (1975) *Acta Neurol. Latinoamer., 21,* 66
14 Christiansen, JC (1977) personal communication, July 20
15 Visscher, BR, Detels, R, Coulson, AH, Malmgren, RM and Dudley, JP (1977) *Am. J. Epidem., 106,* 470
16 Kurtzke, JF (1978a) In *Advances in Neurology. Vol 19* (ed BS Schoenberg). Raven Press, New York, page 55
17 Kurtzke, JF, Beebe, GW and Norman, JE Jr (1979a) *Neurology* (in press)
18 Schumacher, GA, Beebe, GW, Kibler, RF et al (1965) *Ann. N.Y. Acad. Sci., 122,* 552

19 Kuroiwa, Y, Hung, T-P, Landsborough, D et al (1977) *Neurology, 27,* 188
20 Kuroiwa, Y and Iwashita, H (1977) *Asian Med. J., 20,* 335
21 Ben Hamida, M (1977) *Rev. Neurol. (Paris), 133,* 109
22 Ben Hamida, M (1979) personal communication, March 22
23 Detels, R, Visscher, B, Malmgren, RM, Coulson, AH, Lucia, MV and Dudley, JP (1977) *Am. J. Epidem., 105,* 303
24 Dassel, H (1972) In *Multiple Sclerosis. Progress in Research* (ed EJ Field, TM Bell and PR Carnegie). North-Holland Publ. Co., Amsterdam, page 241
25 Kurtzke, JF and Bui, QH (1977) *Trans. Am. Neurol. Assoc., 102,* 54
26 Detels, R, Visscher, BR, Haile, RW, Malmgren, RM, Dudley, JP and Coulson, AH (1978) *Am. J. Epidem., 108,* 386
27 Kurtzke, JF, Beebe, GW and Norman, JE Jr (1979b) *Neurology, 28,* 579 (abstr.)
28 Acheson, ED (1972) In *Multiple Sclerosis. Progress in Research* (ed EJ Field, TM Bell and PR Carnegie). North-Holland Publ. Co., Amsterdam, page 204
29 Nathanson, N and Miller, A (1978) *Am. J. Epidem., 107,* 451
30 Kurtzke, JF (1965) *Acta Neurol. Scand., 41,* 140
31 Dean, G and Kurtzke, JF (1971) *Brit. Med. J., 3,* 725
32 Kurtzke, JF, Dean, G and Botha, DPJ (1970) *S. Afr. Med. J., 44,* 663
33 Dean, G (1967) *Brit. Med. J., 2,* 724
34 Kurtzke, JF (1972) In *Multiple Sclerosis. Progress in Research* (ed EJ Field, TM Bell and PR Carnegie). North-Holland Publ. Co., Amsterdam, page 208
35 Alter, M, Leibowitz, U and Speer, J (1966) *Arch. Neurol., 15,* 234
36 Alter, M and Okihiro, M (1971) *Neurology, 21,* 1030
37 Alter, M, Kahana, E and Loewenson, R (1978) *Neurology, 28,* 1089
38 Dean, G, McLoughlin, H, Brady, R, Adelstein, AM and Tallett-Williams, J (1976) *Brit. Med. J., 1,* 861
39 Dean, G, Brady, R, McLoughlin, H, Elian, M and Adelstein, AM (1977) *Brit. J. Prev. Soc. Med., 31,* 141
40 Kurtzke, JF (1976) *Brit. Med. J., 1,* 1527
41 Kurtzke, JF (1978b) *Acta Neurol. Scand., 57,* 141

195

Chapter 16

MULTIPLE SCLEROSIS IN NORTH-EAST SCOTLAND

D Shepherd

Multiple sclerosis (MS) has long been recognised as a common disorder in north-east Scotland [1]. The first recorded case of cerebrospinal sclerosis, as it was then called, was noted in 1882, and between 1891 and 1908 over 70 patients were admitted to Aberdeen hospitals [2]. No formal epidemiological study had been undertaken until, in 1970 and 1973, I conducted two separate prevalence studies covering the same geographical area. North-east Scotland (Fig. 1) is a compact

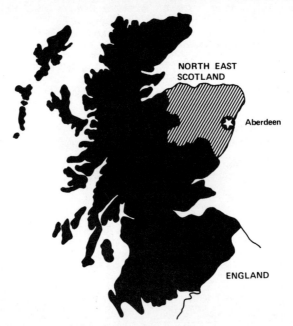

Figure 1 North-east Scotland

region consisting of the City of Aberdeen and counties of Aberdeen, Kincardine, Moray and Banff, which is almost equivalent to the Grampian region. It is ideally suited for epidemiological study by virtue of the stability of the population and the fact that almost all neurological patients pass exclusively through the Aberdeen hospitals.

Patients were located from all possible sources. Neurological, neurosurgical and

196

general medical indices were searched in some instances back to 1933. Every hospital ward in the region was visited, including geriatric, psychiatric and those under the care of general practitioners. All cases obtained from this extensive record surveillance were arranged into practices. Questionnaires were sent to general practitioners detailing patients thought to be under their care and they indicated those alive and in the practice on the chosen prevalence days. In both studies every general practitioner replied with minimal prompting. In the United Kingdom few practices have a comprehensive diagnostic index and, hence, epidemiological studies beginning with a request for possible patients from general practitioners must lead to underestimation of prevalence and incidence figures. Some [3, 4] have questioned the value of contacting all general practitioners in a survey area, but in the present studies their contribution was considerable [5]. The diagnostic classification chosen was that of probable (Group I), early probable and latent (Group II), and possible MS (Group III) in accordance with previous surveys [6, 7]. In the first study, 77 per cent of the patients and all additional patients in the second study were examined. Patients were excluded if they had retrobulbar neuritis alone, if they were living outside the study area, or if they had died prior to the respective prevalence days. For the study of geographical distribution, north-east Scotland was divided into 28 area units based on the administrative districts but combining adjacent districts, where necessary, to produce unit populations exceeding 10 000 in almost every instance. I also studied the distribution by county in north-east Scotland (Fig. 2).

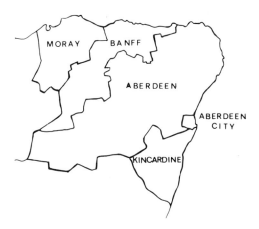

Figure 2 The Counties of north-east Scotland

Prevalence and Incidence

In the first study in 1970, 557 patients with MS were living in north-east Scotland. The overall prevalence was 127/100 000 population and for Groups I and II the prevalence was 105/100 000 (Table I). Among women, the prevalence was considerably greater than among men. By 1973 57 patients had died, 23 had left the

197

area and the diagnosis was no longer acceptable in five. In the interim, 162 additional patients had been diagnosed and 50 of these had been alive and in north-east Scotland in 1970 with sufficient symptoms and signs to have permitted a diagnosis of MS. An adjusted prevalence for 1970, therefore, would be 138/100 000 population. The overall prevalence of 144/100 000 population in 1973 (Table I) is the highest ever recorded in an area of comparable population size and has been exceeded only in Orkney and Shetland [9, 10] and in the small Massachusetts community of Duxbury [11].

TABLE I Prevalence in north-east Scotland according to Group and Sex

	1st December 1970		1st December 1973	
	No. of patients with MS	Prevalence/ 100 000 population*	No. of patients with MS	Prevalence/ 100 000 population*
All Groups	557	127	634	144
Groups I and II	464	105	517	117
Group I	310	70	324	81
All women	342	149	402	175
All men	215	102	232	110

* Population in 1971 [8] was 440 176: Women 229 926, Men 210 250

The mean duration of the disease in 1973 was 15.3 years which is longer than in any previous MS prevalence study [12-14]. Five patients had had MS for more than 50 years, the longest survival being 59 years, and 12.2 per cent had survived more than 30 years. The mean age of all patients in 1973 was 48.6 years (range 14-87). Age and sex specific prevalence rates (Fig. 3) have been calculated for the north-east population using the percentage distribution of age and sex in the whole Scottish population [8, 15]. The highest rate for men 282/100 000 population was recorded for those aged 50-59 and for women a rate of 384/100 000 was obtained for those aged 40-49 years. Among the 104 000 people aged 40-59 in north-east Scotland, one in every 306 had MS on 1 December 1973. It seems unlikely, however, that MS is becoming more common in north-east Scotland. The mean incidence between 1956 and 1973 was 5.2/100 000 population (Fig. 4) based on the date of disease onset of patients from both studies. Lower rates were recorded for the earlier period because of the premature death of patients prior to 1970, and for the later period because some patients had yet to present [16].

Geographical Distribution

The prevalence rates of MS in the 28 areas according to address on 1 December 1970 showed a distribution highly significantly different from that expected (Table II). In the City of Aberdeen (Fig. 5) three adjacent areas (7, 8 and 10) had rates more than 25 per cent above the mean for the whole region. This may well have been related to social class (*see* below) since 45 per cent of the patients from these areas belonged to social classes I and II compared with an expected

198

23 per cent in the general population [17]. The highest prevalence, 250.7/100 000, occurred in area 16 in rural Aberdeenshire (Fig. 6) and this same area had the highest prevalence in 1973. This area also had the highest prevalence according to

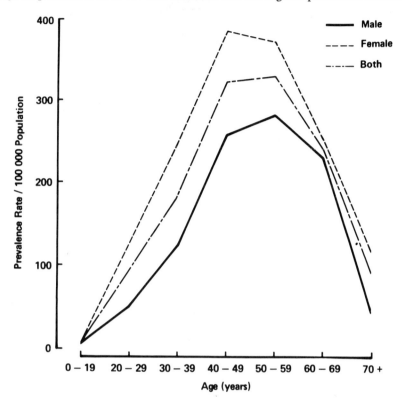

Figure 3 Age and sex specific prevalence of MS in north-east Scotland on 1 December 1973

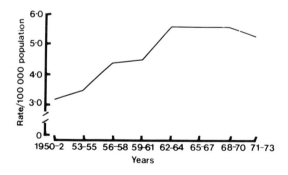

Figure 4 Incidence rates per 100000 population in three-year periods for north-east Scotland

199

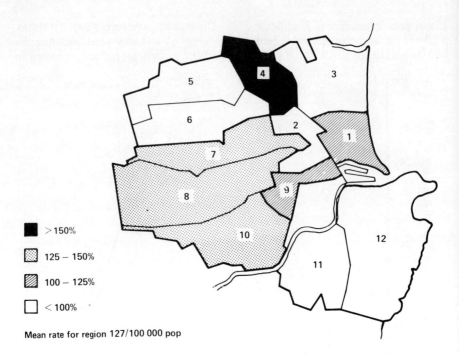

> 150%

125 – 150%

100 – 125%

< 100%

Mean rate for region 127/100 000 pop

Figure 5 Prevalence of MS in City of Aberdeen according to area of residence 1 December 1970. Key indicates relationship to mean prevalence in the whole region

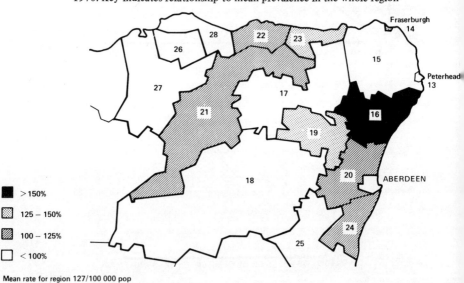

> 150%

125 – 150%

100 – 125%

< 100%

Mean rate for region 127/100 000 pop

Figure 6 Prevalence of MS in north-east Scotland according to area of residence on 1 December 1970. Key as for Figure 5

200

TABLE II Prevalence of MS by area in which patients were living on 1 December 1970

Area No.	Population*	No. of patients with MS	Expected No. of patients	Prevalence/100 000 population	χ^2
1	9 623	13	12.2	135.1	0.007
2	9 923	8	12.7	80.6	1.445
3	18 121	11	22.9	60.7	5.675
4	11 768	23	14.9	195.4†	3.877
5	17 392	20	22.0	115.0	0.102
6	21 439	15	27.1	70.0	4.965
7	15 748	29	19.9	184.2†	4.631
8	14 507	27	18.4	186.1†	3.566
9	11 160	17	14.1	152.3	0.409
10	16 248	27	20.6	166.2†	1.690
11	19 875	22	25.2	110.7	0.289
12	15 349	18	19.4	117.3	0.042
13	14 160	13	17.9	91.8	1.082
14	10 606	19	13.4	179.1†	1.941
15	20 415	16	25.8	78.4	3.352
16	10 768	27	13.6	250.7†	12.236
17	17 027	20	21.5	117.5	0.047
18	14 635	18	18.5	123.0	
19	14 220	24	18.0	168.8†	1.680
20	36 130	50	45.7	138.4	0.404
21	15 242	22	19.3	144.3	0.251
22	16 537	21	20.9	127.0	0.008
23	11 724	19	14.8	162.1†	0.925
24	11 913	18	15.1	151.1	0.381
25	14 146	9	17.9	63.6	3.942
26	20 050	25	25.4	124.7	
27	16 343	19	20.7	116.3	0.070
28	15 107	7	19.1	46.3	7.045
Total	440 176	557	557.0	126.5	60.062

* Obtained from 1971 Census [8]. † More than 25% above mean prevalence. DF = 27; P < 0.001.

birthplace [5, 15] and clearly whatever the environmental factor implicated in the aetiology of MS, it has been operating in this geographical area for many years. The distribution of MS in the north-east counties (see Fig. 2) according to residence on both prevalence days was not significantly different from expected (Table III). Lower rates were recorded in the more peripherally placed counties and this may indicate that some patients were investigated in adjacent regions. In 1973 no county prevalence was less than one per thousand population.

Clustering

In the only formal statistical analysis involving MS patients, no evidence of clustering was found by the methods used [18, 19], but Millar [20] described two high risk areas in Northern Ireland. One further instance was found in north-east Scotland. In a relatively isolated valley, 12 people who later developed MS had lived there at some time between 1913 and 1966 (Fig. 7). Two houses at separate times

TABLE III Prevalence of MS in north-east Scotland by county distribution

		1 December 1970			1 December 1973		
	Population*	No. of patients with MS	Expected No. of patients	Prevalence/ 100 000 population	No. of patients with MS	Expected No. of patients	Prevalence/ 100 000 population
Aberdeen City	181 153	230	229.2	127	257	260.9	142
Aberdeen County	137 961	187	174.5	136	226	198.8	164
Banff County	43 503	62	55.0	143	59	62.6	136
Kincardine County	26 059	27	33.0	104	31	37.5	119
Moray County	51 500	51	65.3	99	61	74.2	118
	440 176	557	557.0	127	634	634.0	144

$$\chi^2 = 6.01$$
P NS

$$\chi^2 = 7.46$$
P NS

* 1971 Census [8]

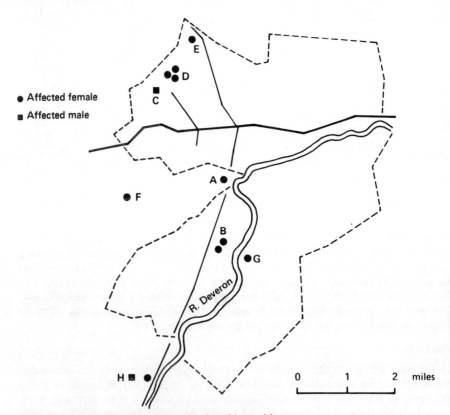

● Affected female

■ Affected male

Figure 7 Location of patients in an Aberdeenshire parish
B – unrelated women living in the same house consecutively
D – mother, daughter and maid living in same house concurrently
H – affected brother and sister

202

had each contained two unrelated people who later developed MS. Although no patients were living in this valley either in 1970 or 1973, 7 had been born there between 1913 and 1930. During this period 291 children were born in the valley and survived at least one year. Of these, one in 70 boys and one in 30 girls later developed MS [15, 21]. The most likely explanation is that this finding in common with those of Millar [20] and Campbell and his co-workers [22] represents a chance environmental occurrence.

Familial Occurrence

In north-east Scotland in 1970, the 557 patients belonged to 541 families and 50 of these (9.2%) contained two or more affected members. In 1973, among the 614 families 9.8 per cent had two or more affected and 2.1 per cent had three or more affected. These familial rates are higher than those found in the large series in north-east England [23] and Northern Ireland [24], but lower than those found in the smaller series in Orkney and Shetland (11.7%) and Denmark (16.7%) [25, 26]. Mackay and Myrianthopoulos [27] have suggested that there are genetically 'high risk' families and two such examples were located in north-east Scotland (Figs 8, 9). Two instances of conjugal MS were found, but in common with most

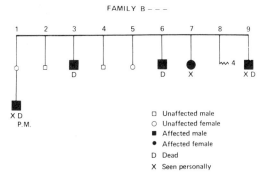

Figure 8 *Familial MS:* four siblings and nephew affected. Four other unaffected siblings died in infancy as indicated

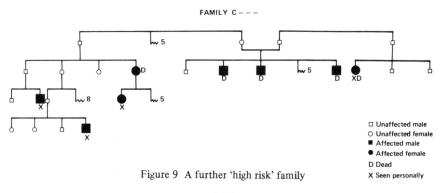

Figure 9 A further 'high risk' family

203

previous reports [28, 29] onset in all four patients had occurred after marriage. These are the only two occurrences in north-east Scotland among over 1000 patients and probably represent a rate little different from the general MS prevalence.

Social Class and Occupation

Among the economically active men at onset of MS aged 15 years and over, the social class distribution was significantly different from expected (Table IV). There was a marked excess of social class I in common with Miller and his associates [31] and Russell [32], but these authors also found an excess of social class II. The Registrar-General's Decennial Supplements for England and Wales [33-35] contain information on the social class status of MS patients. No consistent pattern emerges, but this may be because analysis was by social class at death rather than disease onset and a chronic disorder such as MS often leads to downgrading in social class status.

TABLE IV North-east Scotland 1970 Study

Economically active men at onset of MS aged 15 years and over

| Social class | MS patients | | Regional census* |
	No.	%	%
I	15	7.1	3.1
II	34	16.2	19.5
III	102	48.6	41.8
IV	45	21.4	27.9
V	14	6.7	7.7
	210		

χ^2 corrected = 16.02   P $<$ 0.01

Area comprising 'Remainder of the Northern Division' [30]

Half a century ago agricultural workers, carpenters and woodworkers were thought to have an excess occupational risk of MS [36, 37], but control population information was lacking. In contrast, Sutherland and Wilson [38] were unable to find any vulnerable occupation among 173 men in Glasgow. North-east Scotland provided an opportunity of comparing the occupations of all known MS patients with accurate occupational information from the whole population [39]. Among woodworkers there was a highly significant excess of MS patients [40] and this was even more striking among joiners and carpenters alone [15]. One in every 258 joiners and carpenters had MS compared with one in 632 of the male working population of north-east Scotland (P $<$ 0.001). Among the economically active women with MS 12.9 per cent were nurses compared with an expected 5.4 per cent (P $<$ 0.001). Thus, one in every 200 nurses had MS and this excludes several women with onset prior to starting nursing.

204

Mortality Rate

Although Scotland has the ignominious distinction of having one of the highest death rates from MS in the world over at least two decades [41-43], the rates are considerably less than the incidence rates mentioned earlier for north-east Scotland. Analysis of only underlying cause of death reveals 75-85 per cent of all certificates mentioning MS in the United States, Denmark and Norway [44,45]. In Scotland, however, in 1974 and 1975 only 50 per cent of certificates mentioning MS included it as the underlying cause of death. The mortality rate for these years in the Annual Reports of the Registrar-General for Scotland [46, 47] is 1.9/100 000 population, but the rate would be 3.8/100 000 if all certificates mentioning MS were analysed. A similar picture emerges in north-east Scotland (Table V). In fact the official statistics reveal only 38 per cent of deaths of known MS patients in north-east Scotland in this five-year period.

TABLE V Deaths from MS in north-east Scotland 1971-1975

	No.	Rate/100 000* population
Reported by Registrar General	39	1.8
All certificates mentioning MS	87	4.0
All known MS deaths	103	4.7

* 1971 Census [8]

Conclusions

These consecutive prevalence studies have revealed that MS affects more than one per thousand of the population in north-east Scotland. Although the occurrence is not spread homogeneously when considered by small geographical units, there is no significant variation by county distribution. The familial occurrence is higher than in many previous studies but cannot account for the high prevalence. Although there is an excess social class I risk and a possible occupational risk for certain categories, again this has a negligible effect on the overall excess. The significance of the HLA association with MS at present remains uncertain, but in north-east Scotland the general population has a high percentage of B7 antigen [5] and an even higher percentage has been found in Orkney and Shetland [48]. This indicates perhaps that these populations contain a larger pool of susceptible individuals than elsewhere.

Chronic disorders such as MS rarely cause death *per se*. Underlying cause of death alone is an unsatisfactory measure of the true occurrence of these disorders in the community. Analysis of all certificates mentioning MS would provide a more accurate estimate. The mortality rate of MS in north-east Scotland is comparable with the rate for the whole Scottish population (Table VI). Multiple sclerosis probably affects, therefore, more than one per thousand of the population throughout Scotland with the exception of the Western Isles.

TABLE VI Death rates/100 000 population* 1964-1973

	Crude rate	Age adjusted**
Scotland	2.3	2.1
North-east Scotland	2.2	2.0
Northern Ireland***	2.0	1.9
England and Wales***	1.7	1.5

* 1971 Census [8, 49]
** Age adjusted to USA 1950 Census population [50]
*** 1964-1972

Acknowledgements

This work was supported by funds from the Maggie Whyte Bequest, Aberdeen University.

I am grateful to the *British Medical Journal* for permission to use Table II and Figures 5 and 6, and to Mrs Christine Walton for secretarial assistance.

References

1 Campbell, AMG (1947) *Quart. J. Med., 16,* 312
2 *Aberdeen Royal Infirmary Reports* (1882-1909) The Aberdeen University Press Limited, Aberdeen
3 Brewis, M, Poskanzer, DC, Rolland, C and Miller, H (1966) *Acta Neurol. Scandinav., 42,* suppl. 24, 9
4 Stazio, A, Paddison, RM and Kurland, LT (1967) *J. Chron. Dis., 20,* 311
5 Shepherd, DI and Downie, AW (1978) *Brit. Med. J., 2,* 314
6 Alter, M, Allison, RS, Talbert, OR and Kurland, LT (1960) *World Neurol., 1,* 55
7 Broman, T, Bergmann, L, Fog, T, Gilland, O, Hyllested, K, Lindberg-Broman, A, Pedersen, E and Presthus, J (1965) *Acta Neurol. Scandinav., 41,* suppl. 13, 543
8 General Register Office, Scotland (1974) *Census 1971 Scotland, Population Tables,* HMSO, Edinburgh
9 Fog, M and Hyllested, K (1966) *Acta Neurol. Scandinav., 42,* suppl. 19, 6
10 Poskanzer, DC, Walker, AM, Yonkondy, J and Sheridan, JL (1976) *Neurology, 26,* No. 6 part 2, 14
11 Deacon, WE, Alexander, L, Siedler, H and Kurland, LT (1959) *New Engl. J. Med., 261,* 1059
12 Poskanzer, DC, Schapira, K and Miller, H (1963) *J. Neurol. Neurosurg. Psychiat., 26,* 368
13 Leibowitz, U, Halpern, L and Alter, M (1964) *Arch. Neurol., 10,* 502
14 Penelius, M (1969) *Acta Neurol. Scandinav., 45,* suppl. 39, 7
15 Shepherd, DI (1976) In *Multiple Sclerosis in North-East Scotland.* MD Thesis, University of Aberdeen
16 Shepherd, DI (1979) *Acta Neurol. Scandinav.* In press
17 General Register Office, Scotland (1963) *Census 1961 (Scotland), County Reports.* HMSO, Edinburgh
18 Ashitey, GA and Mackenzie, G (1970) *Brit. J. Prev. Soc. Med., 24,* 163
19 Hargreaves, E and Merrington, M (1973) *J. Chron. Dis., 26,* 47
20 Millar, JHD (1966) *J. Irish Med. Assoc., 59,* 138

21   Downie, AW and Shepherd, DI (1980) In *The Ecology of Disease in Urban Societies.* Symposium of the Society for the Study of Human Biology (in press)
22   Campbell, AMG, Herdan, G, Tatlow, WFT and Whittle, EG (1950) *Brain, 73,* 52
23   Schapira, K, Poskanzer, DC and Miller, H (1963) *Brain, 86,* 315
24   Millar, JHD and Allison, RS (1954) *Ulster Med. J., 23,* suppl. 2, 29
25   Allison, RS (1963) *Proc. Roy. Soc. Med., 56,* 71
26   Thygesen, P (1953) In *The Course of Disseminated Sclerosis. A close-up of 105 attacks.* Rosenkilde and Bagger, Copenhagen, page 119
27   Mackay, RP and Myrianthopoulos, NC (1966) *Arch. Neurol., 15,* 449
28   Luban-Plozza, B (1964) *Schweizer Arch. Neurol. Neurochir. Psychiat., 94,* 63
29   Cendrowski, WS (1965) *Acta Neurol. Scandinav., 41,* 557
30   General Register Office, Scotland (1966) *Census 1961 Scotland.* Vol. VI Occupation, Industry and Workplace. Part I Occupation Tables. HMSO, Edinburgh
31   Miller, H, Ridley, A and Schapira, K (1960) *Brit. Med. J., 2,* 343
32   Russell, WR (1971) *Lancet, ii,* 832
33   The Registrar-General's Decennial Supplement (1938) *England and Wales 1931.* Part IIa Occupational Mortality. HMSO, London
34   The Registrar-General's Decennial Supplement (1958) *England and Wales 1951.* Occupational Mortality. Part II, Volume 2 Tables. HMSO, London
35   The Registrar-General's Decennial Supplement (1971) *England and Wales 1961.* Occupational Mortality Tables. HMSO, London
36   Dreyfuss, H (1921) *Z. Ges. Neurol. Psychiat., 73,* 479
37   McAlpine, D (1927) *Brit. Med. J., 1,* 269
38   Sutherland, JM and Wilson, DR (1951) *Glasg. Med. J., 32,* 302
39   General Register Office, Scotland (1966) *Census 1961 Scotland.* Occupation and industry. County tables, Aberdeen City and Counties of Banff, Kincardine, Moray, Nairn and Aberdeen. HMSO, Edinburgh
40   Swinscow, TDV (1976) *Brit. Med. J., 2,* 166
41   Limburg, C (1950) In *Multiple Sclerosis and the Demyelinating Diseases,* Volume 28. Williams and Williams Co, Baltimore. Page 15
42   Kurland, LT, Stazio, A and Reed, D (1965) *Ann. N.Y. Acad. Sci., 122,* 520
43   Stocks, P (1971) *J. Hygiene, 69,* 373
44   Kurland, LT and Moriyama, IM (1951) *J. Amer. Med. Assoc., 145,* 725
45   Kurtzke, JF (1972) *Acta Neurol. Scandinav., 48,* 148
46   Registrar General, Scotland (1975) *Annual Report 1974.* Part 1. Mortality Statistics. HMSO, Edinburgh
47   Registrar General, Scotland (1976) *Annual Report 1975.* Part 1. Mortality Statistics. HMSO, Edinburgh
48   Roberts, DF (1979) Personal communication
49   General Register Office (1974) *Census 1971 Great Britain.* Age, Marital Condition and General Tables. HMSO, London
50   United States 1950 Census Population (1955) In *United Nations Statistical Office Demographic Year Book.* International Publications Services, New York. Page 396

Chapter 17

MULTIPLE SCLEROSIS IN
THE ORKNEY AND SHETLAND ISLES

D F Roberts

The interest of the Orkney and Shetland Isles for the study of mutliple sclerosis, and particularly for its genetic analysis, stems from the work of Sutherland (1956) [9]. In a survey carried out in 1954 he was the first to note the high prevalence, about twice that farther south in Scotland, and interpreted the difference in terms of population ancestry, particularly the Norse influence in the islands. The 'unusual concentration of cases, certainly much greater than that known in any other region of Europe, or North America' (Allison, 1963) [1] was again emphasised in the follow-up study by Allison, Fog and Hyllested carried out eight years later in 1962, and noted again in Poskanzer's survey of 1970 (Poskanzer and associates, 1976) [2]. Sutherland also drew attention to the higher familial incidence (i.e. the occurrence of the same disease in a relative of the patient) in Orkney and Shetland, and suggested some genetic element in the aetiology. He stated that 18.2 per cent of the positive cases in Shetland and 17.6 per cent in Orkney showed a familial incidence. Allison noted the same unusually high familial incidence of cases, 9.6 per cent of his Orkney cases and 13.7 per cent of his Shetland. The opportunity offered to investigate the genetic component in multiple sclerosis appeared unique so, in collaboration with Dr Poskanzer of Harvard, we initiated a genetic study of the disorder in the two island groups. This paper reports some of the preliminary work, particularly that relating to the prevalence of multiple sclerosis.

Orkney consists of a group of about 70 islands, extending some 50 miles NNE from the northernmost tip of Caithness, from which the nearest island is separated by the Pentland Firth, 6½ miles wide at its narrowest point. Of the total island area of 376 square miles, and total population of 17 077 (1971), most is located on the largest island of Mainland, with an area of 207 square miles and a population of 12 747. The remainder of the inhabitants is distributed throughout the other islands, the smallest populations being found on Swona and Papa Stronsay with three inhabitants each. About 40 per cent of the population are in the two towns, Kirkwall and Stromness, both on Mainland. The islands lie between latitudes 58°45' and 59°25'N.

Further north-east, between latitudes 59°50' and 60°50'N, lies Shetland, a group of rather more than a hundred islands, extending about 70 miles in their long axis aligned north-north-east, and 36 miles across. The total area is some 552 square miles, and the population was 17 327 in 1971. Only 19 of the islands are inhabited, the largest (Mainland) containing 12 944 inhabitants in its 378 square miles, the smallest (Noss) containing 3. There is only one urban area, Lerwick.

The two island groups have in common a high northern latitude, a generally mild and equable though windy climate, and an almost complete absence of tree cover. Both were settled by Norse colonists who displaced or submerged earlier inhabitants. Formerly distinct linguistically, there still remain Norse words in the dialect, and particularly many place names have clear Norse origin, and indeed Norse was spoken in Foula as late as the year 1774. In 1468, the islands were attached to Scotland as a pledge for the dowry of the Princess of Denmark on her marriage to James III—a pledge that was never redeemed—and this was followed by settlement of Scots and suppression of many features of the earlier Scandinavian culture. Both Orkney and Shetland attained their maximum population about a century ago, nearly double the present numbers. However, there are differences between the two island groups. Orkney, except for the island of Hoy with its impressive cliffs, consists of low softly rolling hills with many freshwater lochs, some areas of peat and moss, but mostly cultivable. Shetland by contrast is much more rugged; the long narrow arms of the sea (the Sounds and Voes) penetrate deep into the islands so that no point is more than three miles from the sea, and only one-sixth can be used for farming other than rough hill grazing.

Methods

In analysing a disorder such as multiple sclerosis, uniformity in diagnosis is essential. For that reason, observed cases were only accepted as such when they had been investigated by Dr Poskanzer, who classified them according to established international criteria into 'probable', 'possible' or 'not multiple sclerosis'. He examined all cases surviving that had been included among the patients listed in the previous surveys, all new patients reported since, as well as those previously diagnosed as possible or doubtful, and, from surveys among all general practitioners in the islands, included any others thought to be affected. For each case a contiguous control was selected who was not a member of the same immediate family, who was born in the same parish in the same year, was of the same sex, resided in the same area for the first 15 years of his life, and was not affected. Where a control was subsequently found himself to have a neurological disorder or to be a first or second-degree relative of the patient to whom he was matched, a replacement control was obtained. In addition, a discontiguous control was selected, of the same sex, born in the same year, but not in a parish in which the patient had been born nor contiguous with it.

Each patient on the list provided by Dr Poskanzer, and each contiguous control, was interviewed. A full family history was obtained, including the necessary identification of his parents, their dates and places of birth, the maternal maiden name, and relevant details of the immediate relatives, including information on any disorders that had occurred in them, where diagnosed and treated, with particular attention to suspected neurological disorders, to give a comprehensive view of the family over three or four generations. This was verified from documentary sources (e.g. death certificates, hospital notes).

Prevalence

Our study series therefore consisted of all patients with multiple sclerosis in the Orkney and Shetland Isles alive on 1st December 1974. These were all those diagnosed and accepted by Dr Poskanzer as probable or possible cases on that date, and were the subjects notified to us by him. There were, apparently, a few further possible cases, for instance where the local family doctor preferred not to give permission to see the patients, and other individuals regarded as doubtful on that date but in whom the diagnosis was only confirmed later; these were not included in our prevalence estimates. The number of cases in Orkney on prevalence day was 51, of whom 45 were diagnosed as probable and 6 as possible; there were 30 females and 21 males. In Shetland there were 33 cases, of whom 28 were probable and 5 possible, 18 females and 15 males. In Orkney, the prevalences per 100 000 population therefore are 292, and 179 in Shetland. They remain apparently the highest in the world.

Secular Trends

On account of the previous studies that have been made in the islands, it is possible to examine the change in prevalence. The islands are one of the two areas in the world where the prevalence has been studied on four occasions and where a secular trend can be sought. Shetland shows a slight but steady increase in prevalence over the 20 years, from 134 in 1954, 165 in 1962, 177 in 1970, and 179 in 1974. Orkney, too, shows a rise, but one that is much more acute, from 111 in 1954, 178 in 1962, 233 in 1970, to 292 in 1974. Whereas in 1954 prevalence in Shetland appeared greater than in Orkney, the position is now reversed. The same trend appears if only probable cases are considered (Fig. 1).

How then to account for the increase in prevalence? The latest figures are certainly not overestimates artificially inflated but rather the reverse; if the additional cases that were confirmed by 1976 and those possibles not seen are included, the prevalences rise to 309 for Orkney and 184 for Shetland. It is possible that some identified cases were not included in the earliest studies, yet this seems unlikely. Sutherland [3] sent a questionnaire to all practitioners asking for the names and addresses of all cases suspected of suffering from multiple sclerosis in their practices and, when necessary, a reminder was sent; replies were finally received from all but two practitioners in the whole of northern Scotland. Sutherland states that 'although it cannot be claimed that all cases of multiple sclerosis living in the region have been seen, I am satisfied that the investigation embraces the vast majority'. It may, however, be that some cases were not recognised by the then practitioners.

There is no evidence that the increasingly high rates in Orkney and Shetland are the results of immigration or re-immigration to the islands of patients with multiple sclerosis. Of all the cases, 48 of the 51 in Orkney and 31 of the 33 in Shetland had been born in the respective islands and, if those born elsewhere are omitted, the prevalences remain high. Instead, comparison of the rates of elimination from the population by death and the occurrence of new cases suggests an actual increase. In Orkney in the 20-year period 1954-1974, 66 new cases were diagnosed, and in

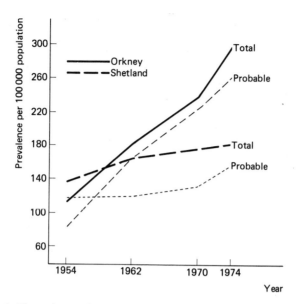

Figure 1 Change in prevalence of multiple sclerosis in Orkney and Shetland

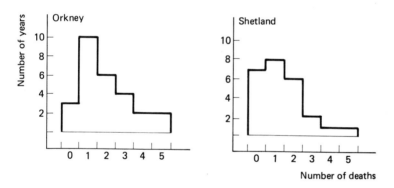

Figure 2 Number of deaths per year in MS patients 1950–1974

Shetland 39, rates respectively of 3.3 and 2.0 new cases per annum. Deaths in multiple sclerosis patients (Fig. 2) occurred in 35 cases in Orkney and 30 in Shetland in the same period, giving rates of 1.8 and 1.5 deaths per annum. It appears that the progressive increase in the prevalence of multiple sclerosis is attributable to the fact that the patients are not dying out of the population at the rate that new cases are emerging. This is quite compatible with the increased control of morbidity in multiple sclerosis these days, not so much of the disease itself but of the associated disorders, e.g. infections which led to the deaths of so many patients

211

formerly. If this hypothesis is correct, one would expect to see similar increases in prevalence in other areas where modern health measures are available.

A contribution perhaps comes from the change in demographic structure of the population. The populations today contain more elderly individuals, as part of the general demographic changes taking place in western Europe with reduced fertility, and as part of the overall population decline peculiar to Orkney and Shetland over recent decades. Since multiple sclerosis is essentially a disorder of middle and later life, any change in the age structure of the population would be reflected in the prevalence. Such change alone, however, is insufficient to account totally for the rise in prevalence.

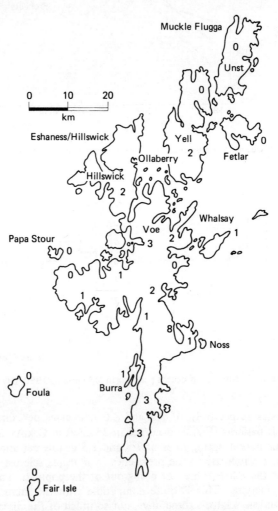

Figure 3 Distribution of cases by birthplace, Shetland

212

Differences Between the Islands

Distribution. Differences that may be relevant to the aetiology are distinguishable between the two island groups in some biological features and not in others. The local distribution of the cases by birthplace in Shetland (Fig. 3) appears fairly even, with a slight concentration per unit population in the northern parishes of Mainland (Delting and Northmavine). In Orkney (Fig. 4) there is a somewhat less even distribution, with a peripheral concentration per unit population in the parishes of Eday, Rousay, Birsay, South Ronaldsay and Westray. There is little similarity in the environmental features of these two zones of suggested higher density in the two island groups.

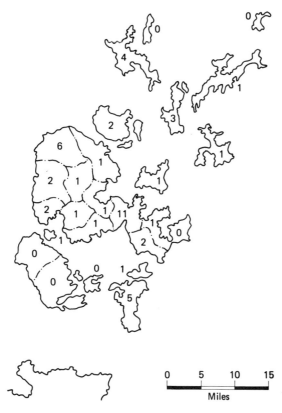

Figure 4 Distribution of cases by birthplace, Orkney

The sex distribution of cases is very similar in both, females accounting for 58.8 per cent of the cases in Orkney, and 58.1 per cent in Shetland. These are very similar to the proportions given for other populations elsewhere. There appears, however, to be a difference between the islands in age of onset. The mean in Orkney is 29.0 years, but is slightly but significantly later in Shetland at 33.6

213

years. This would give rise, assuming similar life expectancy, to an upward shift in the distribution of patients' ages in Shetland. Such was indeed noted by Fog and Hyllested (1966) [4] with a Shetland mean at 49.4 years and Orkney at 45.5, but in the present data does not occur (Shetland 49.5, Orkney 52.7).

Although variation in parental age at the birth of patients is important in a number of disorders, as yet there is no evidence that this is relevant in multiple sclerosis. Table I and Figure 5 show the parental age at the birth of patients and controls. There is no significant difference between patient and control groups in the mean ages of mothers and fathers at the birth of the subjects. However, the age of the mother at the birth of the patient is significantly lower in Orkney than in Shetland.

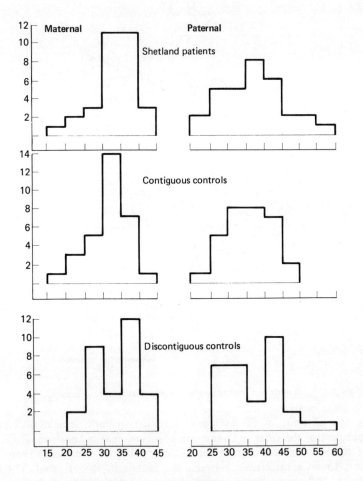

Figure 5 Parental age at birth of subjects and controls

214

TABLE I Parental Age (years) at Birth of Subject

	Mother			Father		
	m	n	SD	m	n	SD
Shetland						
Patients	34.23	31	6.39	37.58	31	8.30
Contiguous controls	31.80	31	5.36	36.02	30	6.40
Discontiguous controls	33.40	31	5.89	37.26	31	7.70
Orkney						
Patients	30.70	51	6.97	36.16	51	7.95
Contiguous controls	31.85	48	6.51	35.74	48	8.72

Immunoglobulins. As a pointer to the possible role of immunopathological mechanisms, serum immunoglobulin levels were examined in all patients and in 408 Orkney and 223 Shetland normal healthy subjects. The normal Shetland mean levels of IgG, M, A and E are consistently and significantly above those of Orkney (Table II). All assays were carried out in the same laboratory by the same procedures, by the same personnel, and specimens were examined at approximately similar intervals after arrival, though the Shetland analysis was carried out several months later than the Orkney (early spring 1975 and autumn 1974 respectively). While the apparent difference between the two island groups may be an artefact, it is also possible that it reflects a difference in the environment of the two island populations.

TABLE II Serum Immunoglobulin Levels in Orkney and Shetland

		Not affecteds			Patients		
		mean	SE	SD	mean	SE	SD
IgG	Orkney	1138	± 12	252	1112	± 38	273
mg/100 ml	Shetland	1266	± 13	190	1260	± 40	225
IgM	Orkney	128	± 2	54	114	± 8	59
mg/100 ml	Shetland	150	± 4	55	157	± 12	67
IgA	Orkney	215	± 2	55	209	± 7	53
mg/100 ml	Shetland	244	± 4	66	256	± 13	73
log IgE	Orkney	2.122	± 0.023	0.316	2.191	± 0.02	0.380
nu/ml	Shetland	2.187	± 0.015	0.223	2.162	± 0.05	0.273

Shetland patients showed no significant difference from the normal levels in any of the four immunoglobulins examined. However, in Orkney there was a slight suggestion of a reduced mean IgM in the patients and a slightly elevated mean IgE. Log IgE levels in rural patients were significantly elevated over those in rural controls ($P < 0.02$), but there was no difference in the urban dwellers. The elevated

215

IgE overall stems from the occurrence of five patients with pronouncedly elevated levels; three of these are reported as having experienced an allergic reaction in the past, but all five had lived on farms with exposure to farm animals, domestic pets and presumably parasites. In any case, past exposure to allergens may not be relevant, for ongoing or recent stimulation may have caused the elevation; perhaps it is in response to some abnormal breakdown product in the patients themselves, though there was no difference when the patients with the chronic progressive form were compared with the exacerbating/remitting type. But whatever the explanation, there is a suggestion here that the environments of the two island populations may be different, and so may be the response of the patients to them.

Genetics. The similarities in the history of the two groups of islands do not necessarily imply that the populations are genetically similar. To examine their genetic constitutions, in the course of the present investigations, blood specimens were obtained from unaffected, outwardly healthy individuals, numbering 413 in Orkney and 323 in Shetland. There emerge highly significant differences between the Orkney and Shetland populations in several bloodgroup systems. In the ABO bloodgroup system, the frequency of the bloodgroup B gene is higher in the Orkney islanders, whereas that of the O gene is lower. They also have, in the MNSs blood-group system, a lower frequency of the gene S while the MNSs phenotype combinations also differ—in Orkney it is particularly the MS haplotype that is less frequent. They also appear to have a lower frequency of the phenotype Le^{a+}. Differences in the other systems tested did not attain significance. These quite pronounced differences indicate that the populations are today distinct genetically. They are sufficiently different to preclude the combination of the two groups of islands in any aetiological analysis.

Associations of multiple sclerosis with several serogenetic characters have been postulated, particularly with HLA antigens [5, 6] but also with the ABO bloodgroups [7]. Such associations of course cannot account for the changing prevalence, but it is worth enquiring whether they may contribute to the high prevalence by comparison with that elsewhere in Britain or to the island differences. The higher group O frequency in Shetland than farther south is not sufficient to account for the greatly enhanced prevalence, and indeed the Hebrides with still higher O frequencies show considerably fewer multiple sclerosis cases. Group O frequencies in the Orkney population are rather lower, so again cannot account for the higher prevalence. Another possible association for which the evidence is much less clear is that suggested with the rhesus haplotype cde, and here neither the Orkney nor Shetland population show any elevation in frequency, but rather the reverse. For HLA types testing was carried out only on specimens from 100 normal Orkney subjects (Table III). These indicate an elevated frequency of A2, A11, and B7 and indeed they appear to be ultra-European in the direction of these differences. What is interesting, however, is that the B7 level is some 70 per cent greater than the normal British frequency [8] and if the association of multiple sclerosis with this HLA antigen is valid, this elevation is high enough to contribute appreciably to the high prevalence of the disorder, though not completely.

216

TABLE III HLA Antigen and Gene Frequencies in a Normal Orkney Sample

HLA Antigen	Phenotypes %	Gene frequencies
A 1	34	0.188
2	60	0.368
3	25	0.134
9 (incl. 23, 24)	9	0.046
10 (incl. 25, 26)	13	0.067
11	20	0.106
W 19 (incl. 29, W30, 31, 32)	17	0.089
28	1	0.005
B 5	13	0.067
7	39	0.219
8	24	0.128
12	31	0.169
13	6	0.031
14	10	0.051
W 15	14	0.073
W 16	1	0.005
W 17	9	0.046
W 18	3	0.015
W 21	2	0.010
W 22	2	0.010
W 35	2	0.010
27	12	0.062
W 40	11	0.057

Conclusion

The prevalence of multiple sclerosis in Orkney and Shetland remains very high, still the highest reported in the world. In both groups of islands it is increasing, at a rate that is particularly high in Orkney. It is argued that this increase is due to improved survival of patients. There is sufficient evidence to show that for genetic analysis of multiple sclerosis the data from Orkney and Shetland should not be combined, the evidence for genetic differences between the two populations being particularly strong. However, there are also suggestions that differences in the environment in the two island groups may be important. The latter suggestions derive from the evidence of the immunoglobulin levels, the maternal ages, and the local distribution of cases, while the disorder itself appears to show differences between the two island groups, notably in age of onset, prevalence, and presence of possible associations with immunoglobulin levels in the one and not the other.

Acknowledgements

Acknowledgement is gratefully made to Dr D C Poskanzer for making available lists of patients and controls and the blood specimens taken during the course of the survey; to Dr Mary Mack and Mrs Catherine Kemp for their invaluable field surveys among the families; to Mr C K Creen, Dr S S Papiha and Dr S K Al-Agidi for their laboratory assistance; to Mrs M J Roberts and Mrs J A Cowie for their assistance with the vital record analysis; and to the Multiple Sclerosis Society of Great Britain and the National Institutes of Health, Bethesda, for financial support.

References

1 Allison, RS (1963) Some neurologic aspects of medical geography. *Proc. Roy. Soc. Med.*, *56*, 71–76

2 Poskanzer, DC, Walker, AM, Yonkondy, J and Sheridan, JL (1976) Studies in the epidemiology of Multiple Sclerosis in the Orkney and Shetland Islands. *Neurology, 26*, 14

3 Sutherland, JM (1976) Observations on the prevalence of Multiple Sclerosis in Northern Scotland. *Brain, 79*, 635

4 Fog, M and Hyllested, K (1966) Prevalence of disseminated sclerosis in the Faroes, the Orkneys, and Shetland. *Acta Scand. Neurol.* (Suppl), *19*, 9

5 Naito, S, Namerow, N, Mickey, MR and Terasaki, P (1972) Multiple sclerosis: association with HL-A 3. *Tissue Antigens, 2*, 1

6 Bertrams, HJ and Kuwert, EK (1976) Association of Histocompatibility haplotype HLA-A3-B7 with Multiple Sclerosis. *J. Immun., 117*, 1906

7 MacDonald, JL, Roberts, DF, Shaw, DA and Saunders, M (1976) Blood groups and other polymorphisms in Multiple Sclerosis. *J. Med. Genet., 13*, 30

8 Bodmer, J (ed) (1975) The ABC of HLA. In *Histocompatibility Testing 1975* (ed F Kissmeyer-Nielsen). Munksgaard

9 Sutherland, JM (1956) *Brain, 79*, 635

Chapter 18

MULTIPLE SCLEROSIS IN THE OUTER HEBRIDES

Geoffrey Dean, Allan Downie and John Goodall

The Orkney and Shetland Islands have been reported to have a surprisingly high prevalence of multiple sclerosis (MS), 309 per 100 000 in the Orkney Islands and 184 per 100 000 in the Shetland Islands when probable and possible MS cases are taken together, and 258 in the Orkneys and 152 in the Shetlands per 100 000 for probable MS alone [1] (*see* Chapter 16).

A recent epidemiological study of MS in north-east Scotland also showed a high prevalence of 127 per 100 000 for probable MS which is greater than in any other surveyed area with a comparable population, 440 000 people [2] (*see* Chapter 16).

Sutherland (1956) [3] was the first to point out that the prevalence of MS appeared to be at least twice as high in the Orkney and Shetland Islands than in the highland areas in the west of Scotland and postulated that there might be a disadvantageous genetic factor in the north-eastern area of Scotland and the Orkney and Shetland Islands where the people are largely of Scandinavian origin, in comparison with the west of Scotland and the Hebrides where the people are often still Gaelic-speaking and are of largely Celtic origin.

The geographical distribution of MS is associated to some extent with the presence of HLA antigens A3 and B7. The prevalence of B7 in north-east Scotland is higher than elsewhere which may partly explain the high prevalence of MS in this area. Because of the higher prevalence of MS in north-east Scotland, the Orkneys and Shetlands, and the reported lower prevalence in south-west Scotland we undertook to ascertain the prevalence of MS in the largely Gaelic-speaking islands of the Outer Hebrides—the Western Isles.

Method

A search was made for all possible and probable patients with multiple sclerosis through the records at the General Hospital, Stornoway, and through the neurological records at the hospitals in Glasgow and Aberdeen. All the doctors on the islands were visited and their co-operation with the study was obtained. Of the 31 000 residents on the islands 24 000 live on the islands of Lewis and Harris. There are seven general practitioners in the only town of the Western Isles, Stornoway, with six doctors in practice in the rest of Lewis and Harris. There is one doctor in North Uist, two in Benbecula where there is an army base, two in South Uist and one in Barra. The visiting ophthalmologist from Inverness who holds clinics throughout the Western Isles also co-operated with the study.

Results

All patients who were suspected of having MS were examined personally by the team either in the hospital at Stornoway or in their homes with the exception of one patient who has not yet been available and is included as possible MS only. The majority of patients had extensive hospital records and some were admitted to hospital in Aberdeen for further investigation. On prevalence day, 1 January 1977, there were 19 patients diagnosed as having probable MS, 10 males and 9 females (Table I). There were 4 additional patients with retrobulbar neuritis only and 2 patients with possible MS. When probable and possible MS and retrobulbar neuritis are taken together, 25 patients, there would be a prevalence rate of 8.1 per 100 000. For probable MS the distribution age standardised to the population of England and Wales the prevalence would be 61.6 per 100 000.

TABLE I Multiple Sclerosis in the Outer Hebrides (The Western Isles) 1976

	Population	GPS	Probable MS	Possible MS	Retrobulbar neuritis
Stornoway	12 878	7	4 (4)	–	1
Rest of Lewis	8177	6	2 (2)	1	3
Harris	2655	2	7 (4)	–	–
North Uist	1618	1	6 (5)	1	–
Benbecula ⎫		2	–	–	–
⎬ 4051					
South Uist ⎭		2	–	–	–
Barra	1464	1	–	–	–
Total	30 844		19 (15)	2	4

Note: The number in brackets is the number of families affected

Of the 19 patients with probable MS, 4 lived in Stornoway, 2 in the remainder of Lewis, 7 in Harris in 4 families—in one family there were twin brothers affected and a sister, in another family a brother and a sister, and 6 in North Uist in 5 families—in one family a brother and a sister were affected. No MS patients were found in Benbecula, South Uist or Barra. The mother of one of the patients also had MS but she was not living on the islands.

The mean age at onset for the MS patients was 35.2 years (36.6 male, 33.7 female) and the mean age on prevalence day 1977 was 44.5 years (46.9 male and 41.9 female).

220

Discussion

The prevalence of probable multiple sclerosis found in the Outer Hebrides is similar to that found in the north-west of Scotland [3], in Northern Ireland (64.2 per 100000) [4], and in the Republic of Ireland (65.5 per 100000) [5]. With the small population and the detailed study that was possible in the Outer Hebrides there is every reason to believe that very few, if any, patients with multiple sclerosis have been overlooked. The prevalence of 81.1 per 100000 for probable and possible MS can be compared with the rate of 127 per 100000 found in the large population studied (440000), in north-eastern Scotland [2]. It is only one-third of that reported in the Orkneys, 258 per 100000 [1].

Genetic factors may be partly responsible for the lower prevalence of MS in the Outer Hebrides, in comparison with the north-east, the Orkneys and Shetlands and a study of the HLA antigen distribution among the MS patients and controls in the Outer Hebrides is being undertaken but will not be completed until late 1979. A report on this study is being prepared for publication.

This study is being supported by the Scottish branch of the Multiple Sclerosis Society of Great Britain and Northern Ireland.

References

1 Poskanzer, DC, Walker, AM, Yonkondy, J and Sheridan, JL (1976) *Neurology, 26,* 6, Part 2, 14
2 Shepherd, DI and Downie, AW (1978) *Brit. med. J., 2,* 314
3 Sutherland, JM (1956) *Brain, 79,* 635
4 Millar, JHD (1977) *Multiple Sclerosis: A Disease acquired in childhood.* Charles C Thomas, Illinois
5 Brady, R, Dean, G, Secerbegovic, S and Secerbegovic, AM (1977) *J. Irish Med. Assoc., 70,* (17), 500

Chapter 19

MULTIPLE SCLEROSIS IN NORTHERN IRELAND

J H D Millar

Northern Ireland is a high risk area for multiple sclerosis. The prevalence in 1961 was 81 per 100 000 of the population (Table I) with a sex ratio of three females to two males. The average age of onset was 33 years for females and 31 years for males.

The incidence, the number of cases per 100 000 with an onset in each year, varied slightly. Between 1943 and 1965 the rates per year were 3.0, 2.9, 2.9, 3.0, 3.3, 4.5, 4.4, 3.4, 3.1, 2.9, 3.4, 2.2, 3.6, 2.8, 3.6, 4.1, 3.7, 5.0, 4.9, 3.6, 2.9, 3.5 and 4.4.

TABLE I Prevalence of Multiple Sclerosis in the Population of Northern Ireland
(Calculations are based on the 1961 census figures)

Age group	Males			Females		
	Total No.	Number affected	Prevalence per 100 000	Total No.	Number affected	Prevalence per 100 000
0 – 4	75354	0	0	71165	0	0
5 – 9	68096	0	0	64348	0	0
10 – 14	68130	1	1	65041	0	0
15 – 19	60287	1	2	59950	8	13
20 – 24	46875	16	34	46877	23	49
25 – 34	83200	69	83	88520	111	125
35 – 44	85545	128	150	90460	193	213
45 – 54	81691	134	164	87377	198	227
55 – 59	34357	52	151	38185	83	217
60 – 64	29435	31	105	36290	43	118
65 – 74	39986	21	53	52285	31	59
Over 75	21268	4	19	30320	1	3

Date of birth unknown in 10 other cases

Summary	694224	457	66	730818	691	95
Overall	1425042	1158	81			

As it seems likely that the disease is acquired in childhood it was decided in 1968 to relate date and place of birth [1, 2]. The group selected for study was born between 1901 and 1925. It was thought that many cases born before 1901 would have died and so would not have been available for the register of cases which

222

started in 1948, and that cases born after 1925 would not necessarily have developed the disease, or at least the disease might not be advanced enough to make a diagnosis possible.

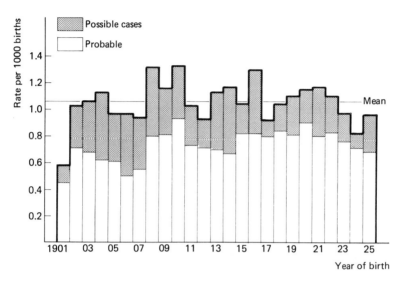

Figure 1 Ascertained MS cases born in N. Ireland per 1000 registered live births (1901–1925)

TABLE II Multiple Sclerosis Cases/1000 Live Births in Belfast and the Counties of Northern Ireland for Five Quinquennial Periods 1901–1925

Year of Birth	Belfast Co. Bo.	Co. Antrim	Co. Down	Co. Armagh	Co. Fermanagh	Co. & Co. B. Londonderry	Co. Tyrone	Northern Ireland
1901–05	0.8	1.1	1.4	1.1	1.1	0.5	1.0	1.0
1906–10	0.8	1.5	1.5	1.2	1.1	1.1	1.4	1.2
1911–15	0.7	1.4	1.6	1.6	2.2	0.5	1.0	1.1
1916–20	0.6	1.2	1.7	1.5	1.7	1.1	1.6	1.1
1921–25	0.6	0.9	0.7	1.7	1.5	0.9	2.4	1.1
Overall rate 1901–25	0.7	1.2	1.4	1.4	1.5	0.8	1.5	1.1

Figure 1 shows the rate for 1000 live births for each year. The mean is 1.1 probable and possible cases and is fairly constant over the 25 years. There was no evidence of an epidemic year. Table II shows the rate for Belfast City and the six

223

counties, for the five quinquennial periods. The rate for the six counties is about twice that for Belfast except for County Londonderry which included the City of Londonderry, where the rate was similar to that for Belfast. These differences were statistically significant (P < 0.001).

Using various statistical techniques, Ashitey [3] could find no clustering of cases by date or place of birth for the rural areas.

Duration of the Disease

In 1973 I analysed the duration of the disease of 482 patients whose year of birth, year of onset and year of death were known (Table III) [4]. The average duration of disease in all patients was 21.5 years with an average age of onset of 32.5 years. The expectation of life in the general population at the age of 32 in 1940 was 42 years, so that the expectation of life in multiple sclerosis patients is about half that of the general population at the onset. There appeared to be no difference between the sexes, and marriage and presumably childbirth did not appear to worsen the outlook.

A small proportion of cases have a benign course. Between 1948 and 1951, 700 cases were diagnosed as suffering from multiple sclerosis. When reviewed in 1973, 220 (31%) were alive and of these 44 (6½%) were only minimally affected.

The longest duration to date in Northern Ireland was 62 years. A man in whom the diagnosis was confirmed at autopsy died aged 82 years with an onset of symptoms at 20 years of age [5].

TABLE III

	Year of birth	Year of onset	Year of death	Duration	Age of onset	Expectation of life
All (482)	1908	1940	1962	21.5	32.5	42
Men (223)	1907	1940	1962	21.6	33.0	40
Women Married (167)	1908	1941	1962	21.1	33.3	44
Unmarried (92)	1910	1939	1961	22.1	29.5	44

Occupation

The census for Northern Ireland in 1961 showed 16 socioeconomic groups for the population over the age of 15. The occupation was known for 427 males suffering from multiple sclerosis (Tables IV and V). There was a highly significant correlation with groups 13, 14 and 15 which were farmers and managers (13), farmers, own account (14) and agricultural workers (15). There was no evidence, as has been found in other centres, that social Class 1 was most at risk.

224

TABLE IV Distribution of Male Population of Northern Ireland (1961 Census) by Socio-economic Group* and Status re Multiple Sclerosis

Socioeconomic group	Known to have MS		Not known to have MS		Total	
1, 2, 3	23	(5.4%)	34 800	(7.6%)	34 823	(7.6%)
4, 5, 6	71	(16.7%)	67 947	(14.9%)	68 018	(14.9%)
7, 8, 9	100	(23.5%)	125 634	(27.5%)	125 734	(27.5%)
10, 11, 12	107	(25.0%)	134 679	(29.5%)	134 686	(29.4%)
13, 14, 15	118	(27.5%)	87 087	(19.0%)	87 205	(19.1%)
16	8	(1.9%)	6 968	(1.5%)	6 976	(1.5%)
Total	427	(100%)	457115	(100%)	457542	(100%)

$$\chi^2 = 25.9 \text{ (5 d.f.)} \qquad P < 0.001$$

*Classes 'Indefinite' and 'Not Applicable' excluded

TABLE V Distribution of Male Population of Northern Ireland (1961 Census) by Socio-economic Group* and Status re Multiple Sclerosis

Socioeconomic group	Known to have MS		Not known to have MS		Total	
13, 14, 15	118	(27.6%)	87 087	(19.1%)	87 205	(19.1%)
All other groups	309	(72.4%)	370 028	(80.9%)	370 337	(80.9%)
Total	427		457 115		457 542	

$$\chi^2 = 20.3 \text{ (1 d.f.)} \qquad P < 0.001$$

*Classes 'Indefinite' and 'Not Applicable' excluded.

Genetic Factors

The familial incidence in Northern Ireland is 6.58 per cent. The incidence of the disease in the sibs of the propositi is five to fifteen times greater than that in the general population [6].

There were, in 1977, ten first cousin marriages in the parents of 840 cases. All were born outside the two cities of Belfast and Londonderry (Table VI). When the figures were analysed by county (Table VII) the observed rates were very much greater than expected rates in all but County Armagh. However the expected rates may not be very accurate [7] but the differences are so great that genetic factors may explain in part the increased prevalence of the disease in rural areas. Six of the ten cases were closely connected with farming.

Environmental Factors

In recent years interest has been revived in the possibility that contact with household pets such as dogs or cats might have a part to play in the causation of multiple sclerosis. In 1977 I asked 50 consecutive outpatients suffering from multiple sclerosis if they had been exposed to dogs or cats in childhood. The control was the next outpatient. The 50 controls comprised 28 patients suffering from epilepsy, five from Parkinson's disease and the remainder from miscellaneous disorders. The 50 multiple sclerosis patients had been exposed to 37 dogs and 35 cats and the controls to 39 dogs and 28 cats. Four multiple sclerosis patients and six controls had been exposed to neither a dog nor a cat.

TABLE VI Consanguinity of MS in N. Ireland

	Not related	First cousins	%
Total patients	840	10	1.2
Born in 2 cities	257	0	0
Born outside 2 cities	512	10	1.9
Born outside N. Ireland	81	0	0

TABLE VII Consanguinity of MS in N. Ireland

County	Not related	First cousins	Expected %	Observed %
Antrim	117	2	0.069	1.68
Armagh	71	0	0.066	0
Down	138	4	0.034	2.78
Fermanagh	45	1	0.075	2.17
Londonderry	39	1	0.032	2.50
Tyrone	102	2	0.049	1.90

Soil

To date it has not been possible to relate the disease to the geology of the province [1]. A provisional geochemical survey of Northern Ireland was carried out in 1973 by the Imperial College of Science and Technology, London. Twenty trace elements were studied but I could see no obvious relationship of any to the disease. Selenium was not studied in this survey.

Comment

There is no evidence that the incidence of multiple sclerosis is either increasing or decreasing. There appear to be no epidemic years. The increased rural risk is probably due in part to genetic factors. The risk of 'inbreeding' in Northern Ireland is increased because the community tends to be divided into two separate religious and cultural groups. Mixed marriages are not encouraged and occur only rarely.

If the environmental factor is a virus it must be a common virus, or more than one common virus.

References

1   Millar, JHD (1971) *Multiple Sclerosis, a Disease Acquired in Childhood.* Charles Thomas, Springfield, Illinois
2   Ashitey, GA and Millar, JHD (1970) *Ulster Med. J., 39,* 55
3   Ashitey, GA (1969) MD thesis, the Queen's University, Belfast
4   Millar, JHD (1975) *Multiple Sclerosis Research.* HMSO, p 226
5   Allen, Ingrid V, Millar, JHD and Hutchinson, MJ (1978) *Neuropath. applied Neurobiol., 4.* 279
6   Allison, RS and Millar, JHD (1954) *Ulster Med. J., 23* (2)
7   Nevin, N (1979) Personal communication

Chapter 20

MULTIPLE SCLEROSIS IN THE FAROE ISLANDS*

John F Kurtzke

In 1956, Sutherland reported the results of his survey of MS in seven counties of north-western Scotland [1]. Prevalence was 113 per 100 000 population in the Shetland Islands, 80 in the Orkneys, and 79 in Caithness. Rates in the other counties ranged from 34 to 51. The Shetland-Orkney rates were by far the highest recorded to that date.

Shortly thereafter, Allison of Northern Ireland and Mogens Fog of Denmark undertook to carry out an intensive survey of MS in the Shetland-Orkneys and in the Faroe Islands, utilising the same field workers in both communities. The Faroes were chosen as an area similar in size, location, occupation and ethnicity to the Scottish Isles, and with the clinical impression that MS was rare among Faroese. Unfortunately, only brief reports of that work were ever published. Allison alluded to his Shetland-Orkney prevalence rate of 143 for 1962 [2], the same year for which Fog and Hyllested recorded a prevalence of 37 in the Faroes [3].

One feature that was striking in the latter series was that most of the Faroese patients were quite young and seemed to have short durations of illness at prevalence day. In 1966 I had commented to Hyllested on that point, but nothing further was done until the question was again raised in 1972. When the original case records of the 1962 series were then reviewed, though, it did seem that something unusual was present: no patient was found with onset of MS before the end of the 1940s. At that point Dr Hyllested and I began this work, which continues to be the most fascinating aspect I know of in this disease.

The Faroes are a group of small islands which lie between Norway and Iceland at 62° north latitude and 7° west longitude. The name of these islands in Danish is Faerøerne, and in Faroese Føroyar, both of which are generally translated as 'sheep islands'. Despite the etymological redundancy, the official English name is Faroe Islands. Until 1948 they were a county (*amt*) of Denmark, and they are still a semi-independent unit of the Kingdom of Denmark. The Faroese have their own language, flag, stamps, currency, and even a navy. They are a Nordic people, and theirs is a Scandinavian language, closest to Icelandic. In 1978 the population was more than 42 000. The capital is Tørshavn with over 13 000 inhabitants. Klaksvík, at some 5000 population, is the second largest town. Medical care has in the past been provided completely by Denmark, and it has long been the custom to send problem cases, including neurological ones, to the University Hospital (Rigshospitalet—RH) in Copenhagen. Since 1929 RH has had an independent

*Supported by the Veterans Administration and the National Multiple Sclerosis Society

Department of Neurology. Since 1933 there has been a nationwide Disability Compensation law in Denmark (including the Faroes), and since 1947 there has been the nationwide Danish MS Registry under Dr Hyllested, which also includes the Faroes.

Beginning in 1972, Hyllested and I have made an intensive search for all instances of known or suspected MS that had occurred on the Faroes. Sources of potential case material were: the Danish MS Registry files; death certificates for Faroese, 1920-76; Rigshospitalet Neurology Department records, 1929-76; the Disability Compensation files; the records of the major hospital on the Faroes, Queen Alexandrine Hospital (DAH) from the 1920s on. For all of these any diagnosis of 'suspect', 'possible' or 'probable' MS was the starting point for a full review by each of us independently of the complete medical records. In addition, the complete files of all three Faroese hospitals (DAH, Klaksvík Hospital, Tvøroyri Hospital) have been reviewed in detail for the period 1960-76 inclusive by Dr Paul Joensen of the Faroes, and all instances of neurological signs or symptoms that could possibly reflect MS were listed. From Dr Joensen's roster we reviewed the complete medical records of all such cases.

There were 78 potential cases found as of July 1977. Except for two instances (patients 55 and 58), all surviving patients up to case 60 were neurologically examined especially for this study in the 1974-77 period. Almost all of these examinations were performed jointly by us both. For almost all patients up to case 60 who had died, relatives were jointly interviewed by us as to residence, family, and neurological histories. We had assigned patient-numbers in such a manner that patients 60-78 were clearly to be discarded as even possible instances of MS; for these only record reviews were performed.

Our full report has been recently published [4]. Table I from that work provides a listing of the 25 native-born resident Faroese who comprise the entirety of the accepted cases of MS known as of July 1977. All patients save one met all requirements of the Schumacher Committee for definite MS [5]. The exception (patient 41) had a recurrent, but varied, myelopathy with three remissions. For this series, the mean age at onset was 26 years, and it was the same for each sex. The sex ratio was equal, with 13 males and 12 females. The clinical characteristics were typical of MS in general [4]. It was only when we looked at these cases over time that we began to find anomalies. Taking the living cases at various dates, there were marked variations in the prevalence rates. In 1950 the rate was 40.9 per 100 000 population; in 1961 it was 63.6; in 1972, 38.3; and in 1977 the rate was 33.7 per 100 000 (Table II). For 1939, the prevalence was 0. Even more discrepant from other series were the durations of illness at these prevalence days. There was a mean duration of 4 years in 1950, 10 years in 1961, 20 years in 1972, and 25 years in 1977. The mean ages of the patients also rose with time, though less steeply, from 31 years of age in 1950 to 48 in 1977.

Plotting these cases by calendar year of onset gave good evidence that on the Faroes, MS had suddenly appeared—and suddenly disappeared (Figure 1). All cases but one began between 1943 and 1960. It is these 24 cases of 1943-60 which meet all criteria of an epidemic: disease occurrence clearly in excess of normal expectancy, and likely to be derived from a common or propagated source.

229

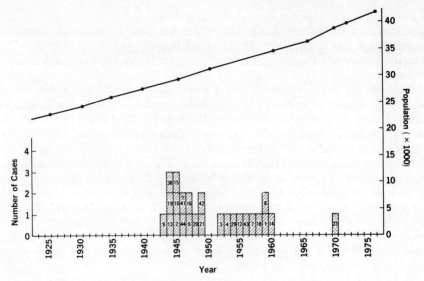

Figure 1 Distribution of MS cases among native-born resident Faroese by calendar year of clinical onset. *Numbers* identify the patients in Table I. Faroese population is recorded (From Kurtzke and Hyllested (1979) [4])

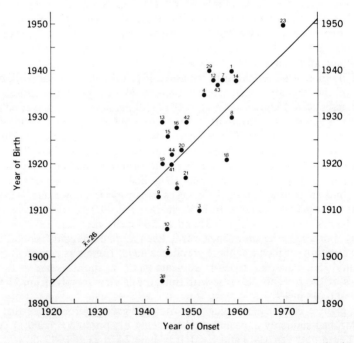

Figure 2 Distribution of MS cases among native-born resident Faroese by calendar years of birth and of onset. *Numbers* identify the patients in Table I. *Diagonal* represents the mean age at onset (From Kurtzke and Hyllested (1979) [4])

230

In Figure 2 we have plotted the cases by calendar year of both birth and onset of symptoms. The diagonal represents the mean age at onset of 26 years, and one would expect cases to cluster about this mean throughout the entire period. The primary conclusion from these data is that the MS of 1943-60 constitute a 'point-source' epidemic, the result perhaps of a single cause that was introduced into the Faroes at a single time before 1943.

In the land of Panum, it was, of course, necessary to compare this epidemic with the occurrence of measles, a need strengthened by the known frequency of elevated measles antibodies in MS. However, measles has been recurrently epidemic there over the last century, and certainly bears no relation to the MS epidemic (Figure 3). We are investigating other diseases and all deaths on the Faroes for the period from 1900 to 1977. All the death certificates have been recoded as to cause, but the results are still to be analysed.

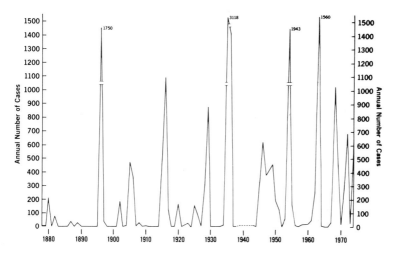

Figure 3 Measles in the Faroes. Annual number of cases reported between 1878 and 1974

The major unusual event that we have found so far on the Faroes was their occupation by British forces for five years in World War II. Denmark was overrun by Germany on 9 April 1940, and on 13 April a detachment of Royal Marines was landed on the Faroes. Within two months they were replaced by the permanent occupation forces. The latter are said to have numbered some 8000 men [6], or almost one Briton for every three Faroese (Figure 4). We have since obtained some 1100 feet of microfilm from the Public Record Office in London, which are copies of all the surviving War Diaries of the occupation forces. A preliminary assessment of these diaries has identified the units listed in Tables III for line forces and IV for support troops. Figure 5 provides the dates wherein these units were on the Faroes. A plus sign instead of an X indicates either an indirect source for the data rather than the unit's own War Diary, or the presence of components (such as RAF Station Vágar) before the official designation of the unit. Details as to specific

231

TABLE I Multiple Sclerosis in Native Resident Faroese, as of July 1977. Total Series by Sex and Calendar Years of Birth, Clinical Onset, and Death. Data of Kurtzke and Hyllested (1979) [4]

Case No.	Sex	Year of birth	Onset	Death
1	F	1940	1959	–
2	F	1901	1945	1966
3	F	1910	1952	1963
4	F	1935	1953	–
6	M	1915	1947	1965
7	M	1938	1957	1966
8	M	1930	1959	–
9	M	1913	1943	1971
10	F˙	1906	1945	–
12	M	1938	1955	–
13	M	1929	1944	–
14	M	1938	1960	1968
15	F	1926	1945	–
16	F	1928	1947	–
18	M	1921	1958	–
19	M	1920	1944	–
20	M	1923	1948	–
21	F	1917	1949	–
23	F	1950	1970	–
29	F	1940	1954	1976
38	M	1895	1944	1945
41	F	1920	1946	1957
42	M	1929	1949	1970
43	F	1937	1956	–
44	M	1922	1946	1970

TABLE II Some characteristics of the MS series, accepted cases, as of various prevalence days. From Kurtzke and Hyllested (1979) [4]

Characteristic	Prevalence day[a]				
	1939	1950	1961	1972	1977
Number of cases	0	13	22	15	14
(number of males)	–	(7)	(12)	(6)	(6)
Prev. rate per 100 000	–	40.9	63.6	38.3	33.7
Mean age @ PD	–	30.85–	35.73	42.67	48.43
Mean age @ onset	–	26.85–	25.32	23.07	23.71
Mean duration (yrs)	–	4.00	10.41	19.60	24.72
Time of onset:					
Mean	–	7/46	11/50	11/52	9/52
Median	–	1946	1949	1951	1951

[a]July 1

232

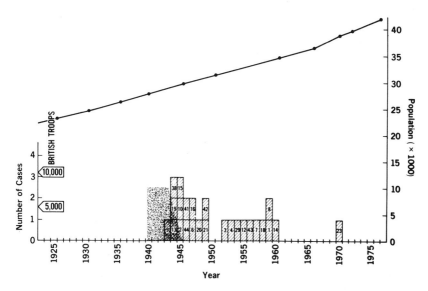

Figure 4 Distribution of MS cases among native-born resident Faroese by calendar year of clinical onset and provisional estimates of British troops during their occupation 1940–45 (*shaded area*) (From Kurtzke and Hyllested (1979) [4])

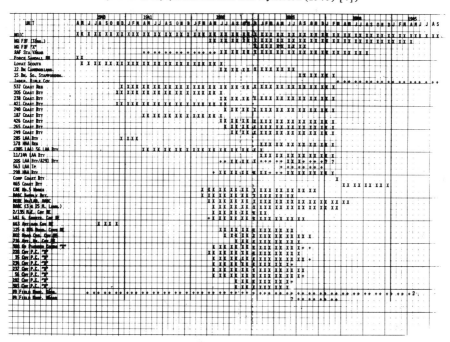

Figure 5 Occupation forces in the Faroes during World War II by units and dates, according to all surviving unit War Diaries available to the Public Record Office, London. A + instead of X indicates either an indirect source of data or the partial presence of the unit

233

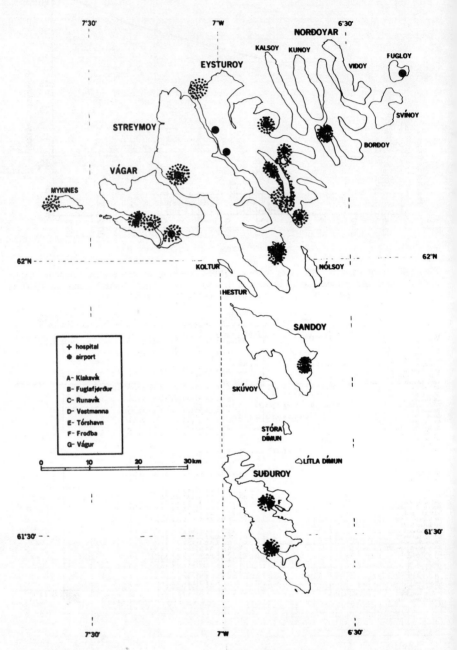

Figure 6 Residences of MS patients during World War II (*large solid circles*) superimposed on locations of British troops (*dotted areas*) during the 1940–45 occupation (From Kurtzke and Hyllested (1979) [4])

234

locations of the troops, and in particular their manning levels at any or all locations, have not been deciphered as yet. However, the locations drawn in Figure 6 have been supported, and thus far no additional sites have been found. The coincidence of the British and the patient residences during the war is, in fact, one of the most striking features of this work [4]. One other point is that many of the units, but not all, seem to be of Scottish origin rather than English. It would certainly be worth the effort if it were possible to identify each individual service man by name and birthplace, even if a follow-up is not feasible.

TABLE III Faroes Occupation WW II: 1. Line Forces

Source	Unit	Dates
Adm 116/5334, 199/671	NOIC	4.40-9.45
WO 176/73, 74	HQ, FIF (Tórshavn)	4.42-4.45
WO 176/75	HQ, FIF 'X' (Vágar)	12.42-9.43
AIR 28/873	RAF Sta Vágar	(4.41-5.42) / 6.42-8.44
Adm 202/432, 199/672	Force Sandall RM	4.40-5.40
WO 176/337	Lovat Scouts	5.40-6.42
WO 176/84	12 Bn Cameronians SR	6.42-7.43
WO 176/85	15 Bn So. Staffordshire Reg	8.43-2.44
–	'Indep. Rifle Coy'	3.44-9.45
WO 176/76	537 Coast Reg	12.40-2.44
WO 176/76	205 Coast Bty	11.40-6.42
WO 176/76	238 Coast Bty	6.42-2.44
WO 176/76	421 Coast Bty	11.40-7.42
WO 176/76	240 Coast Bty	7.42-2.44
WO 176/76	187 Coast Bty	4.41-6.42
WO 176/76	426 Coast Bty	6.42-2.44
WO 176/77, 76	265 Coast Bty	7.42-2.44
WO 176/76	249 Coast Bty	8.42-2.44
WO 176/82	285 LAA Bty (→)	12.40-3.41
WO 176/80, 81, 83	178 HAA Reg	1.43-2.44
WO 176/82	(285 LAA)→56 LAA Bty	4.41-1.43
WO 176/80	11/144 (Ulster) LAA Bty	1.43-2.44
WO 176/83	205 LAA Bty/A291 Bty	(6.42-12.43?)
–	(563 LAA Tp)	(6.43-12.43)
WO 176/81	290 HAA Bty	5.42-2.44
WO 176/79	Comp Coast Bty	3.44
WO 176/78	465 Coast Bty	4.44-12.44

An obvious next question is what has happened with MS in Iceland. The same Norse Vikings settled Iceland at about the same time as the Faroes. Like the Faroes, it had been a county of Denmark, but had attained semi-independence earlier in this century. Also like the Faroes it was occupied in World War II, not only by the British, but also by the Canadians and the Americans. Iceland declared its independence as a nation during that war.

With the late Kjartan Gudmundsson, we have collected all MS cases known in Iceland from 1900-1975 [7]. Figure 7 shows the correlation of these cases by

TABLE IV Faroes Occupation WW II: 2. Support Forces

Source	Unit	Dates
WO 176/86	CRE No 5 Works (Aerodrome) 'X'	3.42–11.43
WO 176/92	RASC Supply Det 'X'	3.42–7.43
WO 176/93	REME Workshop/LAD, RAOC 'X'	4.42–5.44
WO 176/94	RAOC Det (No 3, 25 Mob Laundry) 'X'	5.42–3.44
WO 176/87	No 2 Sec 135 M.E. Coy RE	5.42–2.43
WO 176/88	681 Gen Constr Coy RE 'X'	4.42–9.43
WO 176/337	663 Artisan Coy RE	8.40–11.40
WO 176/89	125 & 856 Quarrying Coys RE 'X'	6.42–7.43
WO 176/90	802 Road Constr Coy RE 'X'	7.42–10.43
WO 176/91	716 Artisan Works Coy RE 'X'	9.42–8.43
WO 176/95	309 Gp Pioneer Corps 'X'	5.42–10.43
WO 176/99	228 Coy Pioneer Corps 'X'	4.42–8.43
WO 176/96	35 Coy Pioneer Corps 'X'	5.42–10.43
WO 176/100	234 Coy Pioneer Corps 'X'	5.42–7.43
WO 176/101	237 Coy Pioneer Corps 'X'	5.42–9.43
WO 176/97	56 Coy Pioneer Corps 'X'	5.42–9.43
WO 196/98	192 Coy Pioneer Corps 'X'	9.42–7.43
WO 176/102	303 Coy Pioneer Corps 'X'	9.42–6.43
(WO 176/337)	9 Field Hospital Tórshavn	6.40–4.45(?)
	4 Field Hospital Vágar	(?)8.43–3.44

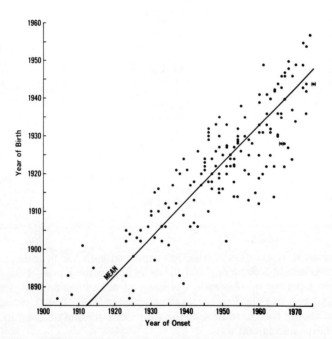

Figure 7 Distribution of MS cases in Iceland, 1900–1975, by calendar years of birth and of onset. *Diagonal* represents the mean age at onset (From Kurtzke et al, in preparation [7])

236

calendar year of birth and onset, the same as with the Faroes in Figure 2. There is certainly no abrupt appearance and no disappearance, but there does seem to be some degree of clustering of cases for ten years or so after 1945. Figure 8 gives the MS cases by year of onset alone. Overall, there seem to be three rather distinct phases in the chronology of MS in Iceland: a low and sporadic occurrence before World War I; a sudden rise in 1923 and then a plateau to 1944; then a sudden rise and an irregular plateau from 1945 on. The war periods are denoted by asterisks in the figure. As stated, Iceland was heavily occupied during World War II, and US military bases are still present there. In World War I Iceland was said possibly to have been a coaling station for the Royal Navy, and may have been a link in the convoys to the UK; but I am not aware of any formal occupation then. In that war its mother country, Denmark, had managed to remain neutral, so that a true occupation by either side would have been inappropriate.

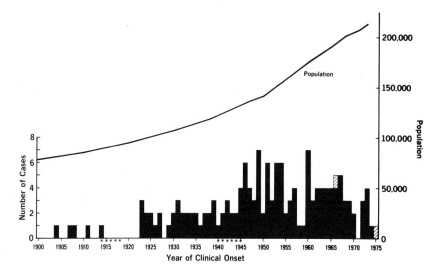

Figure 8 Distribution of MS cases in Iceland, 1900–1975, by calendar year of onset. Icelandic population is noted (From Kurtzke et al, in preparation [7])

However, especially for World War II, and particularly with the steadily increasing population base over time, it is not too unlikely that the disease was reintroduced, or at least reinforced, concomitant with the occupation. We may possibly see here also the 'critical mass' of population required to maintain the disease within a relative geographic isolate. Throughout this century the population of Iceland has been about five times that of the Faroes. While not as definitive, then, as in the Faroes, the Icelandic saga may warrant as detailed scrutiny as we are attempting to accomplish for the Faroes in terms of the introduction and epidemic occurrence of MS.

237

Summary

Up to 1977, Hyllested and I have been able to identify on the Faroe Islands 25 cases of multiple sclerosis among native-born resident Faroese. All but one had clinical onset of MS between 1943 and 1960; one began in 1970. Median year of onset was 1949. The 24 included cases of 1943-60 met all criteria for a point-source epidemic. Measles on the Faroes was not related in time to the MS. Other diseases and causes of death are under investigation, but present evidence as to a source for this epidemic points to the British troops, who occupied the Faroes in large numbers for five years from April 1940. Residences of all but three patients during the war were locations where the troops were stationed, and these three also had direct contact with the British. Available war diaries seem to confirm our earlier data as to the troop locations, but numbers and durations of the occupation forces need clarification. Many of the British units would appear to have been Scottish rather than English in composition.

MS in Iceland *may* have features in common with the Faroese situation. Over time there seem to have been two step-wise increases there in the occurrence of new cases of MS: after World War I; and after World War II, with plateaus following each of these increments.

References

1 Sutherland, JM (1956) *Brain, 79,* 635
2 Allison, RS (1963) *Proc. Roy. Soc. Med., 56,* 71
3 Fog, M and Hyllested, K (1966) *Acta Neurol. Scand., 42* (suppl. 19), 9
4 Kurtzke, JF and Hyllested, K (1979) *Ann. Neurol., 5,* 6
5 Schumacher, GA, Beebe, GW, Kibler, RF, et al (1965) *Ann. N.Y. Acad. Sci., 122,* 552
6 Müller, E (1945) *Fem Aar Under Union Jack,* Gyldendal, Copenhagen
7 Kurtzke, JF, Gudmundsson, KR and Bergmann, S (in preparation)

Chapter 21

MULTIPLE SCLEROSIS AMONG IMMIGRANTS TO ENGLAND

Geoffrey Dean, Hilda McLoughlin, Rosaleen Brady,
A M Adelstein, Joanne Tallett-Williams and Marta Elian

Between 1972 and 1975 a study was undertaken to ascertain the hospitalised prevalence of multiple sclerosis among immigrants to the United Kingdom. They came from areas of the world where the disease is common, such as Europe and Ireland, the old commonwealth countries of Australia, Canada and New Zealand, and from areas of the world where MS is believed to be uncommon, that is, India, Pakistan, Africa and the West Indies. First admissions for motor neurone disease were used as a control. In this study all hospitalised patients in Greater London and the West Midlands were included between the years 1960 and 1972. The majority of immigrants came from countries that are now called the 'new commonwealth countries', which, in the main, are countries that were formerly colonies of the British Empire. Many of them have settled in Greater London and the West Midlands, that is, the area in and around Birmingham and Wolverhampton [1, 2].

First admissions to hospital for multiple sclerosis were as common, or nearly as common, among immigrants from Europe and the old commonwealth countries as in the United Kingdom-born. Among immigrants from Ireland the hospitalised prevalence of MS was two-thirds of that in the United Kingdom-born. This lower risk in the Irish may be because it is really less common among Irish immigrants or it may be that those Irish immigrants to England who do develop the symptoms of MS return to Ireland (Table I).

TABLE I Greater London Residents First Admissions 1960–1972. By birthplace

	Actual	Expected
Europe	152	158.1
Ireland	168	225.3
Old commonwealth	17	24.8
America (N and S)	12	16.5
Cyprus	23	35.0
USSR	4	7.1

The actual and expected number, age-standardised at United Kingdom-born rates, of MS patients born in Europe and resident in Greater London and first admitted to hospital between 1960 and 1972 is shown in Table II. Immigrants

239

from northern and central Europe had the same risk of MS as the United Kingdom-born. Immigrants from Italy, 24 MS patients in London and 27 expected, had almost as high a risk of developing MS as the United Kingdom-born. A high proportion of the Italian immigrants came from southern Italy and Sicily. Immigrants from Spain had a significantly reduced risk of being hospitalised with MS, 8 patients when 16.4 were expected. Also from southern Europe (Table I) immigrants from Cyprus had two-thirds of the risk of the United Kingdom-born, 23 MS patients when 35 were expected.

TABLE II Greater London Residents First Admissions 1960–1972. Europe

	M	F	Total	Exp.
Germany	3	31	34	29.2
Italy	12	12	24	27.2
Poland	18	7	25	25.4
Austria	1	8	9	11.0
France	4	7	11	9.8
Belgium/Luxembourg	0	2	2	3.9
Netherlands	1	2	3	4.3
Hungary	3	4	7	6.1
Spain	0	8	8	16.4*
Other	8	21	29	24.8
Total	50	102	152	158.1

* Only Spain shows a significant difference between actual and expected number (P $>$ 0.05)

In contrast to the high risk of MS among immigrants from Europe, with immigrants from the new commonwealth countries of America (the West Indies), Africa, Asia and Europe (Malta) the risk of being hospitalised with MS is very small. The small number of immigrants with MS who were born in these countries were nearly all of European stock. For instance, there was only one Indian and no Pakistanis among the large number of Indian and Pakistani immigrants from Asia resident in Greater London and there were no Africans with MS. The very low risk of MS among Asian, African and, to a lesser extent, the West Indian immigrants has been confirmed by Adelstein from studies of deaths certified as having MS (see Chapter 22). Among the immigrants born in the islands of Malta there were no hospitalised MS patients, although 10 (9.7) would have been expected in London and the West Midlands if they had had the United Kingdom-born risk (Table III).

The southern Mediterranean area would appear, therefore, to be an area of particular interest as it is at the junction between the high MS prevalence found among immigrants to England from Europe and the negligible risk of MS among African immigrants to England. We have, therefore, undertaken studies of the prevalence of MS in the southern Mediterranean in the island of Sicily (see Chapter 24) and in the islands of Malta (see Chapter 23) on behalf of the Special-

240

ised Working Group—Epidemiology of the European Community. Both Sicily and Malta have been invaded, in turn, by people of Phoenician, Greek, Roman, Carthaginian and Arab stock, as these islands are on the crossroads of the Mediterranean. The people of Malta speak an Arabic tongue and there may well be a difference in the genetic strain of the Maltese people in comparison with those of Sicily, with a more Semitic element in Malta. The HLA blood group composition of the MS patients and of controls in the islands of Malta and of Sicily is now being studied.

Sicily, the Maltese islands and the north coast of Africa are at the meeting point of high and low MS prevalence. Here the genetic and environmental factors associated with MS can be compared and contrasted. Such studies should throw great light on our understanding of the aetiology of multiple sclerosis.

TABLE III Greater London Residents First Admissions 1960-1972. Low MS Areas

	Actual	Expected
New commonwealth		
America (West Indies)	16	130.0
Africa	4 *	25.8
Asia (excluding Cyprus)	13 *	85.7
Europe (Malta)	0	8.4
Burma	1 *	3.9
China	0	2.8
South Africa	3 *	11.5
London and West Midlands		
Malta	0	9.7

* All except one Indian from Asia and one from Africa descendants of European forebears

Acknowledgements

The study on MS among immigrants to Britain was supported by the Multiple Sclerosis Society of Great Britain and Northern Ireland.

References

1   Dean, G, McLoughlin, H, Brady, R, Adelstein, AM and Tallett-Williams, J (1976) Brit. Med. J., 1, 861.
2   Dean, G, Brady, R, McLoughlin, H, Elian, M and Adelstein, AM (1977) Brit. J. Prev. and Soc. Med., 31, 3, 141
3   Dean, G, Grimaldi, G, Kelly, R and Karhausen, L (1979) J. Epid. and Commun. Hlth., 33, 107
4   Vassallo, L, Elian, M and Dean, G (1979) J. Epid. and Commun. Hlth., 33, 111

Chapter 22

MORTALITY FROM MULTIPLE SCLEROSIS, MOTOR NEURONE DISEASE AND CEREBROVASCULAR DISEASE AMONG IMMIGRANTS IN ENGLAND AND WALES

A M Adelstein

Introduction

Comparing disease rates of immigrants with those of populations in home and host countries is a useful way of seeking clues to causes. For such comparisons, analysing causes of death as revealed in routine death certification has many advantages. In England and Wales, immigrants and home population receive similar medical care and medical certification of death.

Scope

In England and Wales there are fairly large numbers of immigrants from Europe and from three main groups of the Commonwealth—West Indies, Indian Sub-Continent, and Africa. There are smaller numbers from the rest of the Commonwealth, from the USA and from other countries outside the British Isles. England and Wales also have large numbers of people born in other countries of the British Isles—Scotland, Northern Ireland and Eire. However, because these immigrants need no formalities to move freely across borders in the British Isles, and because these movements have a long history, selection factors that influence their migration may well be quite different from those that operate in more foreign and distant countries from which entry may be formalised and restricted and may include health checks.

Methods

This analysis of death rates is based on registrations of deaths and, for (some) denominators, on the numbers of persons enumerated in the 1971 Census. For both numerators and denominators an immigrant is a person who was born outside England and Wales (as recorded in the Census or at registration of death).

To estimate numbers of immigrants with Commonwealth ethnic origins (as apart from place of birth) a question in the Census asked for country of birth of parents. But there was no similar question for registrations of deaths. In this paper we use two methods of estimating death rates: first, conventional death rates by country of birth, irrespective of ethnicity (SMR is the percentage ratio of observed number to expected based on national age rates); secondly, proportional mortality rates for various causes in ethnic groups, as judged by their names on death certificates. Expected numbers of deaths for a category of disease (e.g. multiple sclerosis) are calculated by applying the proportion of all deaths attributed to the particular disease in the national figures, to deaths among the ethnic group, age by age.

Cause of Death

This is based on coding of the so-called underlying cause using the *International Classification of Diseases* (8th revision). Dean and Adelstein [1] carried out a prospective check of causes of death attributed to known multiple sclerosis patients in England. Among 168 who subsequently died, multiple sclerosis was stated as the cause, in Part I of the certificate, in 44 per cent, and in Part II (contributory causes) in 27 per cent, while in 29 per cent multiple sclerosis was not mentioned. We have no reason to suspect that there would be significantly different problems of diagnosing cause of death between immigrants and others.

For traditional analysis based on population at risk we analysed deaths over the five year period 1969-73, by country of birth. For ethnic analysis, judged by names, deaths during the 3-year period 1970-72 were used. In all analyses expected numbers of deaths are age standardised.

Figures are shown in Tables I and II. The patterns of mortality rates among the immigrants differ between multiple sclerosis and motor neurone disease. For motor neurone disease there are no significant differences between observed and expected numbers of deaths estimated either by populations or by proportions of all deaths (Table I).

TABLE I Multiple Sclerosis and Motor Neurone Disease Deaths among Immigrants, England and Wales 1969-73. Expected deaths based on age-standardised populations

Place of birth	Multiple sclerosis		Motor neurone disease	
	Actual	Expected	Actual	Expected
Europe (including USSR)	67	69.2	39	44.3
Ireland	84	94.2	59	58.7
India and Pakistan	11	29.9	17	16.6
New Commonwealth Africa	0	4.3	1	1.3
West Indies	3	18.1	6	6.7

However, for multiple sclerosis there are distinctly fewer deaths than expected among persons born in the 'New' Commonwealth: India, Africa or West Indies (Table II). For immigrants from the Indian Sub-Continent and Commonwealth Africa, classified by names into ethnic groups, there are clear differences—ethnic Asians and Africans have a much more clearly marked paucity of death attributed to multiple sclerosis than do people of British (or European) origins. For persons of Asian or African ethnic origin there were no deaths, although over 14 were expected on national rates. Among West Indians (no ethnic separation was possible) there were 2 deaths, and 13 were expected.

243

TABLE II Multiple Sclerosis and Motor Neurone Disease Deaths among Immigrants, England and Wales, 1970-72, by ethnicity expected on proportional rates. Expected deaths based on proportions of all deaths (age standardised)

Place of birth	Multiple sclerosis		Motor neurone disease	
	Actual	Expected	Actual	Expected
Indian Subcontinent:				
Persons of Asian origin	0	11.6	2	4.6
Persons of other origin	6	8.9	5	6.7
All born in India	66	20.5	7	11.3
African New Commonwealth:				
Asian and African origin	0	2.6	0	0.7
Other origin	0	1.1	0	0.7
West Indies	2	13.4	3	4.1
Europe (including USSR)	53	40.4	27	25.6
Ireland	48	70.0	34	43.6

Although rates of mortality among immigrants from Europe are on the whole similar to those of all persons in England and Wales, there are differences between people from separate countries; death rates from multiple sclerosis are higher among immigrants from Germany and from Poland. SMRs are 189 and 173 with 15 and 17 deaths respectively.

Discussion

Mortality rates in England and Wales from multiple sclerosis parallel rates of hospital admissions in that they are extremely low for immigrants from Asia, Africa or West Indies and more especially for the ethnically indigenous people of these countries. Motor neurone disease, showing no such pattern, is analysed as a control group against the possibility that there was a strong selective force preventing potential multiple sclerosis cases from emigrating. The conclusion must be in line with the findings by Dean and others [2] that multiple sclerosis is exceedingly rare among the indigenous people of the New Commonwealth and that this immunity persists after emigration. It is too early to know whether immigrant children will continue to be immune throughout life.

Cerebrovascular Disease

This ICD category (A85) includes haemorrhage, thrombosis and other cerebrovascular disorders. Perusal of SMRs (at ages 20-69) for immigrants from various continents shows that two are outstandingly high, i.e. above 200 in either males or females. These high rates are for immigrants from West Indies and from Africa. For West Indian immigrants, SMRs were 206 and 235 for males and females re-

244

spectively (based on 164 and 129 deaths) and for African Commonwealth immigrants SMRs were 203 and 190, based on 39 male and 23 female deaths.

When deaths of immigrants from Commonwealth Africa are examined by ethnic origin, Africans have a PMR of 177 while the PMR for those of British origin is 129. These are based on relatively small numbers (24 and 15) but, taken together with the high SMR rate for all persons born in Africa, they point clearly to very high rates for immigrant Africans.

In parallel with high rates of mortality from strokes are exceptionally high mortality rates from hypertensive heart disease for both these communities and these, again, are in keeping with high rates of hypertension reported from various communities in Africa, the West Indies and among black people in the USA [4]. However, there does not seem to be clear evidence as to whether these high rates are the result of enviroi ment or heredity. It should be noted that there are large differences in mortality from hypertensive disease and from strokes among social classes in England and Wales; for hypertensive disease rates rise regularly from 71 for men in social class I (professional) to 141 for men in social class V (unskilled labourers). For cerebrovascular disease they range from 75 in social class I to 138 in social class V [3].

Summary

In England and Wales death rates from multiple sclerosis in immigrants from the Indian Sub-Continent, the West Indies, and Africa are very low, especially for those immigrants whose names suggest that they are ethnically Asian or African. Mortality attributed to motor neurone disease is unexceptional among immigrants. Mortality attributed to strokes and to hypertensive disease is very high among immigrants from the West Indies and from Africa, especially if they are ethnically African.

Acknowledgements

I thank the Registrar General for permission to publish, and colleagues for their help. My special thanks to Mr Bulusu for his assistance.

References

1 Dean, G, McLoughlin, H, Brady, R, Adelstein, AM, Tallett-Williams, J (1976) Multiple sclerosis among immigrants in Greater London. *Brit. Med. J., 1,* 861
2 Dean, G, Adelstein, AM, et al (1977) Motor Neurone Disease and Multiple Sclerosis among immigrants to Britain. *Brit. J. Prev. Soc. Med., 31,* 141
3 Occupational Mortality 1970-72 (1978) Office of Population, Censuses and Surveys, HMSO
4 Harburg, E, Gleibermann, L, et al (1978) Skin Colour, Ethnicity, and Blood Pressure 1: Detroit Blacks. *Amer. J. Publ. Hlth., 68* (12), 1177

Chapter 23

MULTIPLE SCLEROSIS IN SOUTHERN EUROPE: PREVALENCE IN MALTA

Luis Vassallo, Marta Elian and Geoffrey Dean

Introduction

The prevalence of MS is known to be high, in the region of 50-60 per 100 000, in north and central Europe and it is believed to be low on the African continent [1]. The prevalence of MS in the islands of southern Europe, for instance in the islands of Sicily and Malta, placed between the areas of suspected high and low MS prevalence, could yield important information on the environmental and genetic factors responsible for the disease. Although the environment would appear to be of major importance in the causation of MS, genetic factors are probably associated with susceptibility to the disease, as shown by the increased frequency of certain histocompatibility antigens (HLA-A3, B7 and DW2), in patients with MS [2], and genetic factors require consideration as well as the environmental factors if any major differences in MS prevalence are found.

Among immigrants to England from Malta (including a small number from the island of Gibraltar) and resident in Greater London and the West Midlands of England, no patients were admitted to hospital with MS between 1960 and 1972, 9.7 being the expected number if they had had the same admission rate as the United Kingdom-born [3, 4]. The absence of hospitalised patients diagnosed as having MS among immigrants from Malta can be contrasted with immigrants from the island of Cyprus among whom there were 23 hospitalised MS patients, 39.3 being the expected number at the United Kingdom-born rates. The absence of MS patients among the Maltese immigrants suggested the need to undertake a survey of the prevalence of MS on the islands of Malta in order to disprove or confirm that MS was uncommon among the Maltese.

The population of the Maltese islands of Malta (297 600–1975) and Gozo (25 000–1975) was approximately 326 000 in 1975. The people of Malta speak an Arabic language and are largely of Semitic origin, although Malta has, like Sicily, been peopled in its time by Phoenicians, Carthaginians, Greeks, Romans and Arabs.

Malta has an excellent health service, largely state supported, with a state teaching hospital and medical school. There has long been a strong alliance between the Maltese and British Medical Associations and medical profession, and many Maltese doctors have studied and practised in England and taken higher English degrees.

Method

A search was made for all patients diagnosed as having possible or probable MS, or other conditions such as encephalitis or retrobulbar neuritis which might have indicated MS. We received the most helpful collaboration from the government, the medical profession and the hospitals. Meetings were held with physicians and ophthalmologists, with general practitioners and also with medical officers of health. The neurological records at the government hospital in Valetta were examined for patients diagnosed as possible or probable MS or retrobulbar neuritis. We also had the collaboration of the medical and records staff of all the Maltese hospitals, including the Naval Hospital, Mtarfa. The list of all those receiving disability benefits on the islands was checked for further cases of possible MS.

Because of the close collaboration between the Maltese and the British health service, patients are frequently sent at state expense for full investigation at the London teaching hospitals, and patients with a neurological condition are frequently referred to the National Hospital, Queen Square. Summaries of the investigations undertaken on patients who had been investigated at the London hospitals were obtained.

The Professors of Medicine in Malta, past and present, the hospital and naval physicians, the ophthalmologists and the government doctors, all collaborated with this study and all patients who might possibly have MS were investigated.

Results

After an intensive search, only 14 patients with probable multiple sclerosis (8 males and 6 females) and 3 with possible multiple sclerosis could be found resident in the islands on the chosen prevalence day, 1 January 1978, and no patients with retrobulbar neuritis only. Of the 14 probable MS, 11 were living on the main island of Malta and 3 on the island of Gozo. Fourteen probable MS patients out of a population of 322 600 is a crude prevalence of 4.3 per 100 000 (5.2 male, 3.6 female per 100 000). Age-standardised for the population of England and Wales, the rate in Malta would be 4.2 per 100 000.

Among the 14 probable MS patients in Malta paraesthesia was the first symptom in 6, paraplegia and retrobulbar neuritis in 3 each and diplopia in 2. The average age on prevalence day was 34.9 years (35.9 for males and 33.5 for females). The average age at onset was 28.3. All the patients had at least partial remission. One of the patients included has been diagnosed as having Devic's syndrome. Of the 14 patients, 9 had also been investigated at a London teaching hospital, and 7 of these at the National Hospital, when the diagnosis of MS had been confirmed. Two of the three patients with possible MS had also been investigated at the National Hospital. It is of great interest that no one was found with a history of retrobulbar neuritis only. None of the MS patients was related, as far as we could ascertain, and all, except one who was born in Italy, were born on the islands of Malta.

Multiple sclerosis was recorded as a primary or contributory cause of death on only 6 death certificates on the Maltese islands between 1967 and 1976. In 5 of

247

these the history and clinical findings confirm the diagnosis and the sixth was probably incorrectly certified. The small number of deaths in which multiple sclerosis (or disseminated sclerosis) is mentioned as a cause of death confirms the small number of patients found to have MS among the living population.

Discussion

After three years' study in close collaboration with the doctors, hospitals and health department in the islands of Malta, only 14 patients have been found to have probable MS and one of these is diagnosed as having Devic's syndrome—a prevalence of 4.3 per 100 000. The low prevalence of MS in Malta is confirmed by the small number of death certificates in Malta in which MS is mentioned, six in 11 years, and by the absence of Maltese patients admitted to hospital in Greater London and the West Midlands (1960-1972) diagnosed as having MS among the Maltese population resident in the United Kingdom. It is possible that we may have overlooked a few undiagnosed MS patients with complete remissions, or a very benign course, living in Malta but they are likely to be few in view of the high level of investigation of neurological disorders that we found in Malta.

The low prevalence of MS in Malta found in this study, 4.3 per 100 000, is less than one-tenth of the expected number at the UK-born rates. It is in great contrast with the high rates found in Enna city in Sicily, 53 per 100 000 [3]. The climate of Sicily and Malta is very similar, although the highland of central Sicily has a colder drier climate than at the coast or on the islands of Malta. The standard of living and way of life of the people in Sicily and Malta are similar but medical attention, with the state health support, is perhaps more available in the islands of Malta.

There are, no doubt, some genetic differences between the populations of Sicily and Malta, with more people of Semitic origin in Malta, and a comparison of the HLA distribution in the populations and in the MS patients will be important. It is also interesting that retrobulbar neuritis, which does not develop into MS, is also uncommon in Malta.

Studies in the islands of the south of Europe, Sicily and Malta, and perhaps in Cyprus and on the north coast of Africa, should add significantly to our understanding of the aetiology of MS and, we hope, lead to its prevention.

Summary

After an intensive survey, only 14 patients have been found with a diagnosis of probable multiple sclerosis in the islands of Malta, which is a low prevalence of 4.2 per 100 000 population. The low MS prevalence is confirmed by the small number of deaths certified as due to MS, 6 in 11 years, and by the absence of Maltese MS patients resident in England among the MS patients admitted to hospital in Greater London and the West Midlands (1960-72). The low prevalence of MS found in Malta can be contrasted with the high prevalence found in Enna city in central

Sicily. The genetic and environmental reasons for this difference in MS prevalence between the neighbouring islands of Sicily and Malta requires further study.

Acknowledgements

The report is published in the *British Journal of Epidemiology and Community Health,* 1979, *33,* 111 and we wish to thank the Editors for their permission to publish in this volume.

We are also grateful to the Committee for Medical Research of the European Economic Community for their support.

References

1 McAlpine, D, Lumsden, CE and Acheson, ED (1965) *Multiple Sclerosis—A Reappraisal.* E & S Livingstone, Edinburgh and London
2 Editorial (1976) *Lancet, ii,* 1286
3 Dean, G et al (1976) *Brit. Med. J., 1,* 861
4 Dean, G et al (1977) *Brit. J. Prev. Soc. Med., 31,* 3, 141

Chapter 24

MULTIPLE SCLEROSIS IN SOUTHERN EUROPE: PREVALENCE IN SICILY

R Kelly

Among the interesting observations that were made by Geoffrey Dean in his useful study of the prevalence of multiple sclerosis among the immigrant population of London [1] was the fact that the high prevalence of multiple sclerosis among Italian immigrants resident in London suggested that the prevalence of multiple sclerosis in Italy as a whole was not greatly different from that in the United Kingdom; and furthermore, that this figure was not artificially boosted because of the high proportion of immigrants from the north of Italy since the majority of immigrants from Italy tend to come from the south and from Sicily. This observation raised in our minds the possibility that the previously reported figures of prevalence in various parts of Italy might be incorrect. As Figure 1 shows, taken

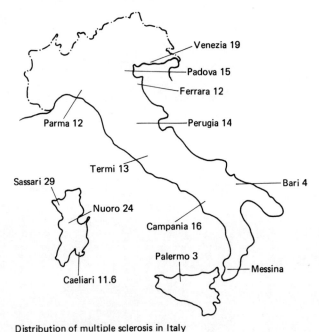

Distribution of multiple sclerosis in Italy

Figure 1   Distribution of multiple sclerosis in Italy (Reproduced from Report of Societa Italiana Di Neurologia, XIX Congresso Nazionale, Genova 3 December 1975)

250

from the report of the Societa Italiana di Neurologia 19th Congresso Nationale, Genova 3 December 1975 [2] it will be seen that everywhere the prevalence has been reported as being very much lower than it is in the British Isles and in Northern Europe, with the highest prevalence apparently in Nuoro and in Sassari of 24 and 29, and the figures in Sicily as low as 3, with a tendency for them to be slightly higher in the north of Italy. It therefore seemed reasonable to try to arrange a personal survey of patients in the south of Italy. We selected Sicily because, as can be seen in Figure 2, it not only represents the most southerly part of Italy and is

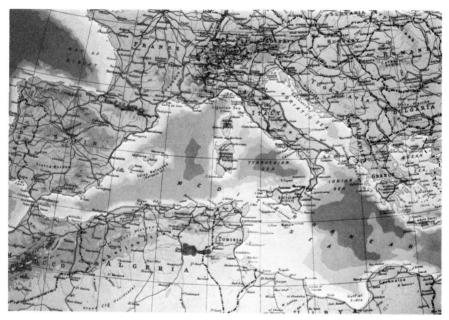

Figure 2 Sicily, the most southerly part of Italy, geographically close to North Africa, and on the same latitude as Malta (Reproduced from Readers Digest Great World Atlas)

geographically close to North Africa, where the prevalence has been reported as being extremely low, but it is also roughly at the same latitude as Malta where Geoffrey Dean [3] demonstrated that there were no patients with multiple sclerosis among the Maltese immigrants in London (*see* Chapter 21). Having settled on Sicily, it was decided first that it would be appropriate to study, if possible, a small self-contained community that was reasonably isolated. For this reason, Enna (Fig. 3) in central Sicily was selected. Secondly, it was selected because it alone had a hospital with an adequate diagnostic index. Enna city had 28 189 residents in 1971, it is a mid-point between the three university cities of Palermo, Catania and Messina, it has a good hospital and neurological service, and at a height of 1000 metres, it is colder than cities at the coast with a winter temperature that averages -1 to +5°C.

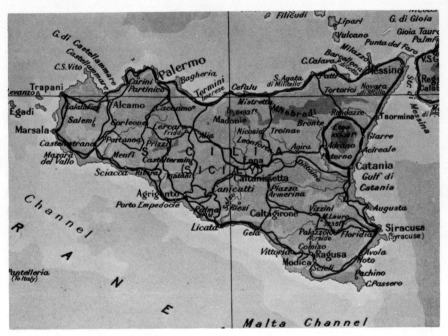

Figure 3   Enna, a self-contained community in central Sicily (Reproduced from Readers Digest
Great World Atlas)

Method

Full co-operation was obtained from the physicians at the Ospedale Umberto I,
Enna and from the 85 general practitioners in the town. Because patients with
multiple sclerosis tend to visit other centres for medical opinion and treatment,
we also obtained a list of patients resident in Enna city and province from the
studies that are being undertaken on the prevalence of multiple sclerosis at
Palermo, Messina and Catania and the multiple sclerosis research centre at
Gallarate, Milan and the collaborative study of the Italian Society of Neurologists.

The records of patients submitted to the neurological department in the
Ospedale Umberto I over a 16-year period was studied. Patients with a diagnosis
of MS, encephalitis, myelopathy or optic neuritis were reviewed and those patients
who had been recorded as 'possible multiple sclerosis' in the hospital records at
Palermo, Messina and Catania and at the MS research centre at Gallarate were
included in the study. All patients who had not died or emigrated were seen by
us and each patient's clinical history was reviewed and the neurological examination repeated.

252

Results

There were 15 patients with probable multiple sclerosis resident in Enna city who had the symptoms of the disease on prevalence day, 1 January 1975. Three of the probable MS patients were male and 12 were female and there were two further patients with a diagnosis of possible MS only (Table I).

TABLE I Numbers of MS Patients found in Enna. Total population 281 189

Prevalence day	Total	Male	Female
1 January 1975	15	3	12

Presenting Symptoms (Table II)

Paraparesis was the first symptom in 7 patients, paraesthesiae in 3, impairment of vision in 3 and the remaining 2 presented with attacks of vertigo or of sciatic pain respectively. The average age of the three males in the study on prevalence day was 36.3 years and of the 12 females 37.5 years. The average age of onset was 26.4: one patient had her first symptom at 8 years and another at 15 years. Of the 15 patients, 14 had at least partial remissions and only one patient had a non-remitting course. In her case, investigation in hospital in Milan and Bologna showed no other alternative pathology than MS to account for her symptoms (Table II).

TABLE II MS in Sicily: Presenting Symptoms

Paraparesis	7	
Paraesthesiae	3	
Impairment of vision	3	
Vertigo	1	
Sciatica	1	
Average age at onset		26.4
Average age on prevalence day		36.3 males
		37.5 females

Of a population of 28 189, 15 patients with probable MS is a true prevalence of 53 (52.9) per 100 000, 22 (21.8) per 100 000 male, 82 (82.1) per 100 000 female. If these rates are age-standardised from the Enna population to the population of England and Wales the expected rate for England and Wales would also be 53 (53.3) per 100 000.

As has been shown, the MS prevalence of 53 per 100 000 found in Enna city is the highest prevalence for MS that has yet been found in any community in Italy and is several times greater than any previously reported in Sicily. It must be stressed that this is a minimum prevalence rate, not only because, no doubt, some patients with multiple sclerosis have been overlooked, but also because some are likely to have been excluded since we adhered to the strictest criteria for máking the diagnosis. No one was included who did not have clear evidence of multiple lesions on history and examination. The true prevalence of MS in Enna is therefore probably higher than we have established.

Studying the history and the clinical condition of the patients presented to us with identifiable disease, we were struck by the fact that it appeared as though multiple sclerosis pursues a less benign course in this part of Europe. For example, all three males examined had a fixed disability, the first after six years, the second after an unidentifiable period, and the third after ten years. Of the 12 females included in the study, 2 (cases 5 and 6) had long remissions, one at 28 and the other 22 years. Only 5 of the 12 had had complete remission. Of the 12 women, 10 had a fixed disability at an average of just over six years after the onset of the illness and, if the two women with long remissions were included, at less than ten years. This is quite contrary to usual experience in the North of Europe, though one would expect to find no evidence of disability whatsoever in over 50 per cent of patients examined six years after the beginning of the illness and very nearly half of the patients when examined ten years after its start. In a series of 335 consecutive patients seen by one of the authors, 183 patients had a history extending back a minimum of ten years without developing a fixed disability and 74 of them (nearly one-fifth of the total patients) had a history of over 20 years [4]. We may, of course, have overlooked some patients resident in Enna who had complete remissions and a more benign course. The minimum prevalence of multiple sclerosis in Enna city—53 per 100 000—is of the same order of magnitude as has been found in studies in Northern Europe; for instance, the reported prevalence of MS in Northern Ireland is 64 [5] and in the Republic of Ireland 65 per 100 000 [6]. As Enna is on high ground and is somewhat colder than the central cities of Sicily a similar study is being undertaken in two small coastal cities.

The fact that we have found a high prevalence of MS in Enna city is no doubt partly due to the fact that an intensive survey has been undertaken in a small population that is provided with a good neurological service. The very low MS prevalence rates reported for many of the other Italian studies may be due to the difficulties in undertaking such studies in large population groups. We feel that intensive surveys in small populations are likely to give more accurate prevalence rates than surveys in large groups. We think it is unlikely that the number we found in Enna was a freak occurrence, and further studies, as yet unpublished, in Agrigento and near Palermo have supported our observations. As mentioned before, the prevalence noted by Geoffrey Dean in his studies on London immigrants supports our figures. A second and more likely explanation, and in my view the more correct explanation, carries implications for the interpretation of all data in epidemiological studies. It has become the established dogma throughout Italy that MS is rare in Italy and rarer in the more southern areas. This prevents the diagnosis being considered in many patients and results in their being indexed, if indeed a diagnostic index exists at all, under some other diagnosis. So, if a survey is carried out by an epidemiologist who depends upon the diagnostic index of someone else, he will net only those patients so diagnosed by the clinician concerned whereas, if a clinician untrained in the epidemiological method carries out a survey, the tendency is to report on those patients referred to him on the assumption that all are seen by him and are correctly diagnosed.

In many cities we have visited in Italy and elsewhere there exists no diagnostic index in the first place. Not only did we study independently all those patients in whom the diagnosis had been made but, by virtue of confining our study to a small circumscribed area of just about 30 000 people, we could rely on identifying nearly every patient in every GPs list who might have spinal cord or cerebral disease. by so doing we were able to identify a number of hitherto undiagnosed cases and we were also able to reject completely a number of wrongly diagnosed cases. It would have been quite impossible to conduct such a survey accurately over a much larger area without having to rely on others' observations. It is for this reason we feel that intensive surveys in small populations are likely to give more accurate prevalence rates than surveys in large groups.

We concluded that there was little reason to believe at present that the genetic background, the level of hygiene, or the way of life of the people of Enna were greatly different from that in other parts of Sicily but we were examining these factors further. A somewhat colder climate is unlikely by itself to account for a high prevalence of MS; for instance, MS is uncommon in Northern Japan which is much colder than Enna. We feel that the studies being undertaken in the southern tip of Europe, in Sicily and in Malta, and one we have already started in North Africa, may be the area where high prevalence and low prevalence MS meet and that the study may, hopefully, throw light on the genetic and environmental factors involved in the aetiology of multiple sclerosis.

Acknowledgements

This work has been published in the *Journal of Epidemiology and Community Health* [7] and we would like to thank the Editors for permission for the paper to be incorporated in this volume. We also wish to thank our many friends who made this study possible, in particular Professor Giorgio Macchi, the President of the Italian Society of Neurologists, Professor Carlo Cazzullo, the Director of the Centro Studi Sclerosi Multipla Gallarate, Professor Raffaelo Gattuso and Professor Francesco Nicoletti of the University of Catania, Professor Agostino Rubino, Dr Giovanni Savettieri and their colleagues at the University of Palermo, Professor Papalia and his colleagues at the University of Messina and Professor Luigi Amaducci of Florence.

We would particularly like to thank Dr Rizzo, Senior Neurologist, and Professor Grimald's Department of Neurology at Enna and the staff of the department, and in particular the Senior Nurse Maria Giuseppina Anzalone. The study was supported by the Committee for Medical Research for the European Economic Community.

This work was done in collaboration with Geoffrey Dean, Giuseppe Grimaldi and Lucien Karhausen, co-authors of the paper published in the *Journal of Epidemiology and Community Health* [7].

References

1 Dean, G, McLoughlin, H, Brady, R and Adelstein, AM (1976) *Brit. Med. J., 1,* 861
2 *Societa Italiana di Neurologia* (1975) XIX Congresso Nationale, Genova, 3 Decembre
3 Dean, G, Brady, R, McLoughlin, H, Elian, M and Adelstein, AM (1971) *Brit. J. Prev. Soc. Med., 31,* (3), 141
4 Kelly, RE (1972) *Pahlavi Med. J., 3,* 518
5 Millar, JHD (1971) *Multiple Sclerosis, A Disease Acquired in Childhood.* Charles C Thomas, Illinois
6 Brady, R et al (1977) *J. Irish Med. Assoc., 70* (17), 500
7 Dean, G, Grimaldi, G, Kelly, R and Karhausen, L (1979) *J. Epid. and Commun. Health 33,* 107

Part IV Paediatric Neuroepidemiology

Chapter 25

FETAL INFECTIONS AND NEUROLOGICAL HANDICAP

Catherine S Peckham

Several agents are known to infect the fetus, and if this infection is widespread and involves the CNS the resultant damage may cause permanent neurological handicap. It is difficult to estimate the true incidence of congenital infection because clinically recognisable maternal infection is the exception rather than the rule and the majority of infections are asymptomatic or lack specific pathognomonic features. The infected infant may be born with obvious neurological damage but in many instances defects may not be recognised or even develop until weeks, months or even years after birth. In the latter case the cause of handicap is unlikely to be known, and it is only from large prospective studies, when congenital infection is diagnosed at birth, that any attempt can be made to estimate the size of the problem of congenital infections and the contribution these infections make to the aetiology of brain damage.

TABLE I Agents Known to Infect the Fetus and Cause Damage to the Nervous System

Rubella	Poliovirus
Cytomegalovirus	*Toxoplasma gondii*
Herpesvirus hominis	*Treponema pallidum*
Varicella-zoster virus	*Listeria monocytogenes*

The agents listed in Table I are known to cause fetal infection and subsequent brain damage. Other infections such as influenza have been incriminated as a cause of neurological handicap but evidence is conflicting and of doubtful significance. Although the contribution fetal infections make to the total problem of handicap is small, they are a particularly important cause of defects because, at least theoretically, preventative measures are more likely to be effective against an infectious disease than against defects that are genetic in origin.

The majority of infections reach the fetus from the maternal circulation via the placenta. Alternatively, some infections reach the fetus from the genital tract by the ascending cervical amniotic route, or infection may occur during delivery. Occasionally, infection may be directly introduced into the fetus, for example, from intrauterine transfusions in the treatment of rhesus disease.

In this chapter, three infections will be considered—rubella, cytomegalovirus, and toxoplasmosis. These are important causes of fetal infection that may result in subsequent neurological damage. Many infants with these congenital infections may appear normal at birth and it is the long-term consequences which highlight the importance of diagnosing infection at birth.

Rubella

Fetal infection results from a primary infection in pregnancy, and reinfection is not considered as constituting a risk. Prevention of defects by rubella vaccination is based on this important assumption. The clinical manifestations of congenital rubella are wide and the major ones are shown in Table II. The CNS is a common site of infection and many neurological defects may be present. These include microcephaly, mental handicap, cerebral palsy, defects of hearing (and speech), retinal changes, and visual disturbance due to cataract and microphthalmos. With the exception of sensorineural deafness other forms of CNS involvement rarely occur in the absence of defects involving other systems. Chess [1] has drawn attention to a high incidence of autistic features in congenital rubella children. These may be due to the reactions of the deaf/blind child with brain damage but a small number who appear not to be deaf or blind have been observed with classic autism.

TABLE II Major Clinical Manifestations of Congenital Rubella

Intra-uterine growth retardation	Pigmentary retinopathy
Failure to thrive	Congenital heart defect
Hepatomegaly/splenomegaly	Sensorineural deafness
Hepatitis/jaundice	Microcephaly
Osteopathy	Cerebral palsy
Thrombocytopenia/purpura	Mental retardation
Cataract(s)	Late onset meningoencephalitis
Microphthalmos	Progressive panencephalitis

The severity of maternal infection has little bearing on its effects on the fetus and, in a high proportion of cases of congenital rubella, there is no maternal history of rubella or indeed of any rash or contact with rubella in pregnancy [2]. Fetal age is important in determining the risk and extent of damage. The earlier that infection occurs in pregnancy the higher the risk of damage; multiple defects result from early gestational rubella whereas infection in the third and fourth month usually results in a single defect which is nearly always sensorineural deafness. Infection after 16 weeks is not usually associated with defects although some causes of deafness have occurred as a result of infection up to 22 weeks.

Prospective studies, where evaluation begins from the time of maternal infection, have been carried out in many countries to estimate the risk of damage. It was concluded from summary of these prospective studies that the risk of damage was of the order of 21 per cent following infection in the first 8 weeks, 18 per cent for the third month, and about 6 per cent for the fourth month of gestation [3]. These estimates are only approximate and have probably been underestimated because they were based on cases of clinically diagnosed rubella, when no account could be made for subclinical infection. As soon as it became possible to diagnose rubella serologically, the majority of pregnancies were terminated if infection in early pregnancy was confirmed and it no longer became feasible to estimate the true risk.

When estimating the risk of fetal damage not only is the time of maternal rubella important but also the age of child at time of assessment. Until recently,

259

congenital rubella defects were considered to be fully established at birth, but it is now apparent that congenital rubella is a potentially progressive disorder and further damage may develop weeks, months, or even years after birth. The most important example of this is sensorineural deafness [4] but other more unusual forms of this late onset disease include pneumonitis, diabetes mellitus, hypothyroidism, growth hormone deficiency and encephalitis [5]. Meningoencephalitis may present in infancy or early childhood, the CSF may contain raised levels of protein associated with a pleocytosis, and rubella virus may be isolated [6]. Infection at this site may be a factor in causing further damage to the nervous system. Several cases of severe neurological disease resembling sclerosing panencephalitis have been observed in patients with congenital rubella, in the second decade of life. Rubella virus has been isolated from the brain in some of these cases and rubella antibody is present in high levels in the CSF [7].

Cytomegalovirus

Cytomegalovirus (CMV) is one of the herpes group of viruses and it is the commonest known cause of congenital infection of the human fetus. In the majority of countries in Asia and Africa nearly all adults show evidence of past infection of CMV, whereas in Europe and North America infection is usually acquired during adolescence or early adult life and about 50 to 60 per cent of adults have CMV antibody, indicating that previous infection has occurred.

It is difficult to assess the frequency of maternal infection since most healthy individuals have no symptoms and infection is rarely suspected. However, seroepidemiological studies suggest that about 40 per cent of women in England and Wales are without antibody when they reach childbearing age and that about 1 to 2 per cent of women undergo serological conversion with CMV complement-fixing antibody during their pregnancy [8]. There is considerable variation in the prevalence of infection among different subsections of the community and primary CMV infection is probably more common in the lower socioeconomic groups and among unmarried mothers [9]. Young mothers and primipara are also more likely to become infected.

In view of the difficulty of identifying maternal infection, the incidence of congenital CMV infection is determined by serological tests on cord blood or isolation of virus from the urine or from nasopharyngeal swabs of newborn infants. Identification of characteristic CMV inclusion bearing cells in urine was originally considered to be a useful method of diagnosis but the percentage of positive results is too low to be of value. It is estimated from various studies [9-13] that between 0.2 and 2.4 per cent of all newborn infants are infected in utero. Mothers who are infected do not necessarily produce infected infants; Stern and Tucker [8] estimated that fetal infection occurred in about 50 per cent of primary maternal CMV infections.

Initially, it was assumed that fetal infection was the consequence of primary infection in pregnancy. However, recent studies in United States [14] and West Africa [15] have shown that a significant number of women, 3.4 and 1.4 per cent respectively, who were known to be seropositive before conception, gave birth to

260

infants with congenital CMV infection. These findings indicate that the presence of maternal antibody does not prevent congenital infection, but the long-term effects of such fetal infections are as yet unknown. In no case of congenital infection in consecutive pregnancies has the second infant shown signs of damage, and it is generally considered that reinfection does not constitute a risk.

For many years congenital CMV infection was recognised as the syndrome of cytomegalic inclusion disease. These affected infants exhibited a constellation of disorders including low birth weight, hepatosplenomegaly and jaundice, purpura, anaemia, microcephaly, intracranial calcification (which is usually paraventricular), mental retardation, cerebral palsy, seizures, chorioretinitis and pneumonia. This severe form of neonatal disease, which carries a high mortality, occurs in fewer than 5 per cent of congenitally infected infants. Those few infants who survive are invariably severely handicapped and often microcephalic and mentally retarded.

A proportion of infants infected in utero have only mild or moderate symptoms and signs at birth. These consist of transient thrombocytopenia with a fleeting purpuric rash, jaundice, enlargement of the spleen and liver and biochemical evidence of hepatitis. This form of presentation is thought to occur in approximately 10 per cent of all infected infants. Follow-up of these infants suggests that the risk of permanent damage to the central nervous system is considerable. The defects may include moderate to severe degrees of mental retardation, with or without microcephaly, and signs of cerebral palsy. More recently, hearing defects have come to be recognised as an important consequence of congenital infection [16].

A number of infants with congenital infection are clinically normal at birth but may later be found to exhibit significant CNS damage including minor degrees of mental retardation, behaviour disturbances, clumsiness and sensorineural deafness. Recent studies [9, 16, 17] have estimated that approximately 20 per cent to 30 per cent of all infants with congenital CMV infection will have some degree of damage. Assuming a birth rate of 600 000 per year and a 0.5 per cent incidence of congenital infection, there would be 3000 infants born in England and Wales with congenital infection per year. If 20 per cent of these infants are subsequently found to have defects, this would represent 600 children born each year with neurological damage resulting from congenital CMV infection. In the United States it has been estimated that 3700 babies born each year will have cytomegalovirus-induced brain damage [18]. CMV may therefore be more important numerically than rubella as a cause of congenital defects. Although the role of CMV in the causation of neurological damage has been well established, the exact risk and the extent of the problem remains to be defined.

There is other circumstantial evidence that CMV may be an important cause in mental retardation of hitherto unknown aetiology. In a hospital study, the serological status of 67 children aged under 3 years with neurological damage of unknown cause was compared with a group comprising 23 children with neurological disease of known aetiology and 23 unselected children. Complement-fixing CMV antibody was present in 21 per cent of the undiagnosed neurological group but in only 4.5 per cent of the other two groups [19]. In another study of 500 mentally retarded children aged under 5 years, the overall prevalence of CMV antibody was not significantly different from that in normal children but, when those children

261

who were microcephalic were considered, the prevalence of antibody was significantly higher than in those without microcephaly [20].

Toxoplasmosis

Infection by the protozoon *Toxoplasma gondii* occurs from ingestion of the cyst forms in meat, or oocysts from cats or infected soil. Undercooked pork and mutton are probably the most common source of infection. Seroepidemiological studies show very marked regional differences in the incidence of past infection in different populations. Fleck [21] reported that between 19 per cent and 25 per cent of individuals in the UK of childbearing age were seropositive, whereas a study in Sheffield [22] reported only 7 per cent of adults to have antibody. Similarly, a striking difference was found between Orkney and Shetland where 45 per cent and 89 per cent of women were seropositive [23]. The incidence of infection in pregnant women varies in different populations according to the risk of exposure. In France, the risk is high, but in the UK toxoplasmosis in pregnancy is uncommon.

Like CMV, the majority of infections in adults are asymptomatic, which makes it difficult to estimate the risk of fetal infection following a maternal infection in pregnancy. Congenital toxoplasmosis was first recognised as a clinical syndrome consisting of chorioretinitis, intracranial calcification, optic atrophy, mental retardation, convulsions, hepatosplenomegaly, jaundice, anaemia and thrombocytopenia. This constellation of defects is, however, uncommon and represents but one end of the spectrum, the other being asymptomatic congenital infection. Less severe manifestations of disease may be present at birth, including low birthweight at term, jaundice, or minor degrees of cerebral disorder.

Clinically normal infants with congenital infection may exhibit abnormalities in the CSF and follow up of such infants may reveal significant abnormalities in brain function. In a prospective study of 378 pregnancies in France [24], where toxoplasmosis in pregnancy is considerably more frequent than in the UK, fetal infection was found to be highest following third trimester infection but congenital disease was more likely to follow first and second trimester infection. Overall, 30 per cent of infants were born with congenital infection and 30 per cent of these had clinical manifestations of the disease.

In this chapter the other agents known to cause fetal infection and neurological damage have not been discussed. However, if it is known that a specific infection may have an adverse effect on the fetus, it is only by regular and carefully controlled long-term evaluation of large numbers of infants, whose infection is detected by routine screening methods at birth, that the full impact of congenital infections can be estimated. These late manifestations of disease, which may include educational backwardness, learning problems, deafness, behavioural disturbance, poor motor co-ordination and even problems presenting much later in life, can be found only at long-term follow-up since they are often not apparent in early childhood. Although the majority of infected infants grow up normally it seems that congenital infections are sufficiently common for those infected to be numerically considerable. Identification of fetal infections, many of which can cause neurological damage, is important because of the possibility of employing preventative measures or treatment with chemotherapeutic agents.

References

1   Chess, S (1971) *J. Autism Child Schizo, 1,* 33
2   Sheppard, S et al (1977) *Health Trends, 9,* 38
3   Dudgeon, JA (1976) *Brit. Med. Bull., 32,* 77
4   Peckham, CS (1972) *Arch. Dis. Child., 47,* 571
5   Marshall, WC (1973) *Ciba Foundation Symposium 10* (new series). Amsterdam, Associated Scientific Publishers, pp. 3-12
6   Desmond, MM et al (1967) *J. Pediat., 71,* 311
7   Johnson, RT (1975) *New Eng. J. Med., 292,* 1023
8   Stern, H and Tucker, SH (1973) *Brit. Med. J., 2,* 268
9   MacDonald, H and Tobin, JO'H (1978) *Develop. Med. Child Neurol., 20,* 471
10 Birnbaum, G et al (1969) *J. Pediat., 75,* 789
11 Starr, JG et al (1969) *J. Pediat., 282,* 1075
12 Melish, M and Hanshaw, JB (1973) *Am. J. Dis. Children, 126,* 190
13 Collaborative Study (1970) *Arch. Dis. Child., 45,* 513
14 Stagno, S et al (1975) *J. Inf. Dis., 131,* 522
15 Schopfer, K et al (1978) *Arch. Dis. Child., 53,* 536
16 Reynolds, DW (1974) *New Eng. J. Med., 290,* 291
17 Hanshaw, JB (1976) *New Eng. J. Med., 295,* 468
18 Medearis, DN (1977) *New Eng. J. Med., 296,* 1289
19 Hanshaw, JB et al (1973) In *Ciba Foundation Symposium 10* (new series). Amsterdam, Associated Scientific Publishers, pp. 23-32
20 Stern, H (1971) In *Proceedings of the XIII International Congress Paediatrics, Vienna,* Vol. 6, Medyiniche Akademia, Vienna, pp. 301-306
21 Fleck, DG (1963) *J. Hygiene, 61,* 61
22 Beverley et al (1954) *J. Hygiene, 52,* 37
23 Williams, H (1977) *Postgraduate Med. J., 53,* 614
24 Desmonts, G and Couveur, J (1974) *Bull. New York Academic Medicine, 50,* 146

Chapter 26

AN OVERVIEW OF CONGENITAL MALFORMATIONS OF THE NERVOUS SYSTEM*

John F Kurtzke

Introduction

For every 1000 total births (live plus stillborn), we may expect to find some 13 infants with major malformations definable at or near birth. Approximately one-quarter of these will be malformations of the central nervous system (CNS). Of this latter grouping about one-third each will be provided by anencephaly, spina bifida aperta, and congenital hydrocephalus (Table I). Alone or in combination, these

TABLE I Percentage Frequencies of Major Congenital Malformations of the Nervous System by type of malformation ascertained at or near birth: Total Births from WHO Study of 24 centres, 1961–64 (Stevenson et al 1966 a, b) [1, 2]; Live Births from US, 1973–74 (Taffel, 1978) [3]

Type of malformation	Total births %	Live births %
Anencephaly alone	34.4 ⎫	20.6
Anencephaly and spina bifida[a]	4.9 ⎬	
Hydrocephalus alone	22.9	16.0
Hydrocephalus and spina bifida[a]	9.7	8.3
Spina bifida alone[a]	20.8	43.0
Occipital meningocele	1.4	–
Other neural tube defects[b]	3.1	4.2
Microcephaly	2.4	5.8
All other nervous system	0.3	1.9[c]
Total	100.0	100.0
(Number of cases)	(1,109)	(5,668)

[a] With or without spinal meningocele
[b] Predominantly encephalocele
[c] Predominantly unspecified anomalies

three states comprise 9 of 10 major malformations of the nervous system identifiable by inspection [1, 2]. If we limit attention to live births alone, the same three entities still provide 9 of 10 CNS malformations, but now with spina bifida clearly predominant [3].

* Supported by the Veterans Administration

264

Should one extend surveillance through the first year of life and include autopsies on almost all deaths, the relative frequencies of the major entities will, of course, decline as more subtle defects are discovered. Table II provides such information from the Collaborative Perinatal Project, a prospective survey of the issue of some 56 000 pregnancies at 12 medical centres in the United States [4]. In that survey the frequency of major malformations was 8 per 1000, of which some 5 per cent were of the nervous system. This frequency for CNS malformations thus differs little from that cited above; the modest excess in fact reflects the 'other cerebral' group of Table II.

TABLE II Percentage Frequencies of Major Congenital Malformations of Nervous System by type of malformation ascertained through first year of life and at autopsy among 53 257 total births from 12 US medical centres of the Collaborative Perinatal Project (Myrianthopoulos and Chung, 1974) [4]

Type of malformation	Alone %	Multiple*%	Total
Anencephaly	9.6	11.5	10.8
Hydrocephalus	21.7	26.2	24.5
Spinal	4.3	19.9	14.1
meningo/myelocele	(4.3)	(17.8)	(12.7)
rachischisis	–	(0.5)	(0.3)
hydromyelia	–	(1.0)	(0.7)
absence sacrum	–	(0.5)	(0.3)
Microcephaly	33.9	24.1	27.8
Encephalocele	0.9	4.2	2.9
Other cerebral	29.6	14.1	19.9
hydranencephaly	–	(1.6)	(1.0)
macrocephaly	(26.1)	(6.3)	(13.7)
porencephaly	(2.6)	(1.0)	(1.6)
abs. corp. call.	–	(0.5)	(0.3)
hypoplasia olfact.	(0.9)	(0.5)	(0.7)
arrhinencephaly	–	(0.5)	(0.3)
frontal hypoplasia	–	(0.5)	(0.3)
agenesis pituitary	–	(1.0)	(0.7)
cyst sept. pell.	–	(0.5)	(0.3)
suboccip. sinus	–	(1.6)	(1.0)
Total	100.0	100.0	100.0
(N)	(115)	(191)	(306)

*With *any* other malformation; multiple entries possible here

It would then seem that limiting attention to the early perinatal period and the three major entities cited would indeed provide us with data referable to the large majority of the important (clinically and numerically) CNS malformations.

Mortality Data

In the Seventh Revision of the *International Statistical Classification of Diseases, Injuries, and Causes of Death*—the ISC—congenital malformations of the nervous system were coded to 750 (monstrosity), 751 (spina bifida aperta), 752 (congenital hydrocephalus), and 753 (other malformations of nervous system and eye) [5]. We shall see that 'monstrosity' was essentially equivalent to 'anencephaly'. Code 751 included meningocele and encephalocele. There were no provisions to handle combinations of malformations, and this was especially important for hydrocephalus and spina bifida. For this reason, the United States devised its own sub-coding to represent, from 1962, either spina bifida with hydrocephalus or spina bifida without mention of hydrocephalus on the death certificate. This change was adopted internationally for the Eighth Revision of the ISC, in effect from 1968-1978 inclusive [6]. There were other changes as well in the Eighth Revision. Code 740 became anencephaly and 741 spina bifida (741.0 with hydrocephalus and 741.9 without). Congenital hydrocephalus was 742 and 'other' malformations were listed under 743; with encephalocele (743.0) and microcephaly (743.1).

In this, as in a number of other aspects for neurology, the Ninth Revision of the ISC is regressive [7]. While 740 and 741 are retained, 742 is 'other congenital anomalies of the nervous system', to *include* hydrocephalus (742.3). And 743 refers to congenital anomalies of the eye [8]. For the present though, 750-753 (7th) and 740-743 (8th) codes provide the sum for congenital malformations of the nervous system. Their status as three-digit codes also makes likely their availability in routinely reported death data.

For the calculation of standard death rates, the denominator is the (living) population at risk, which in this context means the live-born infants and all their survivors at all ages. Accordingly, in mortality data we lose those proportions of CNS malformations found among the stillborn. The age at death varies for these entities. For anencephaly, virtually all are dead before their first birthday, and usually before 28 days of life. For the others, the proportions dying in the first year are 89 per cent for spina bifida, 69 per cent for hydrocephalus, and 61 per cent for 'other' malformations [9].

There are several ways of comparing death rates from congenital malformations. The simplest is the crude death rate (deaths/total population). For these infantile deaths it is far better to use an age-adjusted death rate. Especially for time trends and international comparisons, differences in birth rates will, however, have a major influence on the death rates for all ages, whether age-adjusted or not. To minimise this influence, one may limit comparisons to deaths and population under 1 year of age, which will encompass most of the cases. This will take into account variations in birth rates·in providing the population at risk.

Another 'approach, which permits the assessment of CNS malformation deaths from routinely reported data without special tabulations, is the calculation of the risk of death among the live-born for the same year. For anencephaly this will reflect accurately the entirety of this condition among those born alive. It will equate with the under-1-year death rate which, in turn, includes all cases. For the other malformations it will also include all cases, but it will tend to overestimate risk *if* the birth rate is falling dramatically. The overestimation though will be minimal, especially for spina bifida. Deaths *not* coded as underlying cause will be lost from all these rates, however. Their numbers will be appreciable, though, only for spina bifida and 'other' malformations [9].

266

United States Mortality Data

Secular Trend

Crude annual death rates per 100 000 population for CNS malformations in the United States show an apparent decline from about 3.3 in 1950-53 to 1.8 in 1972. However, the birth rate has also fallen over this interval, from about 2.5 per 100 population to some 1.6. Using the risk of death among the live-born, though, we can confirm a moderate decline from over 1.2 per 1000 births down to almost 0.9 per 1000 (Figure 1). The heavy arrow on the figure indicates the date when the

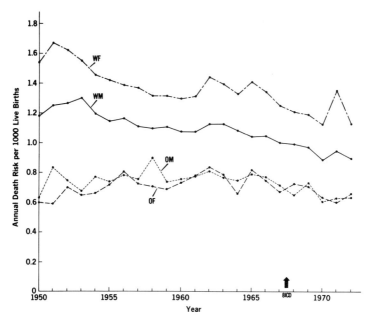

Figure 1 Congenital malformations of the central nervous system: annual death risk per 1000 live births for all CNS malformations by sex and colour; United States 1950-1972 (From Kurtzke (1978) [10])

8th revision of the ISC went into effect. There is a clear difference between the colours, whites being regularly more affected than non-whites (classed as 'other'). Among the whites, females have appreciably higher risk ratios than do males. On the other hand, there is no variation of note between the sexes for non-whites, of whom some 90 per cent would be blacks or Negroes [10].

By type of malformation, the overall death risks for spina bifida and for hydrocephalus have declined between 1950 and 1972, while rates for anencephaly and 'other' malformations of the CNS have not changed, or have possibly increased a little. Note there is no break in the curve for monstrosity/anencephaly at the time when the 8th ISC coding became effective, confirming the essential equivalence of

267

'monstrosity' with anencephaly (Figure 2). However, the use of subcodes for spina bifida with and without hydrocephalus, which became effective in 1962 (open arrow in Figure 2), produced dramatic changes in the death risk ratios: spina bifida increased markedly, while hydrocephalus ratios declined. Both thereafter resumed their modest downward trend, and there was little additional change with the introduction of the 8th revision. There is a modest rise in the 'other' category with the introduction of the 8th revision. This may be because of encephalocele, now 743.0, which had been under the spina bifida code in the 7th revision.

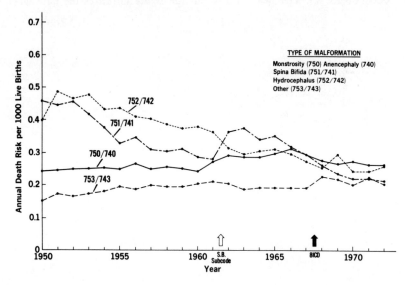

Figure 2 Congenital malformations of the central nervous system: annual death risk per 1000 live births by type of malformation; United States 1950–1972 (From Kurtzke (1978) [10])

Race

In Figure 3 are under-1-year death rates for CNS malformations according to specific race. As inferred from the total non-white grouping (Figure 1), blacks or Negroes are clearly lower than whites, and show no sex predilection. On the other hand, the American Indian rates are almost identical with those of the whites. Rates for Americans of Oriental and 'other' origins may also be low, but numbers are small for Japanese Americans, although the difference is at least suggestive. Cases are too few to place any reliance on the apparent sex differences in the last three groups. The 'other' category would include primarily Aleuts, Polynesians, and Filipinos. Spanish-Americans would be classed as white, black, or Indian as appropriate.

As to which of the malformations contribute to the racial differences, the Negro rates are clearly low for both monstrosity(-anencephaly) and spina bifida (Figure 4). Conversely, hydrocephalus rates are about equal for whites, blacks and Indians,

268

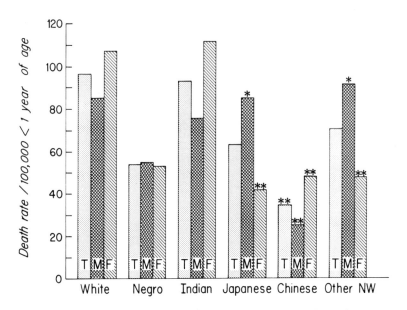

Figure 3 Rates per 100000 live births for deaths under one year of age due to congenital malformations of nervous system by race and sex; United States, 1959, 1960 and 1961. Rates based on less than 20 deaths (*) or less than 10 deaths (**) are thus identified in this and Figure 4 (From Kurtzke et al 1973b [11])

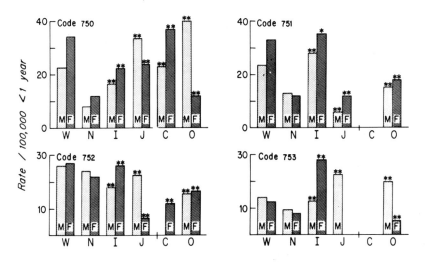

Figure 4 Rates per 100000 live births for deaths under one year of age due to each type of congenital malformation of the nervous system (7th rev. ICS codes 750–753) by race and sex: United States, 1959, 1960 and 1961. (From Kurtzke et al 1973b [11])

269

and for either sex. By type of malformation we can no longer rely on the rates for Orientals.

Type of Malformation

Anencephaly. The secular trend for monstrosity/anencephaly by sex and colour is shown in Figure 5. There is a slight rise in the frequency over time and a marked preponderance among whites. Females are clearly in excess among whites, and generally appear to be slightly higher even among non-whites. Remember that data are limited to deaths among the live-born. For anencephaly, this excludes perhaps the majority of cases. The birth rate for anencephaly in the US has declined from a peak of about 3 per 1000 total births around 1932 to about 0.5 per 1000 in 1975 [10].

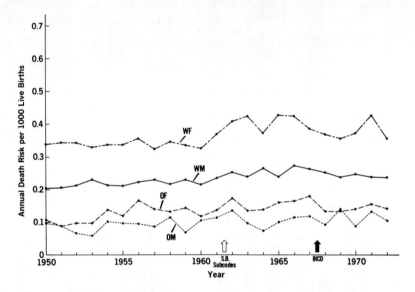

Figure 5   Anencephaly: annual death risk per 1000 live births for monstrosity/anencephaly by sex and colour; United States 1950–72 (From Kurtzke 1978 [10])

Geographically, the anencephaly deaths are concentrated in the north-eastern quadrant of the United States [11]. An east–west gradient is clearly seen for both sexes among the whites, but this distribution is lost for non-whites. Blacks, who have low anencephaly rates, are concentrated in the south-eastern US. Elwood and Mousseau [12] have documented a similar east-west gradient for anencephaly in whites in Canada with both mortality and morbidity data.

Spina Bifida. As with anencephaly, white females are notably more often affected than white males, while the sexes are equal in the non-whites (Figure 6). The striking change resulting from the subcodes for spina bifida with and without hydrocephalus is obvious, and from 1962 on, the subcodes can be compared

270

(Figure 7). Regardless of the concomitant presence of hydrocephalus, there is still the white preponderance, the white female excess, and the equality of the sexes in the non-whites. But the decline over time in the spina bifida risk is almost entirely limited to spina bifida without hydrocephalus. Geographically, the spina bifida death rates show an east-west gradient, but only among whites; similar to that for anencephaly [11].

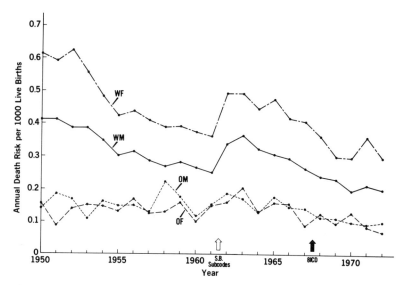

Figure 6 Spina bifida: annual death risk per 1000 live births by sex and colour; United States 1950–1972 (From Kurtzke 1978 [10])

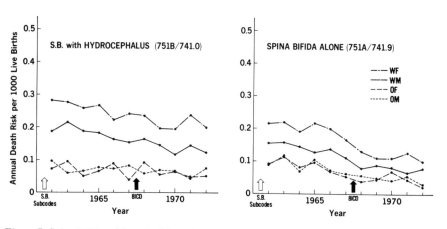

Figure 7 Spina bifida with and without hydrocephalus: annual death risk per 1000 live births by sex and colour; United States 1962–1972 (From Kurtzke 1978 [10])

271

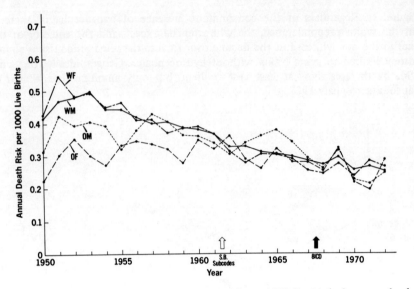

Figure 8 Congenital hydrocephalus: annual death risk per 1000 live births by sex and colour, United States 1950–1972 (From Kurtzke 1978 [10])

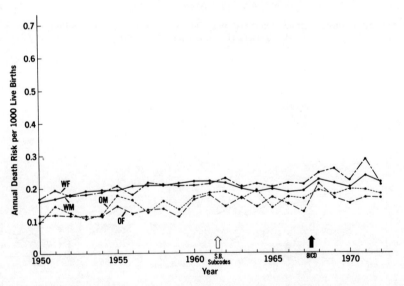

Figure 9 Other malformations of the nervous system: annual death risk per 1000 live births by sex and colour; United States 1950–1972 (From Kurtzke 1978 [10])

272

Hydrocephalus. Congenital hydrocephalus behaves differently from the prior malformations. There is a modest downward trend in the risk of death from hydrocephalus over time, but there is no clear or consistent difference between the sexes or the colours (Figure 8). The drop is a bit more abrupt between 1961 and 1962, when the spina bifida subcodes were introduced. The geographic distribution for deaths *before* the recoding of spina bifida appears to be similar to the prior malformations, but the death rates by state are in fact much more homogeneous [11].

Other Malformations. This is a grouping, of course, of separate entities. There is little to choose between the sexes as to their frequency, and but a trivial white excess is apparent (Figure 9). Over time, there has been little change, though a slight increment can be seen between 1967 and 1968 with the introduction of the 8th revision of the ISC, when encephalocele was removed thereto from prior code 751. Geographically, there is no patterning to the distribution by state. Most of the higher rates are in the east and west coasts, as well as the midwest, but the range is modest [11].

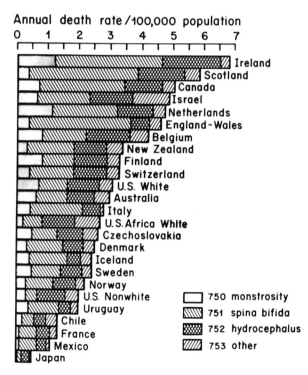

Figure 10 Congenital malformations of the nervous system: average annual age-adjusted death rates per 100000 population by type of malformation; 24 countries, 1951-1958, from data of Goldberg and Kurland 1962 [13] (From Kurtzke et al 1973b [11])

273

Goldberg and Kurland [13] provided a valuable paper on the distribution of neurological deaths among 33 countries. Most of the material was from deaths for five years within the 1951–58 period. Their data are redrawn in Figure 10 [14]. For all CNS malformations combined, the rates vary markedly from 6.8 per 100000 population per annum in Ireland to 0.5 per 100000 in Japan. For US whites the age-adjusted rate was 3.1 versus 2.0 for nonwhites. The few Latin American rates represented are all to the low side: 1.1 (Mexico), 1.3 (Chile), and 2.0 (Uruguay).

Highest by far were Ireland (6.8) and Scotland (5.8). Also high were Canada (5.0), Israeli Jews (4.8), the Netherlands (4.7), England and Wales (4.6) and Belgium (4.2). Conversely, neighbouring France was low (1.3). The Scandinavian countries of Norway, Sweden, Denmark, and Iceland were all between 2.2 and 2.5 per 100000, although Finland's rate was 3.3. All the high rates were from the British Commonwealth (including Ireland) and the Benelux countries. As to the low rates, age-adjustment may not fully compensate for marked differences in the birth rates, which have been low in France and Japan, at least.

Anencephaly death rates were between 0.5 and 1.0 per 100000 in Australia (0.6), Belgium (0.8), Canada (0.7), Finland (0.8), Israel (0.6) and US whites (0.7). They were above 1 per 100000 in Ireland (1.2) and the Netherlands (1.1). Spina bifida death rates ranged from 3.4 per 100000 for Ireland to 0.2 for Japan. Rates over 2 per 100000 were recorded for Canada (2.7), England-Wales (3.2), Ireland (3.4), Netherlands (2.1) and Scotland (3.4).

On the high side for hydrocephalus (over 1.1 per 100000) were Belgium (1.4), Canada (1.2), Ireland (1.9), Israel (1.3) and Scotland (1.5). Below 0.6 per 100000 were Chile (0.3), France (0.5), Iceland (0.4), Japan (0.3), Mexico (0.4) and Uruguay (0.3). Thus, the range for hydrocephalus is quite small, and the variations may reflect more the spina bifida admixtures than congenital hydrocephalus itself. Note that even Japan was not too distant from the others for hydrocephalus.

As to 'other' malformations, all but four countries recorded rates between 0.2 and 0.6 per 100000: Israel (1.1) and Republic of South African whites (0.9) were high, while Italy and Mexico reported rates of 0.1 per 100000. For Israel the excess may be a coding artefact; in other diseases, at least, the 'other' category for coding cause of death is mandatory there without documented proof of a specific cause within the category.

In these data, there was generally a considerable female preponderance for anencephaly and spina bifida, while hydrocephalus and other malformations on the average appeared a little more frequent in males or were equally distributed by sex [14].

Morbidity Data

The frequency of CNS malformations is preferably described as a rate per unit of births, and best when both numerator and denominator include stillbirths (28-week or more) as well as the live-born. The proportions of stillborn malformations among total malformations vary by type, being highest for anencephaly and lowest for spina bifida among the three major types. However, even within a given type, the proportions vary in different series; for example, stillborn anencephalics are under 40 per cent of all anencephalus in Hamburg, Germany [15], but some 85 per cent of the total in England–Wales [16]. To minimise these variations, we shall limit all data presented to rates per 1000 total (live + stillborn) births.

Types of CNS Malformations

From two major prospective series, numbers of CNS malformations and their rates per 1000 total births are described in Table III. Almost all cases will be covered if we subdivide into anencephaly; total spina bifida—meaning SB with or without hydrocephalus; and hydrocephalus alone. Admixtures of anencephaly and SB are almost always coded to anencephaly, and it is in this manner we shall describe the frequencies to preserve three discrete groups.

The average rate for the worldwide survey conducted within 24 centres under the auspices of the WHO was 2.7 per 1000 total births [1, 2], while it was almost twice this value, at 4.8 per 1000, for England and Wales [16]. In each, the

TABLE III Congenital Malformations of the Nervous System: Cases and rates per 1000 total (live + stillborn) births by type of malformation from two large series

	WHO study 24 centres 1961–64[a]		England–Wales 1967–72[b]	
	Cases	Rate[c]	Cases	Rate
Total CNS	1109	2.66	23092[d]	4.80
Anencephaly total	436	1.05	8455	1.76
Anencephaly alone	382	0.92	–	–
Anencephaly-SB[e]	54	0.13	–	–
Spina bifida[e] total	393	0.94	8449f	1.76
SB[e] alone	231	0.55	5593g	1.16
SB[e]-Hydrocephalus	108	0.26	2856g	0.59
Hydrocephalus alone	254	0.61	2875	0.60
Hydrocephalus total	362	0.87	5731g	1.19
Occipital meningocele	16	0.04		
Microcephaly	27	0.06 ⎫		
Other neural tube[h]	34	0.08 ⎬ 0.19	⎫ 3313i	⎫ 0.69
All other CNS	3	0.01 ⎭	⎭	⎭

a Stevenson et al 1966a, b, single births only [1, 2]
b from data of Rogers and Weatherall 1976 [16]
c rate standardised for maternal age
d estimated from 'notifications' (Appendix D) plus 'combined stillbirths and notified livebirths' (Tables 4.1a, b, c)
e spina bifida with or without spinal meningocele
f excludes anencephaly-SB
g estimated from 'notifications' (Appendix D)
h predominantly encephalocele
i 'notifications' only without unreported stillbirths

anencephaly rates were about equal to the total spina bifida rate, while hydrocephalus alone was appreciably lower. The differences between the two surveys lie in the anencephaly and SB rates, hydrocephalus being equal at 0.6 per 1000 total births.

Sex Ratios

Male/female ratios on the incidence rates for CNS malformations are presented in Table IV. Anencephaly is uniformly greater in females, with a male/female ratio of about 1/3 to 1/2. Regardless of which type of malformation is present together with anencephaly, the sex ratio is essentially the same as when it is the sole malformation.

TABLE IV   Congenital Malformations of the Neural Tube: Sex ratios of incidence rates per 1000 total births, and type of malformation

Malformation type	Source			
	WHO study[a] M:F ratio (N)	Rochester, MN[b] M:F ratio (N)	Scotland[c] M:F ratio	England-Wales[d] M:F ratio (N)
Anencephaly				
alone	0.54 (381)	0.08 (14)	–	–
total	0.52 (435)	0.09 (24)	0.36	0.41 (13431)
Spina bifida				
alone	0.82 (229)	0.43 (10)	–	–
with anencephaly	0.42 (54)	0.11 (10)	–	–
with hydrocephalus	0.96 (108)	0.56 (28)	–	–
total	0.79 (391)	0.37 (52)[e]	0.76	0.75–(12900)
Hydrocephalus				
alone	1.33 (252)	0.73 (19)	–	1.12 (4677)
total	1.21 (360)	0.62 (47)	1.04	–

[a] 24 centres, single births 1961–64 (Stevenson et al 1966a, b) [1, 2]
[b] 1935–67 (Gibson & Kurland, 1973) [17]
[c] 1939–46; numbers of cases not available (McKeown & Record, 1951) [18]
[d] 1964–72 (Rogers & Weatherall, 1976) [16]
[e] includes 4 cases with microcephaly

The male/female ratio on the incidence rates for spina bifida is about 3/4 in the three large series. It is lower (under 1/2) when combined with anencephaly, and higher (almost unity) when with hydrocephalus. Hydrocephalus shows a male preponderance with a ratio of about 4/3 when alone, and somewhat near unity when with spina bifida.

Birth Rates for CNS Malformations

WHO Series. The WHO study mentioned covered centres in the Americas, Europe, Asia and Africa. Rates for the individual malformations by type and centre from this study are drawn in Figure 11 [14]. Admixtures of types are represented by the overlapping shading.

276

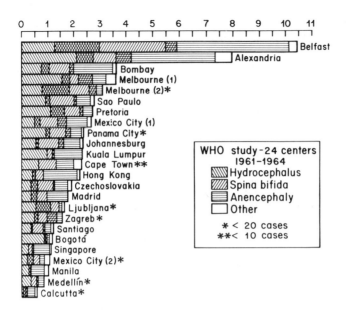

Figure 11 Congenital malformations of the neural tube: Rates per 1000 total (live + stillborn) births by type of malformation and centre within the WHO study of 24 centres 1961-1964; 27 microcephaly and 3 'other CNS' cases excluded from the 1079 malformations among 417000 single births represented by this series; data of Stevenson et al 1966a, b [1, 2] (From Kurtzke and Kurland 1973 [4])

There is a marked excess for CNS malformations in Belfast and in Alexandria, Egypt. Bombay (3.8) and Melbourne are next, but lowest of all is Calcutta (0.6). All other rates lie between 1 and 3 per 1000 total births. The three South African rates (Pretoria, Johannesburg, Cape Town) each reflect the three different racial groups (White, Black, Coloured) and are quite close one to the other. The striking excess in Belfast (10.4) and Alexandria (7.9) is seen for all three main types: anencephaly, spina bifida and hydrocephalus. The Belfast excess is in accord with the death data considered above.

Other Series

In Table V are summarised the incidence rates per 1000 total births for the major CNS malformations. 'Anencephaly' includes anencephaly with or without spina bifida, and 'total spina bifida' refers to SB with or without hydrocephalus. Taking the WHO average of 2.6 per 1000 as the norm, an 'average' rate might be considered as between 1 and 4 per 1000 total births. Toward the lower side then would be Sweden, Finland, Czechoslovakia, Japan and Australia. Hamburg (0.7) appears even lower, but the low proportions of malformations reported there among stillbirths might indicate this is a reflection of incomplete ascertainment. Note that the Japanese rate, from a small series, does not seem exceedingly low, in contrast to the death data.

277

TABLE V Congenital Malformations of the Neural Tube: Total cases and rates per 1000 total (live + stillborn) births, from selected community surveys

Survey area (source)	Survey Years	Total Rate (cases)	Rate per 1000 total births		
			Anencephaly*	Total SB**	Hydroc.alone
WHO, 24 centres (a)	1961-64	2.6 (1079)	1.1	0.9	0.6
England–Wales (b)	1967-72	4.8(23092)	1.8	1.8	0.6
Northern Ireland (c)	1969-73	7.2 (1140)	3.1	3.3	0.8
Scotland (d)	1939-45	6.9 (4526)	2.5	2.3	2.1
Birmingham, Eng. (e)	1940-65	(4.7)(1966)	2.2	2.6	–
Birmingham, Eng. (f)	1950-52	6.6 (375)	2.0	2.8	1.8
Liverpool, Eng. (g)	1960-63	(6.8) (438)	3.3	3.5	–
Liverpool, Eng. (h)	1960-64	7.4 (675)	3.1	3.4	0.6
Northamptonshire, Eng. (i)	1944-55	3.2 (168)	0.9	1.9	0.5
Southampton Bor., Eng. (j)	1958-62	6.0 (90)	2.0	3.2	0.9
South Wales (k)	1956-62	8.1 (835)	3.4	4.1	0.5
Belfast, N. Ire. (l)	1964-68	(8.7) (360)	4.2	4.5	–
Belfast, N. Ire. (m)	1957	8.3 (71)	4.6	2.2	1.5
Northern Ireland (mm)	1974-76	8.6 (686)	3.1	4.0	0.9
Dublin, Eire (n)	1963-66	9.5 (355)	4.2	3.6	1.7
Cork, Eire (o)	1962-66	4.5 (167)	2.1	2.1	0.4
Glasgow, Scot. (p)	1964-68	6.6 (681)	2.8	2.8	1.0
Rochester, MN (q)	1935-67	3.2 (85)	0.9	2.0	0.4
New York, NY (r)	1945-59	2.9 (7403)	0.9	1.2	0.8
Israel (s)	1959-60	2.0 (182)	0.6	0.7	0.6
Budapest, Hung. (t)	1963-67	3.7 (351)	1.1	1.9	0.8
Hamburg, Ger. (u)	1971-75	0.7 (55)	0.2	0.4	0.1
Sweden (v)	1964-69	1.1 (421)	0.4	0.5	0.2
Finland (vv)	1965-73	1.1 (710)	0.3	0.4	0.3
Czechoslovakia (w)	1952-62	1.3 (650)	0.5	0.3	0.5
Victoria, Austr. (x)	1942-57	1.8 (292)	0.7	0.6	0.6
Melbourne, Austr. (y)	1942-57	1.9 (305)	0.7	0.6	0.6
Japan (z)	1948-54	1.1 (70)	0.7	0.2	0.2
Cairo, Egypt (aa)	1963-67	11.6 (114)	5.1	2.1	4.1

*Anencephaly c/s spina bifida
**Spina bifida c/s hydrocephalus
(a) Stevenson et al 1966a, b [1, 2], (b) Rogers & Weatherall 1976 [16], (c) Elwood 1976 [19], (d) Record & McKeown [20], (e) Leck 1963, 1966 [21, 22], (f) McKeown & Record 1960 [23], (g) Smithells 1962, 1964, 1965 [24, 25, 26], (h) Smithells 1968 [27], (i) Pleydell 1957 [28], (j) Williamson 1965 [29], (k) Laurence 1966 [30], (l) Elwood & Nevin 1973 [31], (m) Stevenson & Warnock 1959 [32], (mm) Nevin et al 1978 [33], (n) Coffey 1973 [34], (o) Spellman 1970 [35], (p) Wilson 1970 [36], (q) Gibson & Kurland 1973 [17], (r) Gittlesohn & Milham 1962 [37], (s) Halevi 1967 [38], (t) Czeizel & Révèsz 1970 [39], (u) Höhn 1977 [15], (v) Källén & Winberg 1971 [40], (vv) Granroth et al 1977 [41], (w) Kučera 1965 [42], (x) Collmann & Stoller 1962a, b [43, 44], (y) Stoller & Collmann 1965 [45], (z) Neel 1958 [46], (aa) Karim et al 1968 [47]

The preponderance of high rates in Table V reflects the great interest in the UK and Ireland in malformations of the nervous system. It is obvious that the excess indicated by death data for this region is very well confirmed. The highest rate recorded (9.5) is from Dublin. Cork in the south of the Republic of Ireland is similar, at 4.5, to the rate of 4.8 for all England and Wales. Northern Ireland,

South Wales, Scotland, and several parts of England (Birmingham, Liverpool, Southampton) all have rates between 6 and 9 per 1000 total births.

Of considerable interest is that the highest rate recorded is 11.4 per 1000 from a hospital series in Cairo, Egypt [47]. Recall that Alexandria, Egypt, was in second position (7.9) in the WHO series.

As to the types of malformations, in most series the anencephaly and spina bifida rates run parallel to each other, and together are responsible for the variations just alluded to. Again, Cairo has the highest rate for anencephaly (5.1) but both Dublin and Belfast also are over 4 per 1000. The only other very high rate found was from a Singapore hospital series of 68 anencephalics in 88 000 total births 1953-56 [48]. While the rate there for Chinese was 0.6 per 1000 and 0.7 for 'Other Indians', the rate for Sikh Indians was 6.5 per 1000 for anencephaly (95 per cent confidence interval 2.8-12.8). Thus it is clear that more than a Norse-Celtic background is required for a high risk of anencephaly.

The rates for hydrocephalus, though, are very uniform, hovering nicely about the WHO average of 0.6 per 1000 births. Scotland, Birmingham, Belfast and Dublin are somewhat higher than the rest at between 1.5 and 2.1 per 1000. But the Cairo rate is strikingly high at 4.1 with a 95 per cent confidence interval of 2.9-5.6. In the WHO study, the rate for hydrocephalus alone in Alexandria was 2.0 per 1000. Thus, the Egyptians may well be at high risk for hydrocephalus as well as for the other CNS malformations.

Distribution within England and Wales

We had seen an east-west distribution for anencephaly and spina bifida deaths within the United States and noted similar findings for Canada [19]. Some of the reported rates just considered from within the United Kingdom also suggest intranational variations.

The monograph of Rogers and Weatherall [16] provides this information according to the nine 1965 Standard Regions of England and Wales (Table VI). The northernmost part of England is number 3, North Region. Below the North Region, Regions number 2 in the west and number 5 in the east extend from coast to coast. Below these in a rough line from west to east are Wales (number 1), West Midlands (number 7), East Midlands (number 4), and East Anglia (number 9). The southernmost part of England is divided into number 6 (South West) and number 8 (South East).

As seen in Table VI, the anencephaly and spina bifida rates vary together, and the range is considerable. While the variations for hydrocephalus tend somewhat in the same direction, the range is much less and the gradient clearly less uniform. The maximal rates for all three malformations, though, are to be found in the northwestern sector of the country—Wales, North West, and North Regions. They thus face Scotland to the north and the east coast of Ireland and Northern Ireland to the west. Dublin lies just across the Irish Sea from the northwestern tip of Wales.

As to the cities of England surveyed for malformations (Table V), Birmingham (6.6 per 1000) is in West Midlands, Liverpool (7.4) in North West, Northamptonshire (3.2) in East Midlands, and Southampton Borough (6.0) in South East. Thus,

279

TABLE VI Major Malformations of the Nervous System according to Type and Standard Region of England–Wales, expressed as percentages of the national (mean) rate per 1000 total births for each entity, 1964–72 data of Rogers and Weatherall 1976 [16]

No. Standard region (1965)	Type of malformation		
	Anencephaly	Total spina bifida %	Hydrocephalus alone %
1 Wales	140	147	121
2 North West	131	121	116
3 North	115–	115–	119
4 East Midlands	104	105–	98
5 Yorkshire–Humberside	99	105–	100
6 South West	98	118	94
7 West Midlands	98	99	103
8 South East	80	79	87
9 East Anglia	80	· 65–	92
Total England–Wales	100	100	100
Rate per 1000 births	1.81	1.74	0.63
(Number cases)	(13437)	(12918)	(4677)

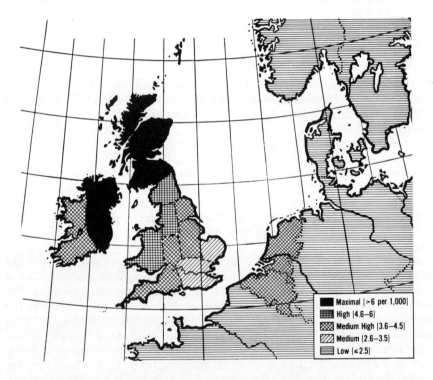

Figure 12 Congenital malformations of the neural tube: Geographic distribution in western Europe according to ranges for rates per 1000 total births

only this last may be discrepant in terms of the Standard Region patterns recorded, and the total rate there is based on only 90 cases.

One could then make a case for concentration of these malformations in the quadrilateral formed by Scotland, Wales and intervening England, and Northern Ireland and the northeastern part of Eire, with considerably lower rates in southern Eire and in southern and eastern England (Figure 12). But even here, 'low' rates are generally in excess of those from most other lands. This high frequency quadrilateral suggests a distribution reminiscent of the Norwegian settlements of the British Isles consequent to their part of the Viking invasions a millennium ago. Recall, however, that the malformation rates in all of Scandinavia at present are low. Nevertheless, a Nordic-Celtic admixture in the background does seem a characteristic of those areas of Europe that are high in CNS malformations: our quadrilateral; then the rest of UK and the Low Countries. This holds primarily for anencephaly and spina bifida aperta, two states that share so many features in time, space, sex and race that their cause(s) might well be common to both.

Summary

Anencephaly, spina bifida aperta and hydrocephalus, alone or in combination, comprise over 90 per cent of major central nervous system (CNS) malformations recognisable at, or shortly after, birth among live or stillborn infants. In the United States these three conditions include over 80 per cent of deaths coded to CNS malformations as the underlying cause of death among the live-born. The risk of death due to CNS malformations among American live births has declined to 3/4 its earlier value between 1950–53 and 1972. This decline was limited to spina bifida and hydrocephalus. From the 1930s to 1975, however, anencephaly birth rates in the US did decrease sharply, from some 3 per 1000 total births to about 0.5. That this decrement is not reflected in the mortality data could be due to an increasing proportion of anencephalics born alive. Not only in the US but also in other lands, anencephaly and spina bifida show marked and concomitant geographic variations, and a female sex predilection; in the US there are low rates for blacks. Highest incidence and/or mortality rates for these two entities are found in Ireland, Northern Ireland, Wales, northwestern England, Scotland—and in Alexandria and Cairo, Egypt. Hydrocephalus appears *relatively* uniform by sex, race, colour and geography, except for high rates in Egypt.

References

1   Stevenson, AC, Johnston, HA, Golding, DR and Stewart, MIP (1966a) *Comparative Study of Congenital Malformations: Basic Tabulations in Respect of Consecutive Post 28-week Births Recorded in the Co-operating Centres.* Medical Research Council Population Genetics Research Unit, Oxford.

2   Stevenson, AC, Johnston, HA, Stewart, MIP and Golding, DR (1966b) *Bull. World Hlth. Org., 34* (suppl), 9

281

3   Taffel, S (1978) *Congenital Anomalies and Birth Injuries among Live Births: United States, 1973-74*. DHEW Publ. No. (PHS) 79-1909

4   Myrianthopoulos, N and Chung, CS (1974) *Birth Defects Original Article Series, X*, 1

5   World Health Organisation (1957) *Manual of the International Statistical Classification of Diseases, Injuries, and Causes of Death, 1955 rev. Vol. 1, Vol. 2*. World Health Organisation, Geneva

6   World Health Organisation (1967, 1979) *Manual of the International Statistical Classification of Diseases, Injuries, and Causes of Death, 1965 rev. Vol. 1, Vol. 2*. World Health Organisation, Geneva

7   Kurtzke, JF (1979) *Am. J. Epidem., 109*, 383

8   World Health Organisation (1977) *Manual of the International Statistical Classification of Diseases, Injuries, and Causes of Death, 1975 rev. Vol. 1*. World Health Organisation, Geneva

9   Kurtzke, JF, Goldberg, ID and Kurland, LT (1973a) In *Epidemiology of Neurologic and Sense Organ Disorders* (ed. LT Kurland, JF Kurtzke and ID Goldberg). Harvard University Press, Cambridge, MA. Chapter 9, p. 169

10 Kurtzke, JF (1978) In *Neurology. Proceedings of the 11th World Congress of Neurology* (ed. WA den Hartog Jager, GW Bruyn and APJ Heijstee). Excerpta Medica, Amsterdam, p 375

11 Kurtzke, JF, Goldberg, ID and Kurland, LT (1973b) *Neurology, 23*, 483

12 Elwood, JM and Mousseau, G (1978) *J. Chron. Dis., 31*, 483

13 Goldberg, ID and Kurland, LT (1962) *World Neurol., 3*, 444

14 Kurtzke, JF and Kurland, LT (1973) In *Clinical Neurology, Volume 3* (ed. AB Baker and LH Baker). Harper & Row, Hagerstown, MD. Chapter 48, p. 53

15 Höhn (1977) personal communication, 7 June, Gesundheitsbehörde, Hamburg, Germany

16 Rogers, SC and Weatherall, JAC (1976) *Anencephalus, spina bifida and congenital hydrocephalus. England and Wales 1964-1972*. Studies on Medical and Population Subjects. No. 32, HMSO, London

17 Gibson, JB and Kurland, LT (1973) Unpublished data cited in Kurtzke et al 1973a [9]

18 McKeown, T and Record, RG (1951) *Lancet, i*, 192

19 Elwood, JH (1976) *Developm. Med. Child Neurol., 18*, 512

20 Record, RG and McKeown, T (1949) *Br. J. Prev. Soc. Med., 3*, 183

21 Leck, I (1963) *Br. J. Prev. Soc. Med., 17*, 70

22 Leck, I (1966) *Lancet, ii*, 791

23 McKeown, T and Record, RG (1960) In *Ciba Foundation Symposium on Congenital Malformations* (ed. GEW Wolstenholme and M O'Connor). Churchill, London

24 Smithells, RW (1962) *Developm. Med. Child Neurol., 4*, 320

25 Smithells, RW and Chinn, ER (1965) *Developm. Med. Child Neurol., 7*, 258

26 Smithells, RW, Chinn, ER and Franklin, D (1964) *Developm. Med. Child Neurol., 6*, 231

27 Smithells, RW (1968) *Br. J. Prev. Soc. Med., 22*, 36

28 Pleydell, MJ (1957) *Lancet, i*, 1314

29 Williamson, EM (1965) *J. Med. Genet., 2*, 161

30 Laurence, KM (1966) *Developm. Med. Child Neurol., suppl. 11*, 10

31 Elwood, JH and Nevin, NC (1973) *Ulster Med. J., 42*, 213

32 Stevenson, AC and Warnock, HA (1959) *Ann. Human Genet., 23*, 382

33 Nevin, NC, McDonald, JR and Walby, AL (1978) *Int. J. Epidem., 7*, 319

34 Coffey, VP (1973) *J. Irish Med. Assoc., 66*, 127

35 Spellman, MP (1970) *J. Irish Med. Assoc., 63*, 339

36 Wilson, TS (1970) *Hlth. Bull.* (Edinburgh), *28*, 32

37 Gittlesohn, AM and Milham, S (1962) *Br. J. Prev. Soc. Med., 16*, 153

38 Halevi, HS (1967) *Br. J. Prev. Soc. Med., 21*, 66

39 Czeizel, A and Révèsz, C (1970) *Br. J. Prev. Soc. Med., 24*, 205

40 Källén, B and Winberg, J (1971) *The Swedish Register of Congenital Malformations 1964-69*. The Swedish Board of Health and Welfare Reports, No. 7, Stockholm

41 Granroth, G, Hakama, M and Saxén, L (1977) *Brit. J. Prev. Soc. Med., 31*, 164

42 Kučera, J (1965) *Annales Pediatrici, 204*, 141

43 Collmann, RD and Stoller, A (1962a) *New Zealand Med. J., 61,* 24
44 Collmann, RD and Stoller, A (1962b) *Am. J. Publ. Hlth., 52,* 813
45 Stoller, A and Collmann, RD (1965) *Med. J. Austral., I,* 1
46 Neel, JV (1958) *Am. J. Human Genet., 10,* 398
47 Karim, M, Yaseen, S, El-Zeniny, A, Badawy, S and Fikry, F (1968) *J. Egyptian Med. Assoc., 51,* 864
48 Searle, AG (1959) *Ann. Human Genet., 23,* 279

Chapter 27

THE CHANGING PROBLEM OF THE NEURAL TUBE MALFORMATIONS IN THE UNITED KINGDOM

K M Laurence

The major neural tube malformations, anencephaly and spina bifida cystica, together with their variants and encephalocele are interrelated and probably all have the same aetiology, namely a polygenically inherited predisposition with environmental trigger mechanisms acting on the fetus during the first weeks of intrauterine development [1]. Complicated spina bifida occulta, i.e. spina bifida occulta involving more than one neural arch, especially if it is associated with widening of the spinal canal, vertebral abnormalities, minor orthopaedic deformities of the legs or feet or some neurological deficit, should also be regarded as part of the spina bifida anencephaly syndrome [2]. Simple spina bifida occulta, on the other hand, usually involving only one segment, seems to be part of normal variation and is probably of no clinical significance. Only about one in 50 cases of spina bifida occulta is of the complicated variety.

Aetiology

The evidence for polygenic inheritance, depending on a genetic variation at several gene loci, is that family aggregation and risks, not confined to brothers and sisters, fit in with those seen in other polygenically inherited malformations and diseases [1] (Tables I and II). The marked ethnic variations in incidence which seem to

TABLE I Risk of Occurrence and Recurrences of Neural Tube Malformations

Risk situation	Approximate risk
Whole population	1 : 200
One previous affected child	1 : 20
Two previous affected children	1 : 10
One parent affected	1 : 25
One aunt or uncle affected	1 : 50
One cousin or great aunt or uncle affected	1 : 100
Other relatives	1 : 200

284

TABLE II Family Patterns of Neural Tube Malformation compared with those of other polygenically inherited malformations (after Carter)

	Cleft lip (± cleft palate)	Talipes equinovarus	Spina bifida and anencephaly	Pyloric stenosis (males)	Spina bifida and anencephaly
	London	Exeter	London	London	South Wales
Birth frequency	0.10	0.12	0.30	0.50	0.77
Family patterns					
MZ co-twins	X 400	X 300	–	X 200	–
1° relatives	X 40	X 30	X 15	X 25	X 7
2° relatives	X 7	X 5	–	X 9	–
3° relatives	X 3	X 2	X 2	X 1½	X 1½

persist to some extent after emigration, the influence of parental consanguinity and the fall of risks of recurrence in a high risk couple when there is a remarriage all seem to point in the same direction [1]. Little is known of the environmental trigger mechanisms involved. The social class, parity and birth order effects are well known and seasonal variations and secular trends have been well documented. Undoubtedly antifolic acid agents [3], used in the past as an abortifacient, increase the risk, as probably do certain hormone preparations which, until recently, have been used as a pregnancy test [4]. Poor diet and vitamin deficiency [5] often associated with low socioeconomic status of the family also seems to be a factor, while dietary counselling given to high risk [6] women seems to reduce the recurrence of risk. In all likelihood there are many causes which may well turn out to be minor hormonal imbalances, minor biochemical changes and minor dietary influences. Whether infection plays a part is still a very open question [7].

Incidence

The incidence of this group of malformations varies greatly in different parts of the world and in different ethnic groups, the Caucasians of North Western Europe having the highest, and the Japanese and Negroes the lowest, rates [8]. The incidence at birth is highest in the British Isles, with rather lower rates in Holland, France, Germany and Scandinavia and apparently still lower rates in the Mediterranean countries. In the British Isles itself, rates vary greatly, Northern Ireland, South Wales and Scotland being the worst affected areas, and the South East and East Anglia the least. There is a suggestion that recently the incidence has been falling. In the mid-Glamorgan area of South Wales, where almost 8 per thousand births between 1956 and 1962 had neural tube defects [9] and about the same number in a survey carried out between 1964 and 1966, the rate in 1976 [10] seemed to be nearer 5 per thousand births, even when the few pregnancies then terminated in mid-trimester are included [11].

In the United Kingdom, neural tube malformations account for almost 20 per cent of perinatal deaths and constitute the commonest serious malformations [12].

285

Fortunately, anencephaly is not compatible with survival but many of the 2000 or more infants with spina bifida cystica born in the United Kingdom each year do survive though often with severe handicaps, both physical and mental, especially when operated upon [13]. It is intended here to show the effects of various management policies for these neural tube malformations but especially those for spina bifida both on the survival rate and the quality of life, making use largely of studies carried out in South Wales.

Changes in Treatment of Spina Bifida

In the past, spina bifida was an almost lethal condition and the few survivors were either so mildly affected that they were able to make their own way in life without much help, or grossly physically handicapped with paralysis and incontinence because of the spinal lesion; they were also often mentally handicapped as a result of hydrocephalus or meningitis [13]. The introduction of antibiotics after the Second World War to some extent reduced the incidence and severity of meningitis, allowing more to survive, but the major change in the survival prospects did not come about until the development of the newer plastics and the introduction of the Spitz-Holter and similar valves and the ventriculo-atrial shunt towards the end of the 1950s [14, 15]. For the first time hydrocephalus, which so nearly always accompanies the more serious forms of spina bifida, no longer seemed to be a barrier to more effective treatment of the condition [16]. However, cases tended to be considered for treatment only after the spinal lesion had become epithelialised; this generally took several months, by which time a considerable proportion of the infants, especially those with the more extensive lesions, would have died of meningitis and also hydrocephalus. In 1963, Sherrard and his coworkers [17] advocated closure of the open spina bifida lesion in the immediate neonatal period with the aim of eliminating much of the infection of the exposed neural plaque and the consequent ascending meningitis and ventriculitis. This policy was adopted by the majority of centres in the United Kingdom and resulted in reducing the mortality from meningitis and in substantially increasing the survival. It probably also reduced additional local neurological damage to the spinal cord tissue, but did not bring back function as was at first claimed. The pendulum had swung from neglect or ineffective management to vigorous interventive treatment with resultant improvement in survival in less than a decade [18].

The survival and quality of life in infants born with spina bifida before 1956 referred to the Hospital for Sick Children, London, was investigated by Evans and associates [19], and those living in South Wales by Laurence and Beresford [20]. Neither of these was a population study and therefore unlikely to be representative of the problem in the community as a whole. Nevertheless, both studies, and especially that of South Wales, suggested that nearly all the survivors had escaped hydrocephalus altogether or that the condition had become spontaneously arrested. Only 34 per cent were moderately or severely handicapped and 30 per cent, mostly true meningoceles, escaped unscathed (Table III). A population and follow up study of spina bifida births between 1956 and 1962 in Glamorgan

286

TABLE III Physical Disability of the
Survivors of Spina Bifida Infants
Born in South Wales before 1956

Disability grade	Number
I	15
II	20
III	16

Grade   I = minimal handicap
Grade   II = moderate handicap
Grade IV = severe handicap

and Monmouthshire by Laurence and Tew [21] gave a clearer picture of the natural history of untreated spina bifida which could be compared with an unselected series of children drawn from the same population treated by the 'new techniques' [13, 22].

Before considering either survival or quality of survival in the two series, it is necessary to emphasise that spina bifida cystica includes meningoceles and myeloceles. The former make up about 5 per cent of the total; they survive, rarely develop hydrocephalus, generally have little or no physical disability, and have a normal distribution of Intelligence Test results. Myeloceles make up the bulk of the cases (90-95%), most of which are open, with an exposed neural plaque. Their chance of survival in the absence of treatment is small. They tend to have limb and sphincter paralysis; 80 per cent have hydrocephalus, and they have a wide spread of mental ability, with a preponderance of dull or dull-normal individuals. There are, however, a few 'closed' cases who have a better prognosis and some with only small lesions who have little physical disability. It is not always possible to distinguish between meningoceles and myeloceles until a surgical exploration has been carried out.

The 'unoperated' series consisted of all the 290 [21] liveborn in Glamorgan and Monmouthshire between 1956 and 1962. As this was before the introduction of the aggressive treatment for the condition, none had any immediate operation for the spinal lesion, though some had 'cosmetic' operations later, and few had surgery for hydrocephalus. They were followed up and, in 1966-7, the survivors were examined and given a Stanford-Binet Intelligence Test, and then followed up again to December 1972 (Table IV). The 'universally operated' group consisted of the 115 liveborn unselected, but episodically ascertained, births with a myelocele and meningocele in Glamorgan and Monmouthshire between 1964 and 1966, being investigated as part of a study of the social and psychological effects of neural tube malformations upon the family. The periods of ascertainment were dictated by the availability of time by the interviewing social worker. The cases were drawn from the 243 liveborn cases, the total ascertained in Glamorgan and Monmouthshire between 1964 and 1966 [10, 23]. All who survived and were fit enough had immediate surgery for their spinal lesion and a Holter valve operation for hydrocephalus if indicated. They have been under continuous surveillance, were given a Wechsler Preschool and Intelligence Test at 5 years and 6 months, and were assessed

287

TABLE IV Survival of the Operated and Unoperated Series of Cases of Spina Bifida. Encephaloceles have been excluded

	Born 1956–62			Born 1964–66	
	Liveborn	Alive 1968	Alive 1972	Liveborn	Alive 1973
Meningocele	18	18*	18	9	9
Myelocele	272	36	31	104	48**
Total	290	54	49	113	57

* one not tested
** two not examined or tested

physically in the spring of 1973. Encephaloceles were excluded from both the investigations. Physical disability was graded into three broad categories of increasing severity taking into account limb function, incontinence, deformity, vision, etc, as used in other studies [13, 21, 24].

1. *The minimally handicapped* included those who had some physical deformity, a squint, slight imbalance, or slight limp. Some of the adults wore surgical supports or boots but were able to walk without aids and were totally continent except when under severe stress.

2. *The moderately handicapped* often had quite severe deformities of the spine or feet, quite marked paralysis of the legs, requiring braces, in some instances extending to the waist. Walking was with a stick or crutches. Some were able to manage only short distances. They were either partially continent usually with incontinence at night or remained dry with appliances or a successful diversion operation.

3. *The severely handicapped* included those who were very severely paralysed and could not ambulate except perhaps for a few steps and were virtually chairbound, or they were totally incontinent without any diversion operation. Most of them were both chairbound and incontinent.

Without operation the majority of liveborn spina bifida infants died, mostly of perinatal causes, then of meningitis and hydrocephalus, mostly in the first six months. A few succumbed later to pneumonia or renal failure. Of the 290 unoperated cases 54 survived to 1968 (19 per cent of the total and 13 per cent of the myeloceles) and only 5 additional cases died by 1972 (Table IV, Fig. 1).

With the more aggressive surgical approach fewer died in the first year; the partial control of infection following immediate closure of the spinal lesion, together with the vigorous use of antibiotics and the relatively successful control of hydrocephalus with shunt operations, were responsible for this. However, more died in the ensuing years of shunt complications and renal failure. Of the 113 liveborns, 57 were known to be still alive in October 1973 (50% of the total and 46% of the myeloceles).

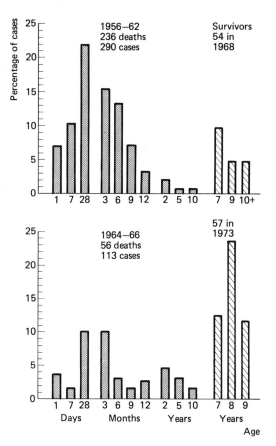

Figure 1 Ages at death and of survivors in unoperated (1956-1962) and operated (1964-1966) series of infants with spina bifida

When these results are converted into life tables, using actuarial methods [25], it is found that, unoperated, 13 per cent of myeloceles (which formed 93% of the total 1956-62 group) can be expected to survive to 10 years (and 11% to 16 years), while, operated, 45 per cent of the myeloceles (which formed 92% of the 1964-6 series) can be expected to reach the same age. This difference is highly significant (p < 0.001). The figures for the total spina bifida group are 16 per cent and 50 per cent for the unoperated and operated groups respectively (Fig. 2).

In 1966-7, when the ages of the survivors of the unoperated group were relatively comparable with those of the operated series examined in 1974, about half the unoperated survivors were almost unscathed (continent and able to get around unaided), and just under one-third were severely handicapped (wheelchair bound and incontinent). Taking the myeloceles alone, one-quarter were relatively unhandicapped, and under one-half were severely affected (Table V). The survivors

289

of the universally operated series include less than one-third mildly handicapped children and over half were severely affected, while less than one-fifth of the myeloceles fell into the mild, and almost two-thirds into the severely affected group. The operated cases were thus significantly more handicapped than the unoperated (p < 0.02).

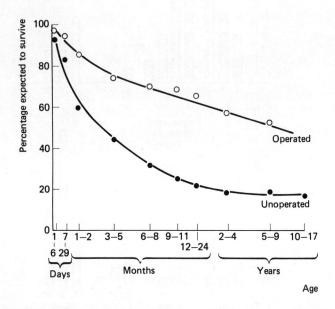

Figure 2 Survival curve drawn from a life table for both the unoperated (1956–1962) and the operated (S1964–1966) series of spina bifida infants. Encephaloceles have been excluded. A semilog scale has been used for the Y axis

TABLE V Physical Disability of the Operated and Unoperated Series of Spina Bifida Children at Comparable Ages. Encephaloceles have been excluded

Disability grade	1956–62		1964–6	
	Total series	Myelocele only	Total series	Myelocele only
	$n = 54$	$n = 36$	$n = 35$	$n = 46$
I	44	25	31	17
II	26	31	15	17
III	30	44	54	65

Figures in percentages
Grade I = minimal handicap; Grade II = moderate handicap; Grade III = severe handicap

290

The unoperated group as a whole had a mean IQ of 89 with the meningoceles and myeloceles having mean scores of 91 and 89 respectively (Fig. 3, Table VI). The operated group, on the other hand, had a mean score of 81 with the meningoceles and myeloceles having scores of 102 and 77 respectively.

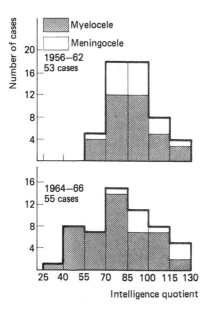

Figure 3 Wechsler, IQ scores of tested survivors of both unoperated and operated series. Meningoceles and myeloceles are shown separately; encephaloceles have been excluded. The mean IQ of the unoperated is 89.4, the operated 80.9

TABLE VI Wechsler Intelligence Quotients in the Operated and Unoperated Series of Spina Bifida Children at Comparable Ages. Encephaloceles have been excluded

	Born 1956–62			Born 1964–6		
	Number	Mean IQ	Standard deviation	Number	Mean IQ	Standard deviation
Meningocele	17	90.8	15.3	9	101.9	13.8
Myelocele	36	88.8	16.6	46	76.8	22.4
Total	53	89.4	16.0	55	80.9	23.1

There were no matched controls available for the unoperated series, but matched control children for 56 of the operated cases had a mean IQ of 104. This accords with the mean Wechsler IQ of a normal British population [26, 27]. The sibs of the

291

operated index cases, who might be expected to be a more accurate guide to the potential IQ of our group, were also examined and were found to have a mean Wechsler IQ of 104 [28]. With immediate operation the series as a whole, as well as the myeloceles alone, seemed to perform less well intellectually than those who were not operated upon, and for the myeloceles the difference reached statistical significance. This was probably due to progressive hydrocephalus, even though usually treated quite successfully by shunting, since over half of the myelocele survivors born between 1964 and 1966 had this complication. In the 1956-62 unoperated group, progressive hydrocephalus was the second most common cause of death, and over two-thirds of the myelocele survivors had either escaped hydrocephalus altogether or had it only mildly with spontaneous arrest [21].

Attainment in terms of reading, spelling, and arithmetic of the unoperated series and also of the operated series was lower than the level expected from the Wechsler IQ results [29]. When both physical disability and intellectual ability were taken together, the results for both groups were even worse, for example, there were children only minimally physically handicapped in the two series but whose IQ results were below normal. There were 11 one-standard deviation (IQ 90), and 5 two-standard deviations (IQ 76), below the mean for a normal population.

The impact of surgical intervention on the quality of life may not be appreciated until the status of survivors after surgery is measured against that of a comparable series of unoperated cases. Without operation, actuarial data indicate that, out of 100 liveborn spina bifida infants, 17 would survive to ten years, with 8 of these either physically normal or relatively unhandicapped and only 5 severely handicapped, chairbound or incapacitated. However, the operative approach without selection, as originally advocated by Sharrard and his colleagues [17] and widely followed in the UK and elsewhere, enabled at least 50 cases in South Wales to survive to ten years with 15 physically normal or near normal survivors, but 27 severely handicapped survivors. Thus, to save 7 relatively unscathed children who might otherwise have died, 22 additional grossly handicapped children will probably live. To save 5 additional good cases in 100 liveborn cases of myelocele, 23 severely affected ones are enabled to survive. When, in addition to the physical handicap, mental handicap is also considered, these figures become even more depressing and they may well be worse still in series where the proportion of operated survivors is greater [30, 31]. The quality of survivors among the South Wales operated cases seems to be very similar to that reported in an operated series by Hunt [32]. It is estimated that in the UK alone, with an average incidence of 2.5 cases of spina bifida per 1000 births, each year about 500 additional families would have to cope with a severely handicapped surviving child, as a direct consequence of the adoption of the aggressive surgical approach to the abnormality.

Although some centres, such as Edinburgh [33] and Oxford [34] had consistently withheld immediate operative closure for the spinal lesion in a considerable proportion of cases, most units in the UK did, in fact, adopt the aggressive approach towards spina bifida advocated by the Sheffield team [17]. This policy obviously resulted in a large number of surviving severely handicapped children, whose lives were not only precarious but made enormous demands on the health services for medical supervision and hospital treatment [35] and later placed considerable burdens on the special education facilities [36]. Their families were under constant stress, often leading to marital disharmony and breakup [37], and they were in need of an enormous amount of social support [22] which was not always forthcoming. Lorber [38], realising the situation, advocated a policy of stringent election which would exclude from surgery and other extraordinary measures more than 50 per cent of all cases referred, including, hopefully, those who would grow up most handicapped. The adverse criteria suggested consisted of gross paralysis, a high (thoracolumbar) lesion, kyphosis with or without scoliosis, cerebral birth injury or unassociated congenital defects and obvious hydrocephalus. Lorber claimed that most of the excluded infants were dead within one month and none survived longer than nine months in spite of normal nursing and feeding, and that nearly all the operated children had survived and were only slightly handicapped. However, this has not been everybody's experience. Although most practised clinicians can accurately predict the degree of paralysis and incontinence a new-born child will suffer later, it seems to be extraordinarily difficult to forecast the likely survival or the degree of mental retardation, largely because of the impossibility of anticipating what complications or therapeutic mishaps might arise [39]. Further, it has been found in several units that a significant proportion of excluded children do not die quickly and some survive [40] (Table VII), as might be

TABLE VII The Fate of Infants Excluded from Surgery in the Neonatal Period

Excluded	Alive at 6 months	Alive at 1 year	Surviving
42	12	6	5

expected from the South Wales follow up study of unoperated cases [21]. Not surprisingly, the selection policy has led to a great deal of discussion, controversy and disquiet about the ethical problems involved within the profession and also some worry in the general public, which fortunately has abated somewhat, since the availability of prenatal diagnosis for neural tube malformations has removed some of the urgency and diverted attention to other aspects.

Prenatal Diagnosis of Neural Tube Malformations in High Risk Pregnancies

The only means of reducing the number of cases had been by genetic counselling in high-risk situations (Table I). Parents tend to act responsibly, and when the risk is high avoid pregnancy and therefore a recurrence [41, 42]. More recently, early prenatal diagnosis followed by selective abortion has become available.

In 1972, Brock and Sutcliffe [43] found that pregnancies of anencephalics and spina bifida fetuses were associated with raised alpha-fetoprotein (AFP) levels in amniotic fluid during the fifth month of gestation. AFP, the serum protein produced by the fetal liver normally up to about 20 weeks gestation, reaches the

293

amniotic fluid via the fetal kidneys [44], to appear in amounts that can be measured by immuno-electrophoretic methods which are within the capabilities of most of the larger biochemical laboratories, or by a more complex radioimmunoassay. Normal adult non-pregnant women have only minute amounts in the serum. 'Open' neural tube lesions such as anencephaly, myelocele and certain other abnormalities that have exposed neural tissue, permit an excessive leak of AFP into the amniotic fluid, which then becomes moderately to severely elevated.

To obtain amniotic fluid for AFP estimation, an amniocentesis, a quite simple and painless outpatient procedure, is carried out between 15 and 19 weeks [45]. It should be preceded by an ultrasound scan, not only to confirm the gestational age from the fetal biparietal diameter, but also to ascertain the position of the placenta, which will determine the precise technique to be used, and to exclude twins, which may make this procedure difficult.

Nearly all cases of anencephaly and 9 out of 10 cases of spina bifida, the 'open' ones, will therefore be detectable from a raised amniotic AFP level. 'Closed' lesions will not be detected. The 10 per cent of undetectable cases consist of encephaloceles, closed myeloceles and meningoceles. Encephaloceles, which are nearly always 'closed', and many of which survive, often with gross handicap, will not be detected. Fortunately, they account for less than 5 per cent of spina bifida. The closed skin covered myeloceles, which are also relatively uncommon, also with a high survival

TABLE VIII Incidence and Detectability of the Various Neural Tube Malformations

Type of lesion	% of total	% of those compatible with survival	Prenatal detection
Anencephaly	50	0	Yes
Exencephaly acrania	0.5	0	No
Iniencephaly	2	0	Usually
Open myelocele	41	87	Yes
Skin-covered (closed) myelocele	1.5	3	No
Small puckered open myelocele	1	2	?
Encephalocele	1.5	3	No
True meningocele	2.5	5	No
Complicated spina bifida occulta	?	?	No
Hydrocephalus without spina bifida	?	?	No

rate but frequently associated with quite severe incontinence and mobility problems, will also not be detected. The true meningoceles, which as a rule do not have any serious sequelae, tend to have a thick membrane and therefore are also not detected. They account for about 1 in 20 cases. The small puckered, partially open myeloceles, generally epithelialised by term or soon after and not associated with severe disabilities, are similarly unlikely to be detected (Table VIII).

The upper limit of AFP in amniotic fluid from pregnancies with normal outcomes, rises rapidly from 14 weeks to reach a peak at 16 weeks, usually not exceeding 40 mg/litre, to fall to single figure amounts after 21 weeks [46] (Fig. 4).

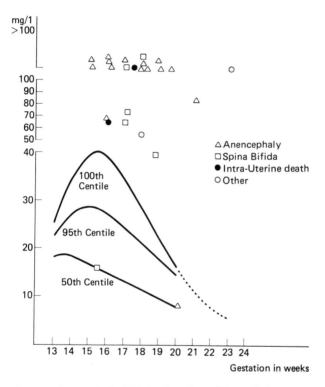

Figure 4 Normal curves for amniotic AFP levels estimated by radio-immunoassay compiled from 796 singleton pregnancies of known gestation length between 13th ana 24th weeks. The *dotted line* in the presumed 'extinction' line was based on very few results. AFP levels in pregnancies associated with abnormal outcomes are added

Anencephalic fetuses, except in the rare 'closed' case, tend to be associated with levels of between 100 and 400 mg/litre. Widely 'open' spina bifida fetuses will have slightly lower levels of AFP, ranging between 70 and 200 mg/litre, but smaller 'open' lesions may have only marginally elevated levels. In the UK, with its high incidence of neural tube malformations, many of the amniocenteses are carried out

295

because the mother has previously had a child affected with a neural tube malformation. A recent Clinical Genetics Society Working Party report on amniocentesis services in the UK [47] analysed over 14 000 amniocenteses carried out by the end of 1976 (Table IX) and found that 4460 amniocenteses carried out because of a previous affected child led to the detection of 132 neural tube defects, an incidence of about one in 34; 458 procedures performed because of a positive family history of neural tube malformation yielded only seven cases, i.e. one case detected in 67 amniocenteses. Anxiety only as a reason for the amniocentesis led to the detection of 3 in 471, i.e. 1 in 150 and the 2025 that had AFP estimations carried out, even though the indication was a chromosomal one, demonstrated 13 neural tube malformations, also about 1 detected in 150, which is only a little above the population incidence. However, the 4786 amniocenteses carried out for a neural tube indication, that also had amnion cell culture and cytogenetics performed, demonstrated 18 chromosome anomalies, 1 in 265, which is about the number of the population incidence expected.

TABLE IX Prenatal Diagnosis of Neural Tube Malformations in the UK up to 1977 (after Ferguson-Smith et al) [47]

Indication	Number of amniocenteses	Number of neural tube defects	Risk
Previous neural tube defect (NTD)	4460	132	1 : 34
Family history of NTD	458	7	1 : 65
Anxiety only	471	3	1 : 150
Chromosome abnormality	2025	13	1 : 150
Raised serum AFP	364	78	1 : 5

Before an amniocentesis is carried out, couples should be counselled so that they are quite clear about the limitations of the tests, that there is an appreciable risk of sequential abortion, put as high as 1.5 per cent by the recently published MRC study [48], and that an abnormal result will lead to the recommendation of a termination. Whether or not an amniocentesis should be agreed to, when the couples refuse to accept a termination on religious, moral or emotional grounds, is a matter of argument. Before 1973, when no practical prenatal diagnostic method was available, fewer than 1 in 20 women who have already had a child with a neural tube malformation, whether dead or surviving, would start a further pregnancy and, in less than one year, almost 50 per cent decided not to have any more children at all, usually opting for sterilisation [46, 49]. Since then, over 50 per cent start a pregnancy within the year and fewer than one couple in five opt to have no further children. These latter tended to be those with a surviving spina bifida child or those who have decided that, after all, their family was complete. Further, while a couple who have an abnormal child unexpectedly at term, are generally greatly upset, those having a planned pregnancy with a planned amniocentesis following an abortion are generally ready to contemplate a further pregnancy after three months.

They seem to be prepared for a possible disappointment and often feel that they took an active part in 'antenatal care'. However, in view of the risks of amniocentesis, an alternative approach should probably be considered for any pregnancy where the risk of neural tube malformation is estimated to be less than 1 in 70. Under these circumstances an ultrasound scan and a maternal serum AFP estimation should be offered, followed by an amniocentesis only if either of these examinations suggest that the fetus may be abnormal.

Maternal Serum AFP Screening

In the UK, only one in ten cases of neural tube malformation is born to women known to be at increased risk [50]. The other nine cases are born to families apparently without any positive history. Population screening to detect the latter, involving a procedure such as amniocentesis with the considerable sequential abortion risk and morbidity that would in all likelihood result when used on a wide scale, could not be justifiable on a population basis, even if the resources to carry out so many were available. Ultrasound, noninvasive and not dangerous to mother or fetus, could only reasonably certainly identify anencephaly but, at best, only a minority of cases of spina bifida. The resources, both in staff and equipment, for performing such careful examinations as would be necessary to detect more cases of spina bifida are at present not to hand. However, population screening has become a possibility with the discovery by the same Edinburgh team that there is an elevated maternal serum AFP level at 16 to 19 weeks, associated with most cases of anencephaly and the majority of open spina bifida [51], a matter confirmed by a UK Collaborative Study [52], involving the collection of more than 18 000 samples of serum from pregnant women in 19 centres. Raised serum AFP levels are also found with multiple pregnancies with threatened or missed abortion and with exomphalos among other conditions. However, in most cases, no cause for the raised levels can be found and this is probably due to a physiological peculiarity in the women allowing the AFP to cross the placental barrier in slightly larger amounts than usual.

Serum AFP screening is now being carried out in quite a number of centres in the UK in addition to those that participated in the UK Collaborative Study. Generally, blood is taken from women attending antenatal clinic between 15 and 19 weeks. Those attending before 16 weeks are asked to return later, while those first attending at 20 weeks or later are usually not screened. If the AFP level is raised, they are offered an ultrasound scan and an amniocentesis, with a view to termination if the amniotic AFP is also raised. In some centres, a second blood sample is tested and an ultrasound scan is performed, before amniocentesis is considered. Those women known to be at high risk of neural tube malformation from their family or obstetric history or for chromosome anomalies, are usually referred directly for counselling, ultrasound scanning and amniocentesis. In the various screening centres, before deciding to recommend amniocentesis, different AFP levels varying from the 95th to the 99th centile are used. Some use multiples of the mean. The 364 amniocenteses that were carried out in the UK up to 1976 because the serum AFP level was raised, led to the detection of only 78 open neural tube malformations, i.e. over one abnormal fetus found in five amniocenteses (*see* Table IX). Serum AFP estimation has been carried out on some pregnancies throughout South Wales since 1974 (Fig. 5), at first as part of the UK Collaborative Study, and is routinely carried out prior to most amniocenteses.

Screening a total population with all its attendant difficulties presents quite different problems from carrying out serum AFP estimations on women from a few selected practices or clinics with dedicated and knowledgeable staff. Popu-

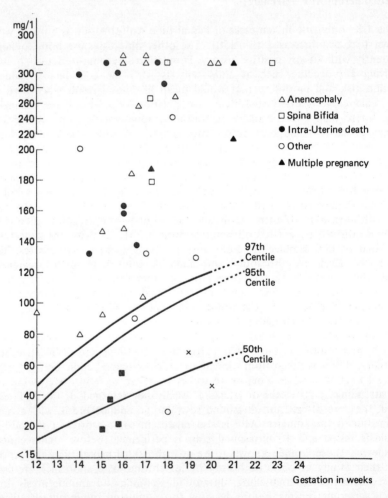

Figure 5 Normal curves for the maternal serum AFP levels estimated by RIA compiled from 1546 singleton pregnancies of known gestation length between the 12th and 20th weeks with normal outcome AFP levels of abnormal outcome added

lation screening is being carried out in very few areas, one possibly being an area around Glasgow, and another is in South Wales, where in Mid-Glamorgan true population screening has been conducted by our team (Professors C J Roberts, B M Hibbard, K T Evans, G Elder and K M Laurence) which has been commissioned by the Department of Health to set up population screening to monitor its operational problems and effectiveness under field conditions [46]. Mid-Glamorgan has been chosen with its high incidence (7.8 per 1000 births in 1965), its relatively scattered population of over 400 000, its 8 antenatal clinics, but no teaching hospital of its own. The aim was to try, in the first instance, to graft on to the existing obstetric services with the least disruption and anxiety to patients and staff, as effectively and economically as possible.

Before effective screening on a large scale can be introduced, solutions to a number of problems will have to be found and it is hoped that our study will do this. An efficient radioimmunoassay laboratory has to be available. How this is to be organised and what size of population it should cater for is not yet certain. A good genetic counselling service, both for 'high risk' couples and for women picked out by the screening programme as possibly carrying an abnormal baby, must also be on hand. While the former should probably be conducted by the genetic advisory service staff, the obstetricians may possibly fulfil the latter. An ultrasound service is vital, as the interpretation of serum AFP levels is dependent on accurate gestational dating. Whether a 'two tier' ultrasound service, one for gestational dating and the other preamniocentesis, is most efficient is uncertain. An efficient amniocentesis service, staffed by skilled and experienced personnel, must be established. Whether this should be concentrated at a 'centre of excellence' or most conveniently conducted in district general hospitals is not known at present. Efficient transportation of specimens and relaying of results, normal and abnormal, is vital to any successful screening. At what sort of level a repeat blood sample is taken, or an ultrasound scan or diagnostic amniocentesis is recommended, is still very much a matter of debate. It is hoped that the investigation will be able to make recommendations here.

Women want sympathetic explanation of screening and its implications. This could be carried out either on the media, in the family doctor's surgery or the antenatal clinic. Whether they should be required specifically to ask for screening before blood is taken for AFP estimation, or whether this is carried out automatically unless they 'opt out', is a matter of argument. However, compliance in the majority of screening schemes in the UK seems to be high. Uptake is, however, invariable and is dependent on the women attending at the doctor's surgery early enough and on the doctor then referring her to the clinic quickly. To achieve high uptake may require both public propaganda and professional education.

With amniocentesis and AFP estimation in mid trimester, now generally available in the UK, a woman known to be at high risk for neural tube malformation can contemplate a pregnancy with relative assurance that an affected fetus will be prevented from reaching term, provided the couple can accept selective termination. However, before amniocentesis is carried out, preferably before the pregnancy is even started, the couple should be counselled so that they are quite clear about the limitations of the tests and made aware that false negatives do occur.

Some women will undoubtedly not want to avail themselves of such a facility on moral, religious, or emotional grounds, or because of the risk of amniocentesis. The same is likely to be true for population screening, which is less firmly based, and decisions about its introduction on a nation wide scale in the UK, even with its relatively high incidence, have yet to be made. In areas with a lower incidence of neural tube malformation it may well be neither feasible nor acceptable. Although from a purely financial point of view, screening may well be cost effective in the UK, the sequential fetal losses following amniocentesis, the possible occasional false positive and the large number of normal pregnancies which will undoubtedly be called to question 'unnecessarily' by the process, may militate against its universal introduction. However, without it, the impact of prenatal diagnosis on the number of neural tube malformations reaching term will be small. On the other hand, with maternal serum AFP screening, it may be possible to reduce by two-thirds the number of spina bifida infants reaching term including, more hopefully, most of the more severe cases and, at the same time, perhaps relieve some of the population's worries about the condition.

Summary and Conclusions

The treatment for spina bifida has seen considerable changes since World War II, from inactivity or ineffective intervention with a high mortality that left a few less handicapped survivors, to active interventive treatment between 1963 and 1973 that resulted in numerous survivors who were grossly handicapped physically, and often mentally as well. Since then, the consensus of opinion has swung again towards inactivity for a large proportion of cases leaving, once more, fewer survivors who are on the whole somewhat less handicapped.

Since 1974, prenatal diagnosis by means of an amniocentesis and amniotic AFP estimations has been available for pregnancies known to be at increased risk for neural tube malformation. However, even if all such pregnancies are monitored and abnormal ones terminated, this would have only a marginal effect on the numbers of spina bifida babies that reach term. To reduce the numbers substantially, population pregnancy screening by means of maternal serum AFP estimation would have to be carried out. Even if 90 per cent of all pregnancies are screened in this way, perhaps 20 per cent of 'open', and therefore serious, spina bifida infants would still be born as well as all the closed lesions, some of which would also be associated with physical disability or mental retardation or both. Therefore the spina bifida problem will certainly not have been eliminated either by selection or by these modern prenatal diagnostic and screening methods, and an appreciable number will still have to be treated and cared for in the foreseeable future in the UK. Finally, prenatal diagnosis followed by selective termination can be regarded only as second best to true prevention, which will not be possible until the trigger mechanisms that set off the malformation in early pregnancy have been identified and hopefully prevented or eliminated.

Acknowledgements

I wish to thank the editor of *The Lancet* for permission to reprint Figure 1 from Laurence [13], and the editor of *Zeitschrift für Kinderchirurgie und Grenzgebiete* for permission to reprint Figures 4 and 5 from Laurence [46].

References

1 Carter, CO (1974) *Dev. Med. Child Neurol., 16,* Suppl. 32, 3
2 Laurence, KM, Bligh, AS and Evans, KT (1968) *Dev. Med. Child Neurol., 10,* Suppl. 16, 107
3 Thiersch, JB (1952) *Am. J. Obstet. Gynec., 63,* 1298
4 Gal, I, Kirman, B and Stern, J (1971) *Nature, 223,* 494
5 Smithells, RW, Sheppard, S and Schorah, CJ (1976) *Arch. Dis. Childh., 51,* 944
6 James, N, Miller, M and Laurence, KM (1979) unpublished data
7 Hurley, R (1978) *Towards the Prevention of Fetal Malformation.* Edinburgh University Press, Edinburgh, p. 101
8 Laurence, KM (1969) *Dev. Med. Child Neurol., Suppl. 10,* 23
9 Laurence, KM, Carter, CO and David, PA (1968) *Brit. J. Prev. Soc. Med., 22,* 146 and 212
10 Richards, IDG and Lowe, CR (1971) *Brit. J. Prev. Soc. Med., 25,* 59
11 Laurence, KM, unpublished data
12 Butler, NR and Bonham, DG (1963) *Perinatal Mortality.* Edinburgh: Livingstone
13 Laurence, KM (1974) *Lancet, i,* 301
14 Nulsen, FE and Spitz, EB (1951) *Surgical Forum, 2,* 399
15 Pudenz, RH, Russel, FE, Hurd, AM and Sheldon, CH (1957) *J. Neurosurg., 14,* 171
16 Doran, PA and Guthkelch, N (1961) *J. Neurosurg. Neurol. Psychiat., 24,* 331
17 Sherrard, WJW, Zachary, RB, Lorber, J and Bruce, AM (1963) *Arch. Dis. Childh., 38,* 18
18 Stark, GD (1976) *Spina Bifida, Problems and Management.* Oxford: Blackwells
19 Evans, K, Hickman, V and Carter, CO (1975) *Brit. J. Prev. Soc. Med., 28,* 85
20 Laurence, KM and Beresford, A (1976) *Brit. J. Prev. Soc. Med., 30,* 97
21 Laurence, KM and Tew, JB (1971) *Arch. Dis. Childh., 46,* 328
22 Hare, EH, Laurence, KM, Payne, H and Rawnsley, K (1963) *Brit. Med. J., 2,* 757
23 Spies, JA (1974), personal communication
24 Richards, IDG and McIntosh, HT (1973) *Dev. Med. Child Neurol., 15,* 292
25 Laurence, KM and Coates, S (1962) *Arch. Dis. Childh., 37,* 345
26 Brittain, M (1969) *Brit. J. Educ. Psych., 39,* 14
27 Rutter, M, Tizard, J and Whitmore, K (1970) *Education Health and Behaviour.* London
28 Tew, BJ and Laurence, KM (1973) *Dev. Med. Child Neurol., 15,* Suppl. 29, 69
29 Tew, BJ and Laurence, KM (1972) *Dev. Med. Child Neurol., 14,* Suppl. 27, 124
30 Mawdsley, T and Rickham, PP (1969) *Dev. Med. Child Neurol., 11,* Suppl. 20, 8
31 Eckstein, HA (1973) *Z. Kinderchir., 13,* 17
32 Hunt, GM (1973) *Lancet, ii,* 1308
33 Stark, GD and Drummond, M (1973) *Arch. Dis. Childh., 48,* 676
34 Hide, DW, Parry Williams, H and Ellis, HL (1972) *Dev. Med. Child Neurol., 14,* 304
35 Brocklehurst, G and Barnett, B (1972) *J. Kentucky Med. Ass., 70,* 860
36 Laurence, ER (1971) *Dev. Med. Child Neurol., 13,* Suppl. 27, 44
37 Tew, BJ, Laurence, KM, Paynce, H and Rawnsley, K (1977) *Brit. J. Psych., 131,* 79
38 Lorber, J (1973) *Brit. Med. J., 4,* 203
39 Laurence, KM, Evans, RC, Weeks, RD, Thomas, M, Frazer, K and Tew, BJ (1976) *Dev. Med. Child Neurol., 18,* Suppl. 37, 150
40 Evans, RC (1979), personal communication
41 Carter, CO, Roberts, AF, Evans, K and Buck, AR (1971) *Lancet, i,* 281
42 Morris, J and Laurence, KM (1976) *Dev. Med. Child Neurol., 18,* Suppl. 37, 157

43 Brock, DJH and Sutcliffe, RG (1972) *Lancet, ii,* 197
44 Laurence, KM (1974) *Dev. Med. Child Neurol., 16,* Suppl. 32, 117
45 Laurence, KM (1976) In *Birth Defects Risks and Consequences.* (ed S Kelly, DT Janerisch and IH Porter). New York: Academic Press, p. 63
46 Laurence, KM (1977) *Z. Kinderchir., 22,* 383
47 Ferguson-Smith, MA, Benson, PF, Brock, DJH, Fairweather, DVI, Harris, R, Laurence, KM, McDermott, A, Patrick, AD, Polani, PE and Walker, S (1978) *Eugenics Soc.,* Suppl. 3
48 UK MRC Amniocentesis Working Group (1978) *Brit. J. Obstet. Gynae., 85,* Suppl. 2
49 Morris, J and Laurence, KM (1976) *Dev. Med. Child Neurol., 18,* Suppl. 37, 157
50 Laurence, KM (1974) *Lancet, ii,* 939
51 Brock, DJH, Bolton, AE and Monaghan, JM (1973) *Lancet, ii,* 923
52 Brock, DJH, Chard, T, Cuckle, H, Ferguson-Smith, MA, Laurence, KM, Peto, R, Polani, PE, Wald, NJ and Woodford, FP (1977) *Lancet, i,* 1323

Chapter 28

ENCEPHALITIS–ENCEPHALOPATHY IN CHILDHOOD

Martin H Bellman

Encephalitis literally means inflammation within the head and implies a no greater degree of diagnostic precision than the equally loose terms nephritis, bronchitis, or arthritis. Indeed, in many cases of 'encephalitis' the inflammatory component of the disorder is doubtful and the even less committal term 'encephalopathy' should be used.

The factors that may play an aetiological role in these disorders are numerous (Fig. 1). A wide range of microbiological organisms of all classes are capable of causing classical acute primary encephalitis by direct effect on the brain. The cerebral matter is infiltrated with the organism by haematogenous spread, often in the course of a generalised infection, and the organism itself may be isolated from a biopsy specimen of brain or sometimes cerebrospinal fluid. The fetal brain may be affected in a similar manner during certain maternal infections such as syphilis, toxoplasmosis, rubella and cytomegalovirus.

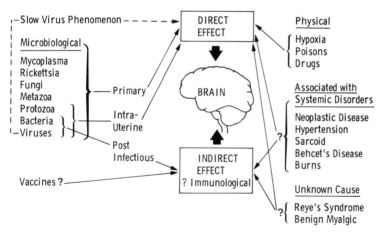

Figure 1 Factors associated with encephalitis–encephalopathy

Some organisms that cause an acute, usually mild, infection in children, e.g. measles, chicken pox, rubella and whooping cough, may give rise to an encephalitic illness after a delay of up to two weeks. This has been termed post-infectious or allergic encephalitis and is thought to be due to an indirect mechanism, probably a hypersensitivity reaction. In contrast to primary encephalitis, the organism is not present in the brain and cannot be isolated from it. In clinical practice it is not always possible to place a case clearly into one category or the other and there is probably considerable overlap between direct microbiological invasion of the brain and immunological reaction. Pathological investigation may be of little help as in many cases of presumed acute encephalitis, especially of viral origin, the organism is not identified, and in some cases of post-infectious encephalitis the virus has been isolated from the brain [1].

Another mechanism for infection of the brain is by the slow virus phenomenon, seen in subacute sclerosing panencephalitis with measles virus [2] and in the spongiform encephalopathies, kuru and Jakob-Creutzfeld disease [3].

Encephalitis is known to occur after administration of smallpox and rabies vaccines and has been alleged to follow whooping cough vaccination. The pathogenesis is probably mediated via immune processes and is analogous to post-infectious encephalitis.

Encephalopathy with or without actual inflammation may be associated with many other factors. Cerebral function may be directly affected by adverse physical conditions, e.g. hypoxia due to acute or chronic airway obstruction or as a result of convulsions themselves, organic and inorganic poisons such as alcohol and lead, and drugs such as phenytoin.

Several systemic disorders may be complicated by encephalopathy, e.g. malignant disease, sarcoidosis, Behçet's syndrome and hypertension. It can also be associated with burns, which may be trivial in themselves, or infection elsewhere in the body, so-called acute toxic encephalopathy [4].

Finally, there are some encephalopathic syndromes in which aetiological factors remain unknown, e.g. Reye's syndrome of acute encephalopathy with disordered liver function [5] and benign myalgic encephalomyelitis or Royal Free disease.

Epidemiological information concerning the many different possible factors is very patchy. It is good in some areas such as those where the aetiology is known, usually, of course, the epidemiology preceding and leading to the understanding of the causal association. As far as micro-organisms are concerned, viral encephalitis is undoubtedly of greatest significance. Knowledge about it is, however, still poor largely because of the difficulty of diagnosis due to the inaccessibility of the brain to direct examination. This position has somewhat improved since the advent of computerised axial tomography [6].

An opportunity to look at some of the encephalopathies in relation to children including Reye's syndrome and virus encephalitis was provided by the National Childhood Encephalopathy Study (NCES) which was set up in 1976. Its primary aim was to investigate the suggested link between whooping cough vaccine and encephalopathy leading to permanent brain damage. Attention was first drawn to the association between these two events in 1933 by Madsen [7] from Denmark, who reported the case of an infant who developed convulsions and died shortly after being given pertussis vaccine. Following this, several more case descriptions appeared and, in 1948, Byers and Moll [8] recorded a series of 15 patients from the Boston Children's Hospital who developed convulsions within 3 days of pertussis vaccination. Two of these children died, 12 had permanent severe neurological problems and one child recovered.

In 1960, Strom [9] described 36 Swedish children of whom 13 had permanent sequelae and entitled his article, 'Is universal vaccination against pertussis always justified?' In 1974 Kulenkampff and colleagues [10] reported 36 children referred over a period of 11 years to the neurological unit at the Hospital for Sick Children, Great Ormond Street, London, who had received pertussis vaccination within 14 days of developing an encephalopathy. Four of these children recovered, two died and 30 were left with long-term residual defects. The debate had up to then remained within medical circles, but was picked up by the mass media and much emotive publicity ensued. The matter was further complicated by widely differing estimates of the risk put forward by various medical experts (Table I), this, of

TABLE I Encephalopathy Following Pertussis Vaccine—suggested incidence

Strom (Sweden) 1960	$1/17\,000 \rightarrow 1/50\,000$ [9, 11]
Prensky (US) 1974	$1/180\,000$ [12]
Stewart (UK) 1977	$1/10\,000 - 1/60\,000$ [13]
Grist (UK) 1977	$1/135\,000$ [14]
Dept. of Health 1977	$1/300\,000$ [15]

course, being the vital piece of information parents wanted to know. The result was that children were not taken for vaccination and the uptake of pertussis vaccine fell from 80 per cent to 35 per cent. National vaccination policy in the UK is determined by the Joint Committee on Vaccination and Immunisation whose members became very concerned about the situation and, through their Subcommittee on Complications of Vaccination, reviewed the available evidence. Because of its anecdotal nature, they found this inconclusive and recommended a controlled epidemiological study to determine whether vaccinated children had a greater risk of developing encephalopathy than unvaccinated children.

The National Childhood Encephalopathy Study requests notification of children admitted to hospital throughout England, Wales and Scotland aged between two months and the third birthday suffering from a defined group of acute neurological problems (Table II). Clinical details are obtained from the hospital, and immunis-

TABLE II National Childhood Encephalopathy Study. Notification Criteria. (Age range: 2 months—3rd birthday)

1 Acute/Subacute Encephalitis/Encephalomyelitis/Encephalopathy
2 Unexplained loss of consciousness
3 Convulsions if – Total duration $>$ ½ hour
                  – Coma $>$ 2 hours
                  – Paralysis or other neurological signs $>$ 24 hours
4 Infantile spasms (West's syndrome) [16]
5 Reye's syndrome [5]

ation histories are supplied by Specialists in Community Medicine (Child Health) who also select control subjects matched for sex and age from children living in the same area. Details about past medical, family and social background are obtained

305

by health visitor home interview. The information can be analysed at a later date by a case-control method. Although the majority of patients recover, we are particularly interested in those who do not. They are defined as children who have not completely recovered by an arbitrary time period of 15 days after their admission to hospital (Fig. 2). They are the 'residual' cases and are followed up with standard neurological and developmental assessments by a member of the research team. The 'non-residual' cases are followed up by letter.

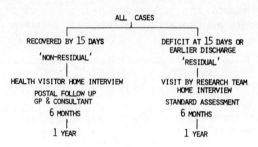

Figure 2 NCES case follow-up

First-Year Results of the National Childhood Encephalopathy Study

In the first year of the Study a total of 387 notifications were received. Of these, 129 were excluded, usually because the child was outside the age range, leaving a working total of 258 accepted cases. There were 132 males and 126 females giving a sex ratio of approximately one to one.

Geographical Distribution

Case reporting was fairly evenly distributed around the country in approximate proportion to the population density. There is no evidence of a regional concentration of cases or a rural-urban difference in distribution.

Social Class

Table III shows a case-control analysis according to the social class of the child's

TABLE III Social Class

	I & II	III	IV & V	Total
Cases	42	85	55	182
	23%	47%	30%	100%
Controls	107	185	73	365
	29%	51%	20%	100%

$\chi^2 = 7.5$; DF = 2; P $<$ 0.05

father. Compared with controls the cases come significantly less often from social classes I and II and more often from classes IV and V. A bias towards the lower social classes is frequently found in hospital patients; however, it is likely that a child with a severe acute neurological illness meeting the Study criteria will be admitted to hospital regardless of social conditions at home and, hence, the gradient demonstrated represents a true association with encephalopathy.

TABLE IV Past History

	Congenital abnormality		Neonatal problem
	Neurological	Non-neurological	
Residual cases	8 (7%)	13 (11%)	21 (18%)
Non-residual cases	2 (1.5%)	3 (2%)	6 (5%)
Total (all cases)	10 (4%)	16 (6%)	27 (10%)

$P < 0.001$

Past History

Table IV shows the distribution of certain features in the past history between residual cases (those children who have a persisting abnormality beyond 15 days after admission) and non-residual cases (children who have fully recovered by 15 days after admission). There is a significant association with the presence of a congenital abnormality or a neonatal problem in the residual cases as compared to the non-residual cases. The association is not confined to neurological defects such as hydrocephalus and microcephaly, but also non-neurological abnormalities which, apart from two cases of congenital heart disease, include mainly minor defects, e.g. cleft palate, dislocated hip, limb anomalies and skin lesions. A similar association is found with neonatal problems such as severe birth asphyxia or respiratory distress and metabolic problems.

Age

The age distribution of residual and non-residual cases is shown in Figure 3. There is a peak in the age incidence of residual cases at five to six months with relatively few occurring over the age of two years. However, the distribution of the non-residual cases is much more evenly spread across the age range. Many children are given their first dose of triple vaccine under the routine immunisation schedule at about six months of age and therefore it would not be surprising if many of them had been recently vaccinated. In order to reach a valid conclusion regarding an association, the incidence of recent vaccination in these cases must be compared with that in a group of control children who do not have neurological disease.

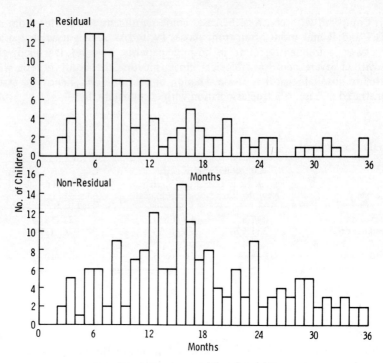

Figure 3 Age distribution of cases

TABLE V History of DPT and OPV Vaccine in Past 28 Days

	Immunised	Not immunised	Total
Cases	16 (6.3%)	239 (93.7%)	255
Controls	33 (6.7%)	463 (93.3%)	496

Not statistically significant

DPT = Diphtheria-pertussis-tetanus immunisation
OPV = Oral polio vaccine

Vaccination

Table V shows the case-control analysis of immunisation with diphtheria–pertussis-tetanus (DPT), and oral polio vaccines (OPV) within the 28 days prior to the admission of the case to hospital. Of 255 cases for whom we have full details, 239 had not been immunised with triple vaccine in this period and therefore immunisation could not have been closely associated with the onset of their encephalopathy. The number of children who had been immunised (16) is very small and the pro-

308

portion of the total (6.3%) is not significantly different from that in controls. Lest vaccine associated cases should be clustered in a shorter time period than 28 days, case-control analyses were carried out for periods of 0-7, 8-14 and 15-28 days, with no significant difference between cases and controls in any group.

Similar analysis of diphtheria–tetanus vaccine without the pertussis component also showed no significant association with cases of encephalopathy.

Diagnosis

The diagnostic categories in Table VI relate to the diagnosis made by the notifying clinician. Of the total of 258 cases notified, 116 (45%) had persisting sequelae (including deaths) and are classed as residual cases. The largest number of children notified, 90, had one or more febrile convulsions with a total duration of at least 30 minutes. They account for 35 per cent of all cases, but only 5 per cent of the residual group.

TABLE VI National Childhood Encephalopathy Study: first year : diagnosis

Diagnosis	All cases		Residual cases	
Febrile convulsions (30 min +)	90	(35%)	6	(5%)
Encephalitis	50	(19%)	23	(20%)
Infantile spasms	41	(16%)	41	(35%)
Encephalopathy	27	(10%)	18	(16%)
Non-febrile convulsions/epilepsy	24	(9%)	10	(9%)
Reye's syndrome	7	(3%)	7	(6%)
Other	6	(3%)	5	(4%)
Not recorded	13	(5%)	6	(5%)
Total	258 (100%)		116 (100%)	

The next most common diagnosis was encephalitis. There were 50 children altogether in this category and 23 of them (46%) had persisting problems contributing one-fifth of the residual cases. Lumbar puncture was performed in 47 cases but the cerebrospinal fluid was abnormal in only 14 (31%). A specific virus was identified in 5 patients and an additional 5 children suffered concurrently from an infectious disease known to be associated with encephalitis. In a further 18 cases the neurological illness was immediately preceded by nonspecific infective features such as rash, runny nose, and cough or diarrhoea. This leaves 22 of the 50 cases (44%) in whom there was no evidence of an infective aetiology for their illness.

There were 41 children with infantile spasms and, because this condition is known to have a poor prognosis, they were all regarded as residual cases. They therefore initially contributed over one-third of the residual group but at one year follow-up four of them appear to be normal.

In 27 cases the diagnosis was encephalopathy. These include three cases of Leigh's necrotising encephalomyelopathy [17] and three cases of Kinsbourne's myoclonic encephalopathy [18] or 'dancing eyes' syndrome. In the remaining 21 cases there were no specific features and no classifiable distinction from the 22

309

cases of encephalitis mentioned above with no diagnostic findings. Cerebrospinal fluid was abnormal in 7 out of 16 patients (30%) which is almost identical with the proportion found abnormal in the encephalitis cases. However, 67 per cent of the encephalopathy cases were in the residual group compared with 46 per cent in encephalitis.

There were 24 cases of prolonged convulsions without fever. Ten of them (42%) had residual problems and it is interesting to compare them with the convulsions associated with fever when only 7 per cent fell into the residual category.

Seven cases of Reye's syndrome were notified and, for the same reason as in infantile spasms, they were all regarded as residual. In fact, one year later one child appears to have fully recovered but four are dead and two severely abnormal. Of the 7 patients, 5 were female and 2 male, in contrast to all the other diagnostic categories in which the sex incidence was approximately equal.

In 6 cases some 'other' diagnosis was made such as 'near-miss' cot death or acute infantile hemiplegia and in 13 cases no diagnosis was recorded.

These are preliminary findings from the first year's data of the Study which is scheduled to run for three years. The numbers of cases reported are not yet large enough to enable definite conclusions to be drawn from case-control analyses, especially for vaccination. However, by the end of the Study period there should be sufficient information for this to be done, not only for vaccination but for a wide range of epidemiological factors.

Conclusion

Encephalitis-encephalopathy has many possible aetiological factors. Particularly in childhood, diagnosis and definition of the illness in many cases remain obscure.

The National Childhood Encephalopathy Study was set up to investigate the problem, particularly in relation to vaccination, which has been under suspicion for many years but has recently assumed topical importance. Risk factors for the development of the neurological disorders reported to the Study include coming from social class IV and V rather than I and II and having a pre-existing neurological problem or congenital defect.

Many different clinical illnesses were included under the headings encephalitis or encephalopathy. However, apart from the cases in which an infective aetiology was identified or a specific diagnosis made, there appears to be much overlap between the two terms. Hopefully more information will come out of this Study but further work needs to be done to increase knowledge and, hence, management of these ill-understood conditions.

References

1   ter Meulen, V, Kackell, Y, Muller, D and Katz, M (1972) *Lancet, ii,* 1172
2   Bellman, MH and Dick, G (1978) *Postgrad. Med. J., 54,* 587
3   Gajdusek, DC (1972) *J. Clin. Path., 25,* suppl. 6, 78

4   *Brain's Diseases of the Nervous System,* revised by Walton, JN. Oxford: Oxford University Press. Page 438
5   Reye, RDK, Morgan, G and Baral, J (1963) *Lancet, ii,* 749
6   Day, RE, Thomson, JLG and Schutt, WH (1978) *Arch. Dis. Childh., 53,* 2
7   Madsen, T (1933) *J. Amer. Med. Ass., 101,* 187
8   Byers, RK and Moll, FC (1948) *Pediatrics, 1,* 437
9   Strom, J (1960) *Brit. Med. J., 2,* 1184
10 Kulenkampff, M, Schwartzman, JS and Wilson, J (1974) *Arch. Dis. Childh., 49,* 46
11 Malmgren, B, Vahlquist, B and Zetterstrom, R (1960) *Brit. Med. J., 2,* 1800
12 Prensky, AL (1974) *Devel. Med. Child Neurol., 16,* 539
13 Stewart, GT (1977) *Lancet, i,* 234
14 Grist, NR (1977) *Lancet, i,* 358
15 Secretary of State for Social Services (1977) *Hansard,* 8 Feb., 925, 1233
16 Jeavons, PM and Bower, BD (1964) *Clin. Devel. Med., 15.* London: Spastics Society and Heinemann
17 Leigh, D (1951) *J. Neurol. Neurosurg. & Psychiat., 14,* 216
18 Kinsbourne, M (1962) *J. Neurol. Neurosurg. & Psychiat., 25,* 271

311

Chapter 29

CEREBRAL PALSY

Eva M Alberman

Definition

Cerebral palsy is not a single clinical or even aetiological entity but comprises numerous very different conditions. A definition frequently used describes the features these conditions have in common, namely a disorder of movement and posture resulting from a permanent, non-progressive defect or lesion of the immature brain.

The constituent conditions can be classified by clinical features or by aetiology, where this is known. There is some overlap between the clinical and aetiological grouping in that patients with certain clinical syndromes tend to have similar birth histories, but there is no consistent relationship between them.

Different Types of Cerebral Palsy

Table I gives the distribution of different types of cerebral palsy in two mutually exclusive geographically based surveys, but carried out by paediatricians who used the same clinical classification. The distribution of the clinical types seen in the two series is fairly similar, and the proportion of hemiplegics (a fairly clear-cut diagnosis, comprising over a third of the total) is almost the same as in the third series reported from Bristol. On the whole this has been found in similar studies from many different places, although differences in classification may shift certain cases from one group

TABLE I Distribution % of Different Types of Cerebral Palsy (from Henderson, 1961 [2])

	Dundee (Henderson [2])	Edinburgh (Ingram [14])	Bristol (Woods, 1957 [15])
Hemiplegia	37.5	36.1	36.6
Double hemiplegia	1.3	3.9	
Diplegia	38.3	38.0	
Ataxic diplegia	2.9	5.8	Different classification
Ataxia	1.7	7.2	
Dyskinesia	8.4	8.2	
Other	10.0	1.0	
	100	100	

312

into another. The problems of the clinical classification are well described by Mitchell (1961) [1].

Birth Factors

Table II gives a broad classification by birth factors, the nearest we can get to aetiology. This is from Henderson's study carried out in Eastern Scotland in 1955 [2]. From the totals it can be seen that low birthweight is certainly an important factor, having occurred in a quarter of the 240 cases of cerebral palsy surveyed, about four times the proportion expected in the population. However, it is in the group of spastics, largely made up by the cerebral diplegics, other than the hemiplegics, that prematurity is clearly very important, making up 40 per cent of the total. This syndrome, in which the legs are always affected more than the arms, has been known to be associated with prematurity for many years, certainly since Little's description in 1861 [3]. In contrast, in 1955, in nearly 40 per cent of the athetoids there had been a history of kernicterus and once these cases were excluded none had been of low birthweight. This is, of course, a condition that is now preventable, and it is a clinical impression, though not substantiated by good data, that frank athetosis is considerably less common than it used to be. In spastic hemiplegia postnatal factors are also of importance, 17 per cent of all cases having followed postnatal disasters such as meningitis, or an acute disease with convulsions in a previously apparently healthy infant. Accidental or non-accidental injury to an infant may also cause spastic hemiplegia, or other forms of cerebral palsy.

TABLE II Birth factors in cerebral palsy of different types (adapted from Henderson, 1961) [2]

	Postnatal (cases of kernicterus in parentheses)		Low birthweight (2500 g or less) after excl. postnatal cases		Abnormalities of labour or delivery (after incl. postnatal and low birthweight cases)		Remainder		Total	
	No.	%	No.	%	No.	%	No.	%	No.	%
Spastic hemiplegia	15	16.9	15	16.9	21	23.6	38	42.7	89	100
Other forms of spasticity (largely cerebral diplegia)	2	2.0	40	40.4	23	23.2	34	34.3	99	100
Athetosis	9(7)	50.0	0	0	4	22.2	5	27.8	18	100
Mixed	3	13.0	0	0	8	34.5	12	52.2	23	100
Other	0		3	27.3	4	36.4	4	36.4	11	100
Total	29		58		60		93		240	100

Henderson did not have a control group with which to compare the frequency of abnormalities of labour, but it has been established from many other retrospective series that a stormy birth history is unduly common in cerebral palsy [4]. Similar findings have also been demonstrated in prospective studies [5]. Multiple births are at particular risk.

The 'Continuum of Reproductive Loss' and Prevention of Cerebral Palsy

It was observations such as these that stimulated Lilienfeld and Pasamanick (1955) [6] to put forward their theory of a 'continuum of reproductive casualty' ranging from perinatal death, to cerebral palsy, to minor forms of neurological defect. Whether or not neonates dying with demonstrable brain damage would have suffered from cerebral palsy had they survived is, of course, unanswerable but intuitively reasonable. Postmortem examination of patients dying in late childhood or adult life are not very informative because often many other pathological changes had been superimposed on the original brain defect. The question of 'continuum' has become an important one in recent years because of the sharp drop in perinatal mortality rates in the developed countries, which has raised the question of whether we are thereby increasing the prevalence of brain-damaged children in the survivors. However, the aetiological heterogeneity demonstrated earlier suggests that, if there is indeed a continuum of casualty, it is unlikely to apply to all types of cerebral palsy, but only to the types commonly associated with stormy perinatal or neonatal histories.

The factor most likely to produce a continuum of reproductive loss is birth weight, and indeed we know that survival of fetuses below 500 g is virtually impossible. Above this weight both mortality and morbidity decrease very rapidly with rising gestational age and therefore birth weight. McDonald (1967) [7] found that the prevalence of cerebral palsy in survivors of 3 lb birth weight or less was 9.2 per cent, but 6.6 per cent in those between 3 and 3½ lb and 5.2 per cent in those between 3½ and 4 lb. This is to be compared with a prevalence of 2 to 2.5 per thousand in the general childhood population. It is precisely in babies of low birth weight 2000 g (4 lb 6 oz) or less that neonatal mortality has fallen very sharply, from 38.8 per cent in 1953 to 23.3 per cent in 1977 (DHSS, Annual Reports on the State of Health of the Nation). If we allow for the increase of survivors of low birthweight, but make the assumption that the incidence of cerebral palsy also has fallen [8], perhaps at the same rate, the overall prevalence of cases due to this cause should have fallen as in Figure 1. The baseline data is as given in Table I, plus the genetic component. Cerebral palsy due to birth injury should also have been reduced, for this complication itself is certainly less common than it used to be, and cerebral palsy due to kernicterus should no longer occur in a well-run neonatal unit. We may speculate that even in the mature births without a history of birth injury cerebral palsy due, say, to intra-uterine infections, may now have become less common.

If these assumptions are all correct there should have been a reduction of 24 per

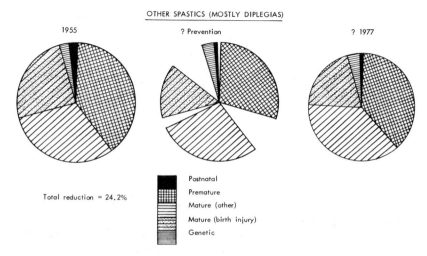

OTHER SPASTICS (MOSTLY DIPLEGIAS)

1955   ? Prevention   ? 1977

Total reduction = 24.2%

Postnatal
Premature
Mature (other)
Mature (birth injury)
Genetic

Figure 1 The possible effects of preventable action on prevalence of cerebral palsy (data adapted from Henderson, 1961 [2])

cent or so in the prevalence of spastic cerebral palsy, other than hemiplegia, between 1955 and 1977 in this country (Fig. 1). Similar predictions can be made for other types of cerebral palsy, using Henderson's data as a base-line.

Incidence and Prevalence

For many reasons, birth incidence of cerebral palsy is impossible to assess with any confidence. The first reason is the high mortality of affected infants and children, which often occurs before a firm diagnosis has been made. In general, many affected children may not be diagnosed until late into their first year or not even until they are in their second or third years of life. Even then it appears that transient signs of cerebral palsy are not uncommon so that apparently affected infants may appear normal neurologically some years later. Moreover, the border-line between the severely clumsy and slightly spastic child is always a difficult one to define, particularly for epidemiological purposes.

Nevertheless, there has been a surprising consistency between age-specific prevalence reported from different surveys (Table III), particularly surprising in view of the heterogeneity of the condition.

Secular Change

The nearest one could come towards a test of the predictions described above would be to use such prevalence studies and to study changes over time, to see

315

TABLE III Reports of the Prevalence of Cerebral Palsy in Great Britain in Children of School Age (adapted from Henderson, 1961) [2]

	Rates per 1000 <1	No. of studies 5
Range of rates reported	1.0–1.4	4
in children of school age	1.5–1.9	4
in 19 studies in UK	2.0–2.5	6
(1948–1957)		
National Child Development Study–1965 [16]	2.4	

whether there had been an inverse relationship between prevalence of certain types of cerebral palsy and perinatal mortality.

The first of such studies, by Hagberg and his colleagues from Sweden [9], suggested that there had been a 41 per cent decrease in incidence of cerebral palsy between 1954 and 1970, mainly among the types associated with perinatal insults. This was in the face of an initially low, and constantly falling, perinatal mortality. A recent report from Western Australia [10] suggests that this relationship does not always hold since, in Australia, the incidence of cerebral palsy, particularly the spastic types, actually rose between 1950 and 1966 while perinatal mortality fell. Since 1966 both have fallen together. In Ireland, too [11] there has been an apparent rise in the spastic quadriplegia and dyskinetic syndromes and no fall in spastic diplegia over two five-year periods, 1966–70 and 1971–75, in the face of a falling perinatal mortality. A different methodology was adopted by Pharoah (1976) [12]. He compared mortality and morbidity in low birthweight babies born in 1966 in two district hospitals with similar maternal age, parity and social class distributions and found a small but not significant excess of births with cerebral palsy in the hospital with the lower mortality.

The general impression of these results up to the present is that, with the improvement of medical care in general, there may be an interim period where the prevalence of brain-damaged children rises, preceding the next stage of improvement where handicap rates fall with mortality.

Other Epidemiological Features

Enough has been said to show that epidemiological descriptions of such features of cerebral palsy as sex ratio, maternal characteristics or severity of defect will vary with the type of cerebral palsy surveyed. In general, there is a small excess of boys among most types of cerebral palsy and, as would be expected, an excess of mothers at high risk of difficulties in pregnancy and labour. Such mothers are at either extreme of the reproductive age span, are having their first baby or babies at high birth rank, or are themselves in poor health or with poor physique. Stanley [10] has pointed out that the secular changes observed may indeed be largely due

316

to differences in the types of mothers giving birth, rather than to medical care factors.

Genetic factors in this country do not seem to be of direct importance except in a small proportion, perhaps 3 per cent or so, but this proportion will rise as the preventable causes are reduced. In certain areas, like the North of Sweden where intermarriage between close relatives is common, the proportion of genetically determined cases is much higher.

Severity and type of handicap also vary considerably. Associated mental handicap is common, about 25 per cent of children having an IQ of below 50, and a further 20 per cent or so an IQ of between 50 and 70 [13]. Visual-hearing and orthopaedic defects are all very common, and add substantially to the burden of handicap. The most severely handicapped as a group are those with spastic quadriplegia, the least handicapped those with spastic diplegia. There is a clinical impression, but again no proof, that in recent years the cerebral palsied children have tended to be less severely handicapped, and this may reflect a shift towards the normal in those resulting from reproductive casualty.

In summary, cerebral palsy is a heterogeneous group of conditions, which until recently was found in about 2.5 per thousand children of school age. Certain types are almost certainly preventable by excellent medical care, the prevalence of others will be reduced if the proportion of mothers at high risk by reason of age, parity or ill-health falls. It is a severely handicapping condition and, therefore, of great importance for both humanitarian and economic considerations, warranting continuing efforts towards its prevention and palliation.

References

1   Mitchell, RG (1961) Chapters IV, VII and VIII. In *Cerebral Palsy in Childhood and Adolescence,* (ed. Henderson, JL). Edinburgh and London: E & S Livingstone Ltd
2   Henderson, JL (1961) *Cerebral Palsy in Childhood and Adolescence.* Edinburgh and London: E & S Livingstone Ltd, p. 18
3   Little, WJ (1861–62) On the influence of abnormal parturition, difficult labours, premature births and asphyxia neonatorum on the mental and physical condition of the child, especially in relation to deformities. *Transactions of the Obstetrical Society of London, 3,* 293
4   Eastman, NJ, Kohl, SG, Maisel, JE and Kavaler, F (1962) The obstetrical background of 753 cases of cerebral palsy. *Obstetric and Gynaecological Survey, 17,* 459
5   Brown, JK, Purvis, JO, Forfar, JO, Cockburn, F (1974) Neurological aspects of perinatal asphyxia. *Developmental Medicine and Child Neurology, 16,* 567
6   Lilienfeld, AM and Pasamanick, KB (1955) The association of maternal and fetal factors with the development of cerebral palsy and epilepsy. *American Journal of Obstetrics and Gynaecology, 70,* 93
7   McDonald, A (1967) *Children of Very Low Birthweight.* Spastic Society Medical Education and Information Unit in Association with William Heinemann Medical Books Ltd
8   Reynolds, EOR (1978) Neonatal intensive care and the prevention of major handicap. In *Major Mental Handicap: Methods and Cost of Prevention.* Ciba Foundation Symposium 59 (new series). North Holland: Elsevier Excerpta Medica
9   Hagberg, B, Hagberg, G and Olow, I (1975a, b) The changing panorama of cerebral palsy in Sweden. 1954–1970. I. Analysis of the general changes. II. Analysis of the various syndromes. *Acta Paediatrica Scandinavica, 64,* 187, 193

10 Stanley, F An epidemiological study of cerebral palsy in Western Australia 1956–1975. Changes in total cerebral palsy incidence and associated factors. *Developmental Medicine and Child Neurology* (in press)

11 Cussen, GH, Barry, JE, Moloney, AM, Buckley, NM, Crowley, M and Daly, C (1979) Cerebral Palsy—A Regional Study: Part II. *Journal of the Irish Medical Association, 72,* 14

12 Pharoah, POD (1976) Obstetric and neonatal care related to outcome. A comparison of two maternity hospitals. *British Journal of Preventive and Social Medicine, 30,* 257

13 Cockburn, June M (1961) Psychological and educational aspects. In *Cerebral Palsy in Childhood and Adolescence,* (ed. Henderson, JL). Edinburgh and London: E & S Livingstone Ltd

14 Ingram, TTS (1955) A study of cerebral palsy in the childhood population of Edinburgh. *Archives of the Diseases of Childhood, 30,* 85

15 Woods, GE (1957) *Cerebral Palsy in Childhood.* Bristol: Wright

16 Davie, R, Butler, N and Goldstein, H (1972) *From Birth to Seven.* Longman in association with the National Children's Bureau, p. 163

Chapter 30

SPECTRUM OF PAEDIATRIC CEREBROVASCULAR DISEASE

Bruce S Schoenberg and Devera G Schoenberg

The initial description of cerebrovascular disease in childhood is attributed [1] to the seventeenth century English physician Thomas Willis, who in 1667, wrote:

'Some time ago a Woman in this City had several children who died of this Disease [convulsions]; at length we dissected the Head of the fourth Child, which died within the first month, like the rest. There was no collection of Serum in the Ventricles; only the substance of the Brain, and its Appendages was moister, and less firm in its Texture than usual. But what was most remarkable, in the Cavity below the Cerebellum, immediately above the Trunk of the Medulla Oblongata, we found a considerable quantity of grumous Blood. But it is uncertain whether that Matter was contained there from the Beginning of the Disease, and so produced the Convulsions, or whether it [was] forced out of the Blood Vessels by the Contraction of the neighbouring Parts during the Paroxysms, and so ought rather to be considered as the effect, than the cause of the Disease'. [2]

Although this condition was recognised more than 300 years ago, there is still much that is not understood about cerebrovascular disease in infants and children. Initially, this phenomenon was considered rare enough to merit case reports which documented the existence of these disorders, and the early publications were followed by case series describing the experience of particular medical institutions. Although a large volume of data was collected on this subject, the magnitude of cerebrovascular disease in a well-defined population of infants and children had never been ascertained. Descriptive epidemiological studies which estimate disease frequency are important for measuring the impact of disease as a health problem in the community. It should be emphasised that investigations based on selected series of cases do not necessarily reflect the experience of the general population.

Several investigations have examined possible risk factors for childhood stroke, although few have measured the frequency of this condition. The role of cerebral hypoxia and acidosis with resultant stasis, thrombosis, and venous rupture in the genesis of subependymal, subarachnoid, and cerebral intraventricular haemorrhages in the newborn has been described in many published reports [3-15].

Cerebral blood-flow studies on newborns have shown that high cerebral blood-flow levels persist in those infants with hyaline membrane disease and that this condition together with apnoea may be responsible for intraventricular haemorrhage [16]. Associated risk factors such as prematurity, low birth weight, hyaline membrane disease, and trauma have been implicated as predisposing conditions [4, 7-10, 14, 17-25]. Recently, agents and procedures (i.e., mechanical ventilation and administration of sodium bicarbonate in alkaline buffer therapy) used to treat the severely distressed premature infant have been questioned as possible aetiologic factors in perinatal intracranial haemorrhage [9, 17, 26-30].

Risk factors for childhood cerebrovascular disease unassociated with birth or trauma have also been identified. These include congenital heart disease [31-35], haematological abnormalities such as the leukaemias, haemophilia, and sickle cell disease [32, 35-40], aneurysms [32, 35], and arteriovenous malformations [32, 35, 41].

In 1965, Leeds and Abbott [42] described a telangiectatic vascular network at the base of the brain associated with distal occlusion of the internal carotid artery in two American-born Japanese children. Other reports on this condition followed [43], and in 1969 the term 'moyamoya disease' was introduced to describe the angiographic appearance of the telangiectatic network of vessels [44]. The word 'moyamoya' in Japanese means 'hazy, like a puff of cigarette smoke drifting in the air'. Although stroke syndromes secondary to infection and trauma have been reported [32], these causes were not included in the epidemiological investigations described later in this review. Moreover, cerebrovascular disease has been reported in otherwise healthy children in the absence of any currently recognised risk factors [45-48].

These early investigations were based on the experience of selected physicians or medical institutions. Although such studies may provide valuable insights into clinical patterns, they also have potentially significant elements of bias. Referral patterns, specialised physician interests, and patient behaviour are such that certain clinicians may see more severe forms of a certain disease. Some physicians may see no cases of a particular disease, while another physician practising in the same community may restrict his practice to patients with that specific disorder. The situation is analogous to blind men examining different parts of an elephant with each coming to an entirely different conclusion as to the characteristics of the beast. To avoid this problem, the neuroepidemiologist attempts to identify all cases of a particular neurological disease in a well-defined population. The remainder of this paper focuses on such epidemiological studies of cerebrovascular disease in well-defined childhood populations.

Descriptive Epidemiology: Disease Magnitude

Descriptive epidemiology characterises observations of disease in human populations [49]. In order to avoid the biases that may be present in data from a single medical institution, Schoenberg and his colleagues [35, 50] studied the entire population of Rochester, Minnesota.

Since the early part of this century, medical practice in Rochester, Minnesota has centred at the Mayo Clinic. The records of this institution and other medical care facilities in the area provided the resources to carry out this investigation of the incidence of cerebrovascular disease in infants and children residing in Rochester. The use of a *unit record system* whereby information on hospitalisations, outpatient care, home visits, and laboratory results is kept together in a single file greatly facilitates epidemiological investigation. In addition, a *records-linkage* system has been established for residents of Olmsted County, Minnesota, which contains Rochester. This includes medical data sources both within and outside the Mayo Clinic, and involves the cooperation of all the medical facilities in the area. Using this system it is possible to locate and review all medical-care records for residents of Rochester. Although the population is relatively small, there is a high level of case ascertainment and follow-up.

Such a records-linkage system provides a rich data base for studies of disease in a well-defined population. Because a large number of Rochester residents work either for the Mayo Clinic or for industries having contractual arrangements with Mayo, this access to medical care is without financial restraint for these individuals. Thus, most health problems are brought to the attention of a physician. The small size of the Rochester population and the ease of data retrieval make it possible to do a fairly exhaustive study without an inordinate expenditure of time or money [51, 52].

Using the facilities of the Rochester, Minnesota records-linkage data resource, Schoenberg and co-workers [35, 50] reviewed the birth, perinatal, and paediatric records for 1965 through 1974 from all medical facilities serving this population. Childhood was defined as up to, but not including, the 15th birthday. For a case of cerebrovascular disease to be included, two reviewing neurologists both had to agree on the diagnosis. Patients with subdural haematoma as the only form of cerebrovascular disease were excluded from further consideration. Beyond the perinatal period cerebrovascular disease secondary to trauma or infection was also excluded. Results are presented in Table I.

TABLE I Frequency of Cerebrovascular Disease in Infants and Children–Rochester, Minnesota, 1965–1974

| | Perinatal Intracranial Haemorrhage | | Stroke Unassociated with Birth, Infection, or Trauma | |
	Live births	All births	Ischaemic	Haemorrhagic
Number of patients	12	13	1	3
Population at risk	10 850 live births	10 952 births	15 834/year	15 834/year
Rate	1.1 cases/1000 live births	1.2 cases/1000 births	0.6 cases/ 100 000 population/year	1.9 cases/ 100 000 population/year
95% confidence interval	0.6–1.9 cases/ 1000 live births	0.6–2.1 cases/ 1000 births	0.0–3.5 cases/ 100 000 population/year	0.4–5.5 cases/ 100 000 population/year

(Reproduced with permission from Schoenberg, BS (in press) In *Advances in Neurology, Vol. 25: Cerebrovascular Disorders and Stroke* (ed. M Goldstein, CL Bolis, C Fieschi, S Gorini and CH Millikan). Raven Press, New York)

Among a total of 10 850 live births in the Rochester, Minnesota population during 1965 through 1974, 12 documented cases of intracranial haemorrhage were found, yielding an average rate of occurrence of 1.1 cases/1000 live births. This figure represents a minimal estimate, since only documented cases are included. In 10 of the 12 individuals, the haemorrhage originated in the germinal matrix, a subependymal layer of the lateral ventricles that is relatively large in premature infants as compared to full-term infants. In two patients who had a non-traumatic lumbar puncture yielding grossly bloody cerebrospinal fluid, the diagnosis was verified before death. All 12 infants had autopsy confirmation of the diagnosis. None of the patients had focal neurological signs. Five infants had one-minute Apgar scores above 8, but soon after birth, manifestations of the respiratory distress syndrome were evident. The remainder had difficulty immediately at birth. In the 12 cases, survival ranged from 1 to 5 days, with a mean of 2.75 days.

In addition to these 12 individuals, one male stillborn infant during the ten-year period had an intracerebral haemorrhage. If this case were to be included in calculating the rate for 10 952 births (live and stillbirths) during this period, the figure becomes 1.2 cases/1000 births.

In considering cerebrovascular disease unassociated with birth, trauma, or infection, records from all medical facilities serving the Rochester, Minnesota population revealed one ischaemic stroke and three haemorrhagic strokes occurring among a mean population of 15 834 resident children. The corresponding average annual incidence rates were 0.6 cases/100 000/year and 1.9 cases/100 000/year, respectively. Two of the haemorrhagic strokes were due to a demonstrated arteriovenous malformation.

If one regards Rochester, Minnesota as a random sample representative of some larger population, one may then calculate confidence intervals for the calculated rates of cerebrovascular disease in infants and children. Since the probability of childhood cerebrovascular disease is rather small, the Poisson distribution was used to establish 95 per cent confidence intervals around the rates. The results are shown in Table I. However, the reader should use great caution in applying these findings to other populations, since Rochester, Minnesota may not be representative of other communities.

On the basis of the Rochester, Minnesota experience it would appear that cerebrovascular disease in the perinatal period is a much more significant problem in terms of magnitude than at later periods of infancy and childhood. Such estimates of disease frequency are extremely helpful in rationally assigning priorities in our search for risk factors.

Analytic Epidemiology: Risk Factors

Studies of potential risk factors for cerebrovascular disease in infants and children require the techniques of analytic epidemiology [53] which involves the study of natural experiments. During the course of our lives, different individuals are exposed to many different factors or conditions, some of which may play an important role in the occurrence of disease. In the case-control investigation, one begins with a group of individuals with the particular disease of interest (cases) and a group without the particular disease (controls). One then explores the present (in a cross-sectional investigation) or past history (in a retrospective investigation) of the two groups for the presence or absence or factors throught to be related to the occurrence of the disease. One looks for factors differentially distributed in the group with the disease as compared to the group without the disease. Recently, three published reports using the case-control study design to investigate perinatal intracranial haemorrhage have appeared [50, 54, 55].

Perinatal Intracranial Haemorrhage

The first such study was carried out by Schoenberg and his colleagues [50] and was based on the 12 cases of perinatal intracranial haemorrhage identified in the Rochester, Minnesota population. Two matched controls were chosen for each case of intracranial haemorrhage (Table II). The controls consisted of the next live birth and the next live premature birth, occurring in the same hospital as each of the cases. Also the parents of the controls had to be residents of Rochester, Minnesota, as were the parents of the cases. Birth, perinatal, pregnancy, and delivery records were reviewed for all patients, as well as for the two sets of matched controls, for all factors outlined in Table III.

TABLE II Perinatal Intracranial Haemorrhage: Selection of Cases and Controls

Case:	Neonates with intracranial haemorrhage (excluding those with subdural haematoma as the only form of intracranial haemorrhage) born during the study decade whose parents were Rochester, Minnesota residents.
Control 1:	Next live birth following each case in the same hospital with parents who were Rochester, Minnesota residents.
Control 2:	Next live premature birth (<37 weeks gestation) following each case in the same hospital with parents who were Rochester, Minnesota residents.

(Reproduced with permission from Schoenberg, BS (in press) In *Advances in Neurology, Vol. 25: Cerebrovascular Disorders and Stroke.* (ed. M Goldstein, CL Bolis, C Fieschi, S Gorini and CH Millikan). Raven Press, New York)

Statistical significance of the association between any of these potential risk factors and intracranial haemorrhage was measured with the Wilcoxon signed rank test [56] for quantitative variables (Apgar score, birthweight, etc.) and with the binomial test [56] for dichotomous variables that are either present or absent (e.g., hyaline membrane disease, caesarean section). Since the statistical techniques employed assume independence among the cases, one patient (the second of a pair of twins) was excluded from this analysis, since data concerning this female infant were not independent of information concerning her twin sister.

Prematurity (defined as a gestational age of less than 37 weeks) [57] was strongly associated with perinatal intracranial haemorrhage ($P < 0.01$). All 12 patients were premature, while none of the first series of controls fell into this category. Factors related to prematurity, such as low birthweight and respiratory

TABLE III Factors Examined in a Case-control Study of Perinatal Intracranial Haemorrhage

Infant	Index pregnancy	Index delivery	Previous pregnancies and deliveries
Sex	Twin pregnancy	Presentation (breech,	Number of previous
Birthweight	Trauma	vertex, etc.)	pregnancies
Gestational age	Bleeding	Type of delivery	History of:
Head size	Infection(s)	(spontaneous/	Miscarriage
Length	Irradiation	induced)	Premature delivery
Apgar score	Anaemia	Forceps	Breech presentation
Hyaline membrane	Diabetes mellitus	High or low	Bleeding during
disease (present/	Drugs (other than	application	previous pregnancies
absent)	vitamins or iron)	Caesarean section	
Use of positive-		Obligate or elective	
pressure assisted		Anaesthesia	
ventilation		Type (general,	
Malformation(s)		epidural, etc.)	
		Anaesthetic agent	

(Reproduced with permission from Schoenberg, BS (in press) In *Advances in Neurology, Vol. 25: Cerebrovascular Disorders and Stroke* (ed. M Goldstein, CL Bolis, C Fieschi, S Gorini and CH Millikan). Raven Press, New York)

distress syndrome, were also strongly associated with perinatal intracranial haemorrhage. To determine whether these factors in themselves were important or whether their relationship to intracranial haemorrhage reflected their correlation with prematurity, a second set of controls was chosen.

This second series of controls consisted of the next live premature birth in the same hospital as the corresponding case with parents residing in Rochester, Minnesota. The same factors listed previously were compared between the patients and the second set of controls. Gestational age was excluded from consideration since this was used to define prematurity. For the reasons already stated, data from the second of a pair of twins were not included in the analysis. Hyaline membrane disease manifested by the respiratory distress syndrome was associated with perinatal intracranial haemorrhage (P < 0.01), as was the use of positive-pressure assisted ventilation (P < 0.05). Although these two factors are related to prematurity, they appear to increase further the risk of intracranial haemorrhage in the premature infant. With such a small number of patients and controls, however, other biologically important risk factors may not have reached statistical significance.

The results of this investigation were supported by two subsequent case-control studies carried out by Leviton and his co-workers [54, 55]. In the first of these studies, the relationship of route of delivery and presence of hyaline membrane disease to eight sites of intracranial haemorrhage was evaluated for 513 liveborn infants who died at a given hospital on or before the 13th postnatal day and underwent a postmortem examination of the brain. Although those delivered by caesarean section were at lower risk for most varieties of intracranial haemorrhage than those who had a vaginal delivery, the differences were not statistically significant. Newborn infants with hyaline membrane disease were at increased risk of intracranial haemorrhage (especially subarachnoid or germinal matrix haemorrhage) when compared to neonates without this condition.

The second investigation dealt with 523 infants who died during the first month of life and underwent a postmortem study of the brain. These infants were derived from the cohort under observation as part of the Collaborative Perinatal Project. Over 1000 characteristics of the 97 infants with ganglionic eminence haemorrhage were compared with corresponding items for the remaining 426 infants without this condition. The most prominent correlate of increased risk was low gestational age. Many of the other risk factors identified were also strongly associated with low gestational age. Although the studies by Leviton and his colleagues have the advantage of large numbers of cases, the patients in their analysis are not derived from a geographically defined population as is the case with the Rochester study. This shortcoming may result in both recognised and unrecognised sources of bias. None of the three study populations represents an unbiased sample of a larger population. Despite these problems, the similarities in the findings are striking.

This Rochester investigation, for the first time, provides an estimate of the magnitude of perinatal intracranial haemorrhage in a well-defined population. In slightly more than 0.1 per cent of all live births in Rochester, Minnesota, this condition developed. The reader should bear in mind that this figure represents a minimal estimate, since only well-documented cases were included. The condition is alarmingly common, especially when considered with regard to the very poor prognosis of infants with intracranial haemorrhage [50]. The disorder is difficult to recognise clinically; the insult of an intracranial haemorrhage on the immature nervous system does not in the majority of cases produce recognisable neurological deficits, especially focal findings. The technological advances available with computerised tomography should improve our ability to identify this condition.

Several recent hospital series, none, however, population-based, have described the use of the computerised tomographic (CT) brain scan to detect the presence of subependymal, intraventricular, and subarachnoid haemorrhages in premature infants [58–60]. In the study by Ahmann and his associates [59], 139 premature (gestational age < 35 weeks) infants who required intensive care were evaluated for the presence of subependymal and/or intraventricular haemorrhages. Of these infants 61 were shown to have suffered a haemorrhage: 52 by CT scan, 5 by ventricular tap, and 4 at autopsy. The CT scan was also used to quantify the amount of blood (an important prognostic marker both in terms of (a) survival and (b) development of progressive hydrocephalus present at the haemorrhage site).

Another hospital series is that of Lazzara and co-workers [60]. Of 81 preterm infants in intensive care units monitored for further signs of distress, 31 demonstrated intraventricular haemorrhage on CT scan. Of these 31, 16 had been predicted clinically. For the 50 infants without a CT-demonstrable intraventricular haemorrhage, 38 had been clinically predicted to be haemorrhage-free.

Computerised tomography was able to diagnose intraventricular haemorrhage in 43 per cent of the consecutive premature infants studied by Burstein and his colleages [61]. In their series of patients, they noted that such haemorrhages may be clinically silent, since 83 per cent of their pre-term infants with haemorrhage were clinically unsuspected.

In light of the results obtained from CT scans, it is apparent that such scans provide valuable diagnostic data on the presence, site, and extent of neonatal intracerebral haemorrhage, as well as the size and distortion of the ventricular system. Moreover, CT scans enable researchers to: (*a*) distinguish intraventricular haemorrhage from subarachnoid haemorrhage; (*b*) confirm the presence of massive intraventricular haemorrhage and so enable the physician to make appropriate prognostic and therapeutic decisions; and (*c*) forewarn of the possible development of hydrocephalus well before clinical signs appear. According to Kirks and his associates [62] long-term CT follow-ups of infants surviving a documented intracranial haemorrhage should detail the ability of such scans to predict psychomotor prognosis based on the initial neonatal event.

As one can see from the above-mentioned studies, cerebrovascular disease is a major concern in the perinatal nursery. But, just how common is this affliction? What is currently lacking is information concerning the population at risk, from which the perinatal intensive care nursery cases, a highly selected population, are derived.

In summary, several case-control studies have been carried out to investigate the association of potential risk factors with perinatal intracranial haemorrhage. Of the characteristics studied, prematurity and hyaline membrane disease manifested by the respiratory distress syndrome emerged as the two most important factors. This is certainly consistent with the findings of published case series. Although agents and procedures used to treat respiratory distress syndrome in the premature infant have been implicated in the aetiology of intracranial haemorrhage, they do not explain all such cases, as noted by the examples given in this review. Intracranial haemorrhage may likewise occur *in utero* as exemplified by the one stillbirth.

Despite the fact that there are no currently available treatments for this important perinatal problem, opportunities do exist for primary prevention. Available data suggest that lowering the frequency of prematurity and hyaline membrane disease would have a significant effect on the occurrence of intracranial haemorrhage in the newborn. Careful perinatal care, including amniotic fluid analysis when clinically indicated, hopefully will help considerably in achieving this goal.

Paediatric Cerebrovascular Disease unassociated with
Birth, Infection, or Trauma

With regard to strokes unassociated with birth, infection, or trauma in paediatric populations, a thorough review of the literature did not reveal any case-control studies of risk factors. In the absence of such an investigation and in order to obtain more current clues to potential risk factors for these disorders, Schoenberg and associates recently reviewed the clinical experience of a large medical centre without regard to the population of origin of the cases [35]. This was necessary in order to obtain a larger number of patients than those occurring in the only well-defined population that has been studied (i.e. Rochester, Minnesota). Therefore, the entire Mayo Clinic experience with these conditions was analysed for cerebrovascular disease (unassociated with birth, infection, or trauma) in children under 15 years of age. The period of study was limited to the decade, 1965–1974. Approximately 1000 potential cases were screened and all accepted cases were independently reviewed by two neurologists.

This review yielded 69 stroke patients during the 10-year period. There were 38 cases of ischaemic stroke, representing some 55 per cent of the total, while there were 31 patients with haemorrhagic strokes, or 45 per cent of the total. The distribution by recognisable cause of these strokes was as follows: of the total, almost 19 per cent were ischaemic strokes with no known predisposing condition; 4 per cent were ischaemic strokes associated with moyamoya disease; 26 per cent were ischaemic strokes with pre-existing heart disease; and about 6 per cent were ischaemic strokes with other associated conditions. Of the total of 69, 10 per cent were haemorrhagic strokes without known predisposing conditions; one patient with heart disease had a haemorrhagic stroke; 19 per cent were haemorrhagic strokes secondary to an aneurysm; 9 per cent were haemorrhagic strokes secondary to an arteriovenous malformation; and 6 per cent were haemorrhagic strokes with other associated conditions.

The results of this investigation demonstrate the value of studies based on a well-defined population and emphasise the need for well-designed case-control studies; for example, infarcts outnumbered haemorrhages in the Mayo Clinic series. The reverse was true in the Rochester, Minnesota population series. This discrepancy results from biases in referral patterns. Although the Mayo Clinic serves a relatively small local population, a large number of patients travel considerable distances to obtain care at this medical facility. Children with intracranial haemorrhage may not survive long enough to be seen at the Mayo Clinic. In addition, the Mayo Clinic cares for many children with congenital heart disease, an important risk factor for ischaemic stroke. This accounts for the apparent excess of ischaemic strokes in the Mayo Clinic series as compared to the population series. Furthermore, the Mayo Clinic series would not be representative of the clinical patterns observed in most large US cities; for example, none of the patients in the group referred to the Mayo Clinic had sickle cell anaemia, a condition associated with paediatric stroke [32] and one that is seen with some frequency in most larger city hospitals.

The descriptive epidemiological study of cerebrovascular disease in children provided an estimate of the magnitude of these disorders. In spite of current levels of medical care, the case fatality rate for stroke in children remains high. One must also consider the quality of life in survivors. Although they may not succumb to the acute event, many are left with residual disability [35]. Available evidence indicates that this group of diseases represents an important cause of death and disability in the paediatric age group. It, therefore, behooves us to carry out carefully designed case-control studies in our search to identify risk factors for these conditions. At our present level of medical knowledge, it would appear that the prevention, early recognition, and treatment of potential precursors of stroke should be of prime concern in our attempt to achieve some measure of primary prevention for these devastating diseases of infancy and childhood.

327

References

1   Von Haam, E (1934) *Am. J. Obstet. Gynecol., 27,* 184
2   Willis, T (1667) *Pathologiae Cerebri et Nervosi Generis Specimen.* In quo Agitur de Morbis Convulsivis, et de Scorbuto. Oxonii excudebat Guil Hall, impensis Ja Allestry, page 49
3   Cole, VA, Durbin, GM, Olaffson, A et al (1974) *Arch. Dis. Childh., 49,* 722
4   Gruenwald, P (1951) *Am. J. Obstet. Gynecol., 61,* 1285
5   Haller, ES, Nesbitt, REL Jr, and Anderson, GW (1956) *Obstet. Gynecol. Surv., 11,* 179
6   Hambleton, G and Wigglesworth, JS (1976) *Arch. Dis. Childh., 51,* 651
7   Harcke, HT Jr, Naeye, RL, Storch, A et al (1972) *J. Pediatr., 80,* 37
8   Larroche, JC (1964) *Biol. Neonat., 7,* 26
9   Ross, JJ and Dimmette, RM (1965) *Am. J. Dis. Childh., 110,* 531
10 Towbin, A (1968) *Am. J. Pathol., 52,* 121
11 Towbin, A (1969) *Science, 164,* 156
12 Towbin, A (1969) *Arch. Neurol., 20,* 35
13 Towbin, A (1971) *J.A.M.A., 217,* 1207
14 Volpe, JJ (1977) *Clin. in Perinatology, 4,* 77
15 Foley, ME and McNicol, GP (1977) *Lancet, i,* 1230
16 Cooke, RWI, Rolfe, P and Howat, P (1979) *Develop. Med. Child Neurol., 21,* 154
17 Anderson, JM, Bain, AD, Brown, JK et al (1976) *Lancet, i,* 117
18 Deonna, T, Payot, M, Probst, A et al (1975) *Pediatrics, 56,* 1056
19 Gilles, FH, Leviton, A and Dooling, EC (1974) *N. Engl. J. Med., 291,* 1088
20 Grunnet, ML and Shields, WD (1976) *J. Pediatr., 88,* 605
21 Leech, RW , Alvord, EC Jr and Kohnen, P (1974) *J. Neuropath. Exp. Neurol., 33,* 194
22 Leech, RW and Kohnen, P (1974) *Am. J. Pathol., 77,* 465
23 Martin, R, Roessmann, U and Fanaroff, A (1976) *J. Pediatr., 89,* 290
24 Rogers, WS and Gruenwald, P (1956) *Am. J. Obstet. Gynecol., 71,* 9
25 Tsiantos, A, Victorin, L, Relier, JP et al (1974) *J. Pediatr., 85,* 854
26 Editorial (1974) *N. Engl. J. Med., 291,* 43
27 Pape, KE, Armstrong, DL and Fitzhardinge, PM (1978) *Pediatrics, 58,* 473
28 Reynolds, EOR and Taghizadeh, A (1974) *Arch. Dis. Childh., 49,* 505
29 Robertson, NRC and Howat, P (1975) *Arch. Dis. Childh., 50,* 938
30 Simmons, MA, Adcock, EW, III, Bard, H et al (1974) *N. Engl. J. Med., 291,* 6
31 Banker, BQ (1961) *J. Neuropath. Exp. Neurol., 20,* 127
32 Golden, GS (1978) *Stroke, 9,* 169
33 Martelle, RR and Linde, LM (1961) *Amer. J. Dis. Childh., 101,* 206
34 Mymin, D (1960) *Arch. Dis. Childh., 35,* 515
35 Schoenberg, BS, Mellinger, JM and Schoenberg, DG (1976) *Neurology (Minneap.), 26,* 358
36 Groch, SN, Sayre, GP and Heck, FP (1960) *AMA Arch. Neurol., 2,* 439
37 Pierce, MI (1962) *Ped. Clin. N. Amer., 9,* 425
38 Campbell, RHA, Marshall, WC and Chessels, JM (1977) *Arch. Dis. Childh., 52,* 850
39 Bennett, M and Sills, JA (1978) *Postgrad. Med. J., 54,* 115
40 Powars, D, Wilson, B, Imbus, C, Pegelow, C and Allen, J (1978) *Am. J. Med., 65,* 461
41 Kelly, JJ, Mellinger, JF and Sundt, TM (1978) *Ann. Neurol., 3,* 338
42 Leeds, NE and Abbott, KH (1965) *Radiology, 85,* 628
43 Schoenberg, BS, Mellinger, JM and Schoenberg, DG (1978) *South. Med. J., 71,* 237
44 Suzuki, J and Takaku, A (1969) *Arch. Neurol., 20,* 288
45 Goldstein, SL and Burgess, JP (1958) *AMA Dis. Children, 95,* 538
46 Sedzimir, CB (1959) *J. Neurol. Neurosurg. and Psychiat., 22,* 78
47 Stevens, H (1958) *Ann. Int. Med., 49,* 1022
48 Wisoff, HS and Rothballer, AB (1961) *Arch. Neurol., 4,* 258
49 Schoenberg, BS (1978) In *Advances in Neurology, Vol. 19: Neurological Epidemiology: Principles and Clinical Applications* (ed. BS Schoenberg). New York: Raven Press, page 17
50 Schoenberg, BS, Mellinger, JM and Schoenberg, DG (1977) *Arch. Neurol., 34,* 570

51 Kurland, LT, Elveback, LR and Nobrega, FT (1970) In *The Community as an Epidemiologic Laboratory: A Casebook of Community Studies* (ed. I Kessler and ML Levin). Baltimore: Johns Hopkins Press, page 47
52 Kurland, LT and Brian, DD (1978) In *Advances in Neurology, Vol. 19: Neurological Epidemiology: Principles and Clinical Applications* (ed. BS Schoenberg). New York: Raven Press, page 93.
53 Schoenberg, BS (1978) In *Advances in Neurology, Vol. 19: Neurological Epidemiology: Principles and Clinical Applications* (ed. BS Schoenberg). New York: Raven Press, page 43
54 Leviton, A, Gilles, FH and Dooling, E (1978) *Neurology (Minneap.), 28,* 333
55 Leviton, A, Gilles, FH and Strassfeld, R (1977) *Ann. Neurol., 2,* 451
56 Siegel, S (1956) *Nonparametric Statistics for the Behavioral Sciences.* New York: McGraw-Hill Book Co. Inc., pp. 36–42, 75–83
57 Cornely, DA (1973) In *Preventive Medicine and Public Health* (ed. PE Sartwell). 10th edn. New York: Appleton-Century-Crofts, page 797
58 Krishnamoorthy, KS, Fernandez, RA, Momose, KJ et al (1977) *Pediatrics, 59,* 165
59 Ahmann, PA, Lazzara, A, Dykes, FD, Schwartz, JF and Brann, AW Jr (1978) *Ann. Neurol., 4,* 186
60 Lazzara, A, Ahmann, PA, Dykes, FD et al (1978) *Ann. Neurol., 4,* 187
61 Burstein, J, Papile, L and Burstein, R (1977) *Am. J. Roentgenol., 128,* 971
62 Kirks, DR, Maravilla, K and Maravilla, AM (1978) *Comput. Tomogr., 2,* 207

Chapter 31

NEUROBEHAVIOURAL ASSOCIATIONS AND SYNDROMES OF 'MINIMAL BRAIN DYSFUNCTION'

Michael Rutter and Oliver Chadwick

Most paediatric neuroepidemiological studies have been concerned with the prevalence of particular neurological syndromes such as cerebral palsy, epilepsy, or hydrocephalus. Many of these categories refer to quite heterogeneous groups of problems; nevertheless even when combined they do not encompass anything like all the neurological disorders of childhood. In the first place, there are many well-defined rarer diseases; for example, metabolic disorders like phenylketonuria or galactosaemia, the cerebral lipoidoses, and the encephalitides, all of which are associated with definite brain pathology. Secondly, surveys tend not to include the mixture of rather ill-defined conditions associated with manifest neurological abnormalities but which do not fulfil the criteria for any of the recognised syndromes [1, 2]. Thirdly, children with severe intellectual retardation are usually omitted in spite of the fact that post-mortem studies have shown that all or nearly all children with an IQ below 50 have demonstrable pathology of the brain [3]. The Isle of Wight epidemiological study [1] showed that if all these various groups are summated, a total prevalence figure of about 6½ per 1000 is obtained for pathological disorders of the brain in childhood. If disorders resulting from lesions at or below the brain stem are added in, the figure rises to about 8 per 1000, and if epileptic conditions are also included a rate of over 13 per 1000 is obtained.

Brain Damage Without Neurological Abnormality

However, even this figure omits many children with indubitable brain injury. It is well recognised that some unequivocal injuries to the brain do not give rise to any signs on neurological examination. This is illustrated, for example, by the study of individuals who have been subjected to pre-frontal leucotomy or temporal lobectomy—clinical examination may reveal no signs of the loss of brain substance. Moreover, children who have had clear neurological abnormalities in infancy may yet appear normal when examined some years later [4]. Similarly, the neurological sequelae of encephalitis may clear up completely as the affected children grow older [5].

It is evident that damage or injury to the brain in childhood may result in impairment which is *not* of a type reflected in the abnormalities of power, tone or reflexes found using the classical neurological examination techniques. An appreciation of this fact led to a variety of new forms of examination designed to detect minor neurological dysfunction [6-8]. Many of these so-called 'soft' signs are highly reliable [1] and are of considerable value as reflections of the child's current functioning with respect to co-ordination, perception, language, etc. Psychometric assessment of the same neurodevelopmental characteristics may add a useful quantitative element to the clinical appraisal.

There is no doubt that all these signs are considerably more frequent in children with independently diagnosed neurological disorders. Nevertheless, for three separate reasons, a neurodevelopmental examination is of quite limited use as a guide to the presence of brain damage in the individual patient. First, the differentiation of children with known physiological brain dysfunction but no structural damage (such as in epilepsy) is quite poor. Second, a substantial proportion of the general population exhibit 'soft' signs of neurodevelopmental dysfunction in spite of a complete lack of history of anything likely to have led to brain injury. This is a consequence of the fact that most of the 'soft' signs reflect developmental functions that show considerable individual variation in rates of maturation. For this reason the presence of 'soft' signs is compatible with normal neurological function; that is, the examination produces a significant proportion of 'false positives'.

However, it also produces a significant proportion of 'false negatives', the third reason for its limited utility. In other words, there are many children with known structural damage to the brain who yet show no abnormalities on a careful neurological examination. For example, together with David Shaffer [9] we studied a group of school-age children with a depressed fracture of the skull, an associated dural tear, and gross damage to the brain substance which had been confirmed at operation. In spite of the fact that the neurosurgeon had seen the damaged brain, some two or more years later a third of the children showed no neurological abnormalities of any kind and a further third showed only dubious signs. Similarly, in a prospective study of head-injured children with a post-traumatic amnesia of at least one week, half showed no abnormalities on a thorough neurological examination by a research neurologist two-and-a-half years later [10, 11]. These findings indicate that there are some children with definite brain damage who show no abnormalities on clinical neurological examination. It is to this group of children that the concept of minimal brain dysfunction may be meaningfully applied.

Cognitive and Behavioural Correlates of Neurological Disorder

The question is how are we to recognise this condition if it occurs in the absence of overt neurological abnormality? The tendency has been to rely on particular patterns of behavioural or cognitive abnormalities [12-14]. But how far is this a valid procedure? To answer that question requires several different steps. First, we need to determine whether the presence of a known brain injury is associated with a definite increase in the rates of psychiatric and cognitive problems. Several studies have clearly demonstrated that it is.

331

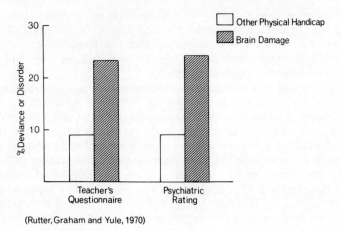

(Rutter, Graham and Yule, 1970)

Figure 1 Brain damage and psychiatric disorder (children IQ 86 or more) [1]

Figure 1 illustrates the findings from the Isle of Wight study [1]. Both as assessed on a teacher's questionnaire and on a clinical psychiatric interview, children of normal intelligence with brain damage were twice as likely as children with other physical handicaps, such as asthma, diabetes or heart disease, to show deviance or disorder. However, as the other physical handicaps were less likely to be accompanied by visible crippling, it was not possible to be sure that the increase in psychiatric problems was due to brain damage per se.

This difficulty was avoided in a study carried out in North London [15]. Thirty-three normally intelligent school age children with cerebral disorders were compared with 42 children with handicapping disorders due to lesions below the brain stem (polio, muscular dystrophy, etc). In spite of the fact that the groups were comparable in terms of visible crippling, psychiatric disorder was found to be much commoner in the group whose physical handicap was attributable to brain damage (Fig. 2). The inference of a *causal* relationship was strong in that the two groups were well matched in other respects. However, longitudinal data showing *changes* in behaviour or cognition following brain injury were necessary before causation could be assumed.

A Causal Relationship?

Such data are available from a recently completed prospective study [10, 11] in which we have compared a sample of children with head injuries which resulted in a post-traumatic amnesia (PTA) of at least a week with an individually matched control group of children with orthopaedic injuries which involved no damage to the head and no loss of consciousness. The parents of both groups were interviewed as soon as possible after the injury to obtain an assessment of the child's behaviour before the accident, and further follow-up assessments were made 4

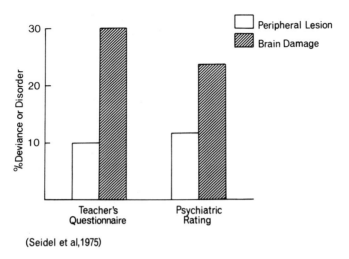

(Seidel et al,1975)

Figure 2 Brain damage and psychiatric disorder [25]

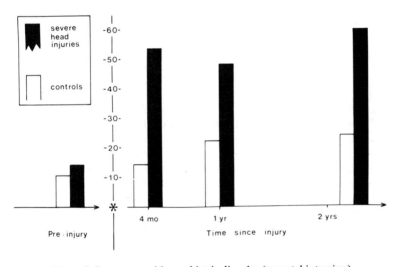

Figure 3 Percentage with psychiatric disorder (parental interview)

months, 1 year, and two to three years after the injury. As Figure 3 shows, the rates of psychiatric disorder were similar in the two groups before the injury but by 4 months after the injury, the rate of disorder in the severe head injury group had greatly increased. It remained high and well above the control group throughout the whole of the 2½ year follow-up. Among the controls without disorder prior to the accident, about one in ten developed a 'new' psychiatric disorder by the 2½ year follow-up, but of the children with head injuries two-thirds did so. The change in the children's behaviour following the head injury indicated a causal connection.

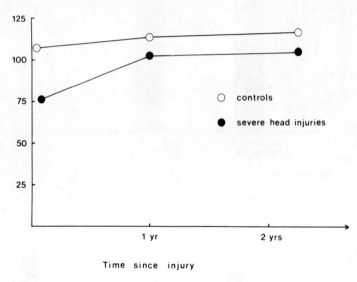

Figure 4 Performance IQ

The pattern of results for cognitive deficits was closely comparable. When first examined shortly after the accident, the children with severe head injuries showed a marked deficit in performance IQ (Fig. 4). However, considerable recovery took place during the year following injury. Here it is this recovery phase which indicates that the cognitive deficit was causally related to the injury. It is clear that brain damage does indeed cause behavioural and cognitive problems.

Psychiatric Disorder, PTA and Neurological Abnormality

However, for this finding to be relevant to the concept of 'minimal brain dysfunction', it is necessary to go on to determine whether this increased rate of disorder is connected with the severity of the injury and, in particular, whether it applies to children who show no residual neurological abnormalities on clinical examination 2½ years later.

These questions may be studied in several different ways. First, the rates of cognitive deficit and of psychiatric disorder after head injury may be related to the duration of PTA. Both types of sequelae were more frequent with longer durations of PTA, confirming the causal connection. Secondly, the frequency of psychiatric disorder may be related to the degree and persistence of cognitive impairment, as shown in Figure 5. Disorder was more frequent in children showing transient or persistent cognitive deficits but the rate of disorder was increased even in those without any identifiable cognitive disability.

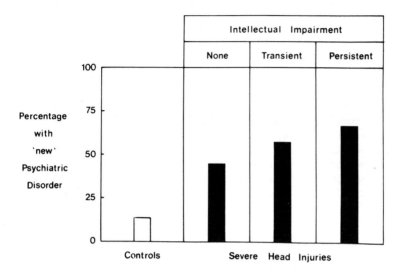

Figure 5 Intellectual impairment

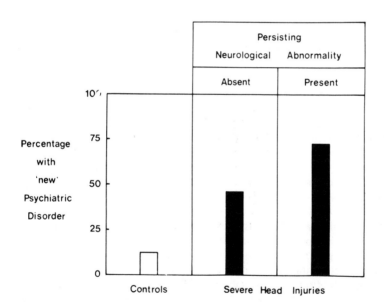

Figure 6 Persisting neurological abnormality

335

Figure 6 shows the association between psychiatric disorder and neurological abnormality within the head injury group. Emotional and behavioural disturbance was more frequent in the children with residual neurological abnormalities (who tended to have had much more severe injuries), but the rate of disorder was still higher than in the controls even for children without any abnormality on a thorough clinical examination at the final follow-up. The finding shows that brain injury (as indicated by a PTA exceeding one week) can lead to psychiatric disabilities even when there are no discernible neurological sequelae. It seems that there are psychiatric disorders due to 'minimal brain dysfunction'.

However, while this is so, it should be emphasised that the conclusion refers to children who have suffered a severe head injury. It cannot be generalised to the very much wider concept of so-called 'MBD', sometimes held to apply to half the child psychiatric clinic population [13]. Moreover, it cannot even be extended to children with milder head injuries (a PTA of over 24 hours but less than one week). These injuries are also associated with psychological impairment but longitudinal data indicate that the cognitive deficit and behavioural deviance probably preceded the injury and, hence, were *not* caused by resulting brain damage [10, 11].

A Distinctive Behavioural Pattern due to Brain Injury?

But these results still leave unanswered the major problem of whether impairment of this kind constitutes a distinctive and recognisable syndrome. The presence of longitudinal data in the case of these children with severe head injuries showed that their psychiatric difficulties were due to brain injury but, of course, such data are not likely to be available in most other instances (as for example when the injuries stem from the perinatal period). Does the particular pattern of behavioural or cognitive abnormalities help? Is there a type of syndrome which, by its form and characteristics, can be identified as a consequence of brain injury?

The issue has been considered in a variety of different neuro-behavioural studies [16] with largely negative findings. It seems that brain damaged children show a heterogeneous range of psychiatric disorders without specific features, except in the case of certain rare conditions. However, this may be because much of the psychiatric disturbance in brain damaged children arises (as with other children) from psychosocial disadvantage and family adversity rather than directly from the brain injury *per se*. It is clear that many mechanisms are involved in the genesis of psychiatric disorder [16]. However, the prospective study of children with head injuries again helps, in that it is possible to isolate disorders arising de novo after severe injuries (and hence those with a high likelihood that the brain injury played a crucial causal role). These disorders were then compared with those occurring in controls or those arising prior to the injury. Very few differences were found and, in particular, the groups did not differ with respect to the hyperactivity features sometimes (and misleadingly) supposed to 'represent' minimal brain dysfunction. The one major exception was disinhibited socially embarrassing behaviour which was quite common in the children with head injuries but rare in the controls. Marked over-eating and enuresis also showed a possible slight association with head injury.

336

However, apart from these symptoms, which are reminiscent of frontal lobe disorders in adults, there was nothing particularly distinctive about the psychiatric disorders arising as a result of brain injury.

Conclusion

We may conclude that above and beyond the major groups of children with identifiable conditions associated with abnormalities on clinical examination, it is certain that there are further children who have suffered undoubted brain injury but who show no neurological signs of that injury. Such damage may result in various cognitive and behavioural sequelae, which might reasonably be considered to constitute syndromes of 'minimal brain dysfunction'. However, although epidemiological and longitudinal studies of children with definite brain damage clearly demonstrate the existence of such syndromes, so far they provide no reliable guides as to their prevalence. Moreover, the same data show that there is not a single brain damage syndrome. Rather, many different syndromes may result and most of these are indistinguishable from those types of behavioural and cognitive disorders that are *not* associated with brain injury. There are important problems here to investigate but as yet we lack the tools to identify most of the syndromes resulting from brain injury. It may be that, in the future, neurometric techniques [17] or new developments in the field of radiological studies may provide the answers but that day has not yet arrived. In the meantime, however, it is clear that there are very substantial neurobehavioural associations with important implications for services and for patterns of therapeutic care.

References

1   Rutter, M, Graham, P and Yule, W (1970) *A Neuropsychiatric Study in Childhood.* London: SIMP/Heinemann Medical
2   Hansen, E (1960) Cerebral palsy in Denmark. *Acta Psychiat. Scand. Suppl.,* 146
3   Crome, L (1960) The brain and mental retardation. *Brit. Med. J., 1,* 897
4   Solomons, G, Holden, RH and Denhoff, E (1963) The changing picture of cerebral dysfunction in early childhood. *J. Pediat., 63,* 113
5   Mayer, E and Byers, RK (1952) Measles encephalitis: a follow-up study of sixteen patients. *Amer. J. Dis. Childh., 84,* 543
6   Ozer, MN (1968) The neurological evaluation of school age children. *J. Learning Disabilities, 1,* 84
7   Touwen, BCL and Prechtl, HFR (1970) The neurological examination of the child with minor nervous dysfunction. *Clinics in Developmental Medicine No. 38.* London: SIMP/Heinemann Medical
8   Touwen, BCL (1976) Neurological developments in infancy. *Clinics in Developmental Medicine No. 58.* London: SIMP/Heinemann Medical
9   Shaffer, D, Chadwick, O and Rutter, M (1975) Psychiatric outcome of localised head injury in children. In *Outcome of Severe Damage to the Central Nervous System.* Ciba Foundation Symposium 34. Elsevier, Excerpta Medica. Amsterdam: North Holland
10 Brown, G, Chadwick, OPD, Shaffer, D, Rutter, M and Traub, M (1979) A prospective study of head injuries in childhood: Psychiatric Sequelae. Paper in preparation

11 Chadwick, OPD, Brown, G, Rutter, M, Shaffer, D and Traub, M (1979) A prospective study of head injuries in childhood: Cognitive Sequelae. Paper in preparation
12 Bax, M and MacKeith, R (ed) (1963) Minimal cerebral dysfunction. *Clinics in Developmental Medicine No. 10*. London: SIMP/Heinemann Medical
13 Wender, PH (1971) *Minimal Brain Dysfunction in Children*. New York: Wiley
14 Kalverboer, AF, Van Praag, HM and Mendlewicz, J (ed) (1978) Minimal brain dysfunction: fact or fiction. *Advances in Biological Psychiatry No. 1*. London: S Karger
15 Seidel, UP, Chadwick, OPD and Rutter, M (1975) Psychological disorders in crippled children. A comparative study of children with and without brain damage. *Dev. Med. Child Neurol., 17*, 563
16 Rutter, M (1977) Brain damage syndromes in childhood: concepts and findings. *J. Child Psychol. Psychiat., 18*, 1
17 John, ER, Karmel, BZ, Corning, WC, Easton, P, Brown, D, Ahn, H, John, M, Harmony, T, Prichep, L, Toro, A, Gersen, I, Bartlett, F, Thatcher, R, Kaye, H, Valdes, P and Schwartz, E (1977) Neurometrics. *Science, 196*, 1393

Chapter 32

EPIDEMIOLOGY OF LANGUAGE DELAY IN CHILDHOOD

Philip Graham, Jim Stevenson and Naomi Richman

Language skills are those involved in all aspects of verbal communication, especially comprehension and expression. Speech refers to those aspects of language that involve verbal expression and articulation. Normal language development in young children proceeds according to a highly characteristic sequence of events. Vocalisation develops during the first year of life, with apparently meaningless babble succeeded by sounds which are increasingly speechlike until the development of the first meaningful word. This occurs in most children by a year or so, but is delayed to eighteen months in about 5 per cent of children [1] and to two years in about 3 per cent [2]. Subsequently, in the second and third years of life, speech normally develops rapidly so that even by two years an average child may be capable of using about 200 words [3]. It is rather less easy to be precise about the development of language comprehension. The capacity to make quite fine auditory discrimination increases rapidly during the first year of life, but the capacity to discriminate two sounds does not necessarily imply an ability to understand differences in meaning between them. However, in general, it seems clear that, in the normal child, comprehension is in advance of expression. Normal language development involves processes which are only grossly subsumed under the headings of comprehension and expression. Both syntactical (grammatical) and semantic (significant or meaningful) aspects of language development have been the subject of study. Utilisation of language skills may provide only a poor guide to an individual's language capacity. Finally, the development of comprehension and expression of written language (reading and writing) is dealt with only peripherally in this chapter since it covers only language delay in the pre-school child; this is clearly important in adaptation to the demands of modern society.

Prevalence of Language Delay

Prevalence, which has been previously summarised by MacKeith and Rutter (1972) [4] is most conveniently considered first in relation to the causes of language delay. One common identifiable cause is deafness. About 2 per 1000 children have deafness to the degree that requires the wearing of a hearing aid [5] and, of these, virtually all will have some degree of language delay produced by their deafness. Quite a large number of others, perhaps 3-4 per cent [6] will have milder or episodic hearing problems produced especially by recurrent ear infection. Such mild or moderate episodic deafness probably makes a significant contribution to language delay, but its extent is unknown. Severe mental retardation, usually produced by brain damage, accounts for approximately 3 per 1000 of the population and, in all children so afflicted, language will be delayed. By contrast, other known causes of language delay are rare. Autism, which is associated with both deviant and delayed language development, occurs in about 0.3 to 0.4 per 1000 children, and developmental aphasia (severe specific developmental language disorder) occurs in about 0.2 per 1000 children. Deafness, autism, aphasia, and severe mental retardation therefore account for language delay in about 5 per 1000 children.

Estimates of the total prevalence of language delay vary according to the criteria used, and, in a recent review of studies of prevalence in children from three to six years, figures between 0.7 per 1000 and 53 per 1000 were cited [7]. In general, the lower figures refer to referral rates for speech therapists and others, while high figures refer to population studies and include immaturities of speech and articulation as well as central language delay. In a total population of 705 three-year-olds carried out in our own department, in which two deaf children and one child with Downs syndrome were excluded [7], it was found that the prevalence of language delay varied markedly according to the criteria used. Severe expressive language delay (defined as language age two-thirds or less of chronological age, i.e. in general about 24 months in the 36-month-old children) occurred in 22 per 1000 (25 per 1000 if the excluded deaf and Downs syndrome children are included). *Specific* expressive language delay (language age less than two-thirds of the non-verbal mental age) occurred in 14 per 1000 children. Finally, specific expressive language delay not associated with general retardation (i.e. a language age two-thirds of mental age in children in whom mental age was at least two-thirds of chronological age) occurred in 5–6 per 1000 children. Approximately 25 per 1000 children have severe expressive language delay, and about 20 per 1000 of these children have such severe delay for reasons other than deafness, autism, aphasia and severe mental retardation. Of these 20, it seems likely that about 5 have specific language delay, i.e. a delay that is not associated with non-verbal retardation nor of such severity and is perhaps not of the same qualitative nature as to be appropriately labelled 'aphasia', while the remaining 15 per 1000 have a delay that is linked to a moderate degree of general mental retardation. To summarise information about prevalence, it seems that the rate of language delay equivalent to two-thirds of chronological age at 3 years is about 25 per 1000. Of these, 2 per 1000 will be deaf, 3 per 1000 will be severely mentally retarded, autism will contribute 0.3–0.4 per 1000 (of which half are severely mentally retarded), aphasia about 0.2 per 1000, specific developmental language delay 5 per 1000, and general moderate developmental delay about 15 per 1000. It should be emphasised that these figures relate to delay at 3 years and are not likely to be applicable to children at different ages.

Associated Factors

Social Class

Deafness, autism, aphasia and severe mental retardation are not particularly linked to low social class; indeed, there is a tendency for autistic children to come differentially from middle-class families. However, our studies suggest that once these conditions have been excluded language delay is strongly linked with social adversity [8]. Of 22 fully assessed children in our language delay group, 85 per cent of the fathers were in manual occupations compared with 65 per cent in the total sample (a non-significant difference). The children with language delay tended to come significantly more often from large families (42 per cent versus 13 per cent, $p < 0.001$), and the housing circumstances of the families in which they lived were significantly more often overcrowded. The language delayed children also had significantly more emotional tension in their home environment. Rates of marital discord and maternal depression were significantly higher than in a control group. The total stress score based on the number of difficulties, financial and otherwise, that the families had experienced in the previous year was also significantly higher in the language delayed than the control group, and significantly more had been in contact with social service departments. Incidentally, these findings in relation to a deviant group contrast with the lack of correlation when age of appearance of first words and first phrases is correlated with social class over the entire range [2].

Sex

Autism and severe mental retardation, though not deafness, is more common in boys. The same is true for developmental language delay, not associated with these conditions. In our study, and this finding is confirmed by the work of others, boys outnumber girls by two or three to one, depending on the criterion of language delay that is taken. This finding contrasts with that in behavioural disturbance at 3 years in which we found a roughly equal sex incidence, but it is in line with findings among antisocial and reading retarded children when examined later in middle childhood.

Behaviour

Children with language delay are much more likely to have a significant behaviour problem than a child in the general population. Our study [9] found that 59 per cent of children with language delay show such behaviour problems compared with 14 per cent in the general population. Incidentally, children with behaviour problems also have a fourfold increase in their rate of language delay compared to those in the general population.

Findings on Follow-up

Our own study [10] and those of others confirm that, although children with developmental language delay do not show the same very poor prognosis of children with severe mental retardation and autism, they are nevertheless more likely to have reading problems and more general moderate learning difficulties later in life. Of children with language delay at 3 years, 45 per cent at 8 years have a reading age 18 months below their chronological age and about one-third (36%) have full-scale WISC IQs below 85, though only 9 per cent have WISC full scale IQs below

70. It is not possible at this stage to be sure whether the persistence of learning difficulties is associated with continuing social disadvantage. Given the nature of the social disadvantage at 3 years, it is likely that this will often persist until at least middle childhood. These figures do not, of course, provide any indication of the value of screening in the pre-school period for later learning problems, but we shall shortly be able to present such information from our own data (Stevenson, in preparation). Other work, however, suggests that a considerable number of learning problems developing later would be missed if reliance were placed entirely on screening examination conducted even as late as five years [11].

Implications of Epidemiological Findings

Delay in the development of language, defined as a language age two-thirds of chronological age at 3 years, occurs in about 25 per 1000 children, or approximately what one would expect from a normal distribution curve if one takes a cut-off point two standard deviations from the mean. However, those children falling into the language delay group are by no means a collection drawn randomly from the general population. Once the deaf, the severely mentally retarded, the autistic and the aphasic (which contribute about 5 per 1000) have been excluded, the remaining 20 per 1000 have been found to be less medically pathological, but to represent, nevertheless, a socially highly deviant group. Indeed, Starte (1975) [12], working from general practice, has suggested that language delay in the 2-year-old is a most effective predictor of social disturbance in the family. Taken together with other work, the aetiological implications of these findings are considerable. They do not suggest that children showing language delay are suffering from a maturational delay produced by immaturity of physiological brain functioning, nor, once the pathological group have been excluded, does it seem as though brain damage or dysfunction is causative. It seems probable that social adversity is more directly responsible for the disability, though the sex ratio suggests that physiological factors may render boys more vulnerable to environmental stress than girls. Whether the language delay is so often the harbinger of later learning difficulties because of continuing social adversity or because, even in favourable circumstances, it is not possible to build scholastic achievement on immature pre-school foundations is unclear. It does seem, however, that both language delay and the later learning difficulties are preventable at least with massive intervention [13]. Whether pre-school or infant school intervention will also provide effective prevention is less certain, but some evidence at least is encouraging [14].

References

1   Morley, ME (1965) *The Development and Disorders of Speech in Childhood.* Edinburgh: E & S Livingstone
2   Neligan, G and Prudham, D (1969) Norms for four standard developmental milestones by sex, social class and place in family. *Dev. Med. and Child Neurol., 11,* 413

3 Rutter, M and Bax, M (1972) The normal development of speech and language. In *The Child with Delayed Speech* (ed M Rutter and J Martin). London: Heinemann

4 MacKeith, R and Rutter, M (1972) A note on the prevalence of language disorders in young children. In *The Child with Delayed Speech* (ed M Rutter and J Martin). London: Heinemann

5 Rutter, M, Tizard, J and Whitmore, K (1970) *Education Health and Behaviour.* London: Longmans

6 Anderson, VM (1967) The incidence and significances of high-frequency deafness in children. *Amer. J. Dis. Child., 113,* 560

7 Stevenson, J and Richman, N (1976) The prevalence of language delay in a population of three year old children and its association with general retardation. *Dev. Med. and Child Neurol., 18,* 431

8 Richman, S and Stevenson, J (1977) Language delay in 3-year-olds: family and social factors. *Acta Paediat. Belg., 30,* 213

9 Stevenson, J and Richman, N (1978) Behaviour, Language and Development in 3 year old children. *J. Aut. and Child Schiz., 8,* 299

10 Stevenson, J (1978) Paper presented to the Association of Child Psychology and Psychiatry, London

11 Bax, M and Whitmore (1973) Neurodevelopmental screening in the school-entrant medical examination. *Lancet, ii,* 368

12 Starte, GA (1975) The poor communicating two year old and his family. *J. Roy. Coll. Gen. Pract., 25,* 800

13 Heber, R and Garber, H (1975) An experiment in prevention of cultural-familial mental retardation. In *Proc. Sec. Cont. Int. Ass. Scientific Study of Mental Retardation* (ed DA Primrose). Warsaw Polish Medical Publishers

14 Arnold, E, Barneby, N, McManus, J, Smeltzer, DJ, Conrad, A, Winer, G and Desgranges, L (1977) Prevention by specific perceptual remediation for vulnerable first graders. *Arch. Gen. Psychiat., 34,* 1279

Chapter 33

EPILEPSY IN CHILDREN

Euan M Ross

'Accurate statistics are notoriously difficult to obtain, especially in a disorder such as epilepsy, that is so often hushed up and that may only appear for a short time in a person's life'

WHO (1957) Technical Report Series No. 130

Introduction

The occurrence of seizures, particularly the first, is most upsetting to parents, who rarely know what to do; in a recent Nottingham Study [1], 30 per cent thought their child was dead or dying. Fits were the commonest single reason for non-planned admissions of children to a large English children's hospital accounting for 15 per cent of doctor- and 23 per cent of parent-initiated admissions [2].

Many attempts have been made to estimate the child population with fits. Burt, in 1937 [3] estimated that 0.25 per 1000 London schoolchildren had epilepsy, a figure that we now know to be far too low. Records of children with epilepsy attending the Mayo Clinic since 1935 [4] show no great change in prevalence in the following years.

Determining the prevalence of epilepsy is not easy; all who work in children's epilepsy clinics realise that there are great difficulties in deciding whether or not a child's problems really have an epileptic basis. Decision rests on clinical judgement; the EEG and other aids are only adjuncts and cannot make the diagnosis. Even in the best clinics some children will be erroneously labelled as epileptic for a time. The label 'epilepsy' may be denied by parents in an attempt to avoid prejudice. There remains a lack of firm agreement between physicians as to what disorders should be regarded as epileptic, and how long freedom from fits can be regarded as cure. These clinical problems are reflected in the diversity of definitions used in recent epidemiological studies. As an illustration, Kurland's [5] definition; 'Any patient whose seizure has occurred *during* the *five years* preceding this day (prevalence day) was included as "active". Any patient who had been on *anticonvulsant medication within five years* of that prevalence day, even if he had been seizure-free during the period, was also included as "active"'. This differs from Pond [6] et al: 'An epileptic was defined as a patient who had had epileptic fits of any sort at some time *during the two years* prior to the time of the survey, or who had been on *regular anticonvulsants during* this period', or Rutter [7]: 'To be regarded as having epilepsy, a child must have had a *definite fit since he started school,* and

344

during the previous *twelve months* there must have been *either a fit* or the child must have taken *regular anticonvulsants'.*

Review of epidemiological studies into epilepsy did not reveal any two that adopted entirely similar definitions of epilepsy or study design.

In an attempt to overcome the great problems of describing the various seizure disorders, an International Classification of the Epilepsies was proposed by the International League Against Epilepsy in 1969 [8], in which epilepsies are divided into partial or generalised types, which may be primary (of unknown cause) or secondary. There is much merit in thinking in terms of aetiology but, sadly, many cases have to be placed in an unclassifiable group. The loss of well-understood and long-used terms, such as petit and grand mal, has limited the appeal of this classification in clinical practice; it is also difficult to find a place for newly recognised forms, such as benign focal nocturnal epilepsy of childhood. It is not surprising that few epidemiological studies have yet been reported using this classification scheme.

Cross-sectional Studies

There is no shortage of recent epidemiological studies into children's epilepsy; Rose et al (1972) [9] reviewed over 30 reports with rates varying from 150/1000 children in the tropical island of Guam to the low figure of 1.5 per 1000 in Japanese schoolchildren. Rose et al contributed a further study based on postal enquiries to parents which yields a high rate of epilepsy by US and European standards at 16 per 1000. Their study, however, yet again illustrates the phenomenon that method and definition dictates findings, a matter discussed in depth by West and Ross [10, 11]. High rates tend to be found where relatively relaxed criteria for epilepsy are accepted. Hospital-based studies exclude those who are solely treated by general practitioners (a type of doctor found in very varying proportions in different parts of the world). There is conflicting evidence concerning the use of hospitals for case-finding purposes. Crombie [12] reported that 75 per cent of patients with epilepsy saw only general practitioners; in contrast, the Carlisle population study [13], carried out in a similar period, found that 78 per cent had seen specialists. General practices tend to exclude the most seriously affected who may be incarcerated in long-term residential institutions. Both types of study have no access to those who do not seek treatment.

Febrile Seizures

The study of epilepsy in the first decade is much complicated by the tendency of pyrexial infants to convulse. Such fits are often dismissed by doctors as trivial; Costeff (1965) [14], from an area of Israel well provided with medical services, reported that many children are never brought to medical attention following fits. His estimate that 19 per cent of children have febrile fits greatly exceeds the rates found in the majority of recent doctor-based studies which yield figures in the

345

range 20-30 per 1000 [15], findings recently updated by Pilling [16] in a comprehensive review of the epilepsies.

Although Lennox [17] described febrile seizures as 'the purest form of epilepsy', it makes prevalence studies much easier if we distinguish febrile from non-febrile seizures and define the latter as 'recurrent paroxysmal disturbances of consciousness, sensation or movement which are primarily cerebral in origin and unassociated with acute febrile incidents'. The rest of this chapter is confined to epilepsy unassociated with fever.

Eight large well-conducted studies of non-febrile epilepsy in the 10-20 age group [5, 7, 11, 12, 18-21] from developed Northern Hemisphere countries were reviewed [11]. In combination, 803 young people of 207054 in the age range 10-20 had epilepsy, giving a rate of 3.9 1000 (Table I).

TABLE I

Investigator		Population	With epilepsy	Rate/1000
Crombie et al	Eng. and Wales (10-14)	22 336	88	3.9
Gudmundsson	Iceland (10-19)	32 872	143	4.3
Cooper	Eng., Scot. and Wales (11)	3 934	23	7.1
Sillanpaa	Turku, Finland (10-15)	108 019	340	3.2
Rutter	Isle of Wight (5-14)	11 865	86	7.2
Kurland	Rochester, USA (10-19)	3 763	13	3.4
Ross and West	Eng., Scot. and Wales (11)	15 496	64	4.1
Ross	Bristol (11-16)	25 165	110	4.3
Total		223 450	867	3.9

Longitudinal Studies

Two large-scale cohort studies from the USA followed children with fits from birth for the first 6 [22] and 7 [23] years respectively, and a further developmental study based on two years births in Geelong, Australia [24] is in progress.

Wallace [25] followed 112 of an original sample of 134 children admitted to Edinburgh hospitals who had febrile convulsions for between 8-10 years, finding 12 per cent had subsequent non-febrile fits. Livingston [26] studied child patients with petit mal through periods between 5-28 years, finding it in 2.3 per cent of 15 102 patients with epilepsy.

Apart from the Mayo Clinic series [4, 5] there are few longitudinal studies of epilepsy from childhood through to adolescence, let alone to adult life. Harrison and Taylor [27] reported a 20-year review of 200 children with fits of all sorts from the Oxford region; Cooper [28], through the National Study of Child Health and Development, followed 27 from birth to age 15. Kiørboe [29] in Funen, Denmark, followed 86 children from age 12 for at least 5 years [15]. Ross followed 64 derived from the National Child Development Study (1958) cohort from birth to 11 and reviewed their progress at 11 [30], and 16 years of age [11]. This data was recorded by school doctors, parents through enquiries made by health visitors and school teachers, at ages 7 and 11. Confirmation of epileptic diagnoses was made through writing to general practitioners and paediatricians. At 11 years the cumulative prevalence was 4.1/1000 of whom half had further fits in the next two years. Two-thirds were educated in normal schools; the remainder, at special schools, were nearly all multiply handicapped, mainly with educational retardation.

Epilepsy in British School Children

Enough, perhaps needlessly many, head counts of children with epilepsy have been carried out. The need is now to assess the quality of life of affected children and document the natural histories of the many types of epilepsies. The Reid Report [31] entitled *People with Epilepsy* lamented 'we were repeatedly confronted with points on which we would have liked to have had factual information of a kind which was not available'. In the course of a study of handicapped children in Bristol [21, 32], 110 in 25 165 (4.3/1000) aged 11–16 years had a history of recurrent fits with at least one occurring within two years prior to the start of the study (Table II). The diagnosis was confirmed by medical examination

TABLE II International Classification of Epilepsy Type (Bristol 11–16 year olds)

	Number	%
Primary generalised	59	53
Secondary generalised	37	34
Undetermined and unclassifiable	12	11
Partial	2	2
Total	110	100

whenever possible together with parental interview and scrutiny of medical notes. This study found there was a slight male excess, and that 15 per cent of children were fatherless, but those in families had a normal social class distribution.

One in five (23/110) had their first attack before their first birthday (Table III); 59 per cent were fit-free in the year before they were interviewed, while aged 11–16 (Table IV). Grand mal was the commonest persisting type of seizure affecting half the children (Table V). Seventeen per cent presented with febrile con-

347

vulsions but it was impossible to tell whether subsequent fits with fever were true sequelae of febrile seizures or misdiagnosis—the well wrapped convulsing child soon develops a fever. 'Pure' petit mal was relatively uncommon, occurring initially in six children but affecting only one in the final year of the study, where it was much more likely to be found in association with other seizure types.

TABLE III Age First Fit (Bristol 11–16 year olds)

	Number	%
Under 1	23	21
1–4	35	32
5–9	39	36
10+	9	8
Not certain	4	3
Total	110	100

TABLE IV Fits in 12 Months Before Interview (Bristol 11–16 year olds)

	Number	%
Grand mal	27	24
Petit mal	1	1
Atypical petit mal	6	6
Psychomotor	1	1
Uncertain whether genuine	3	3
No attacks	65	59
No information	7	6
Total	110	100

TABLE V First Fit (Bristol 11–16 year olds)

	Number	%
Grand mal (afebrile)	57	52
Grand mal (with fever)	19	17
Petit mal	5	4
Atypical petit mal	4	4
Psychomotor/temporal	1	1
Uncertain or mixed	23	21
No record	1	1
Total	110	100

Educational Aspects

Children's epilepsy has important educational implications [33]. In the Bristol study, over a third (38%) were unable to attend normal schools due to a wide variety of handicaps, mainly mental retardation. The progress and future of the child with epilepsy seems to be more dependent on the nature of other physical handicaps than the occurrence of fits *per se.* About half the children (56/110) were regarded as having epilepsy alone while the rest (54/110) had epilepsy with one or more other handicaps. Those with 'epilepsy alone' were much less likely to have missed much schooling or to expect employment problems on leaving school.

A great deal has been learnt about the educational needs and behaviour of school children with epilepsy through detailed studies of the whole child population aged 5-14 in the Isle of Wight [7] and a survey of children in Bedford schools [34]. Taken together, these studies leave no doubt that all children with epilepsy have multiple needs; those in normal education have learning and emotional problems, resulting from epileptic discharges, drug treatment and low expectations. The problems are worse in special school children who usually have other physical and mental handicaps as well as more frequent fits [11].

Hopkins [35] has argued, in the case of adults, that hospital supervision is often ineffective and could well be replaced by high quality general practice. The Bristol study showed a tendency for children with epilepsy to receive little continuity of hospital treatment. Children with 'epilepsy alone' were more likely to attend hospital outpatients than those with multiple handicaps. On average, each child attending hospital had 8 appointments during a 6-year period during which they saw at least four different doctors. At the worst, four children had 20, 23, 25 and 27 appointments in a six-year period being seen by 12, 11, 4 and 22 different doctors respectively.

Conclusion

From all round the world repeated epidemiological studies have documented the great needs, educational, social and medical of all children with convulsive problems. The Court [36] and Warnock [37] reports, if adopted, could result in greatly improved services for children with epilepsy, but professional timidity rules out early action. Not surprisingly, scrutiny of the contents of the major journals suggests that epileptic disorders appeal less to writing paediatricians than to those of the heart, kidney and blood diseases.

Although a great deal has been learnt in recent years there is need for more information concerning the influence of the new anticonvulsant drugs, of education and management policies [33, 38]. In particular, there is a clear need for every Area Health Authority to keep simple descriptive statistics of their children with epilepsy. These facts need to be gathered and then disseminated along the same lines as perinatal or child abuse data through regular local meetings of concerned professional workers. Effective usage of simply gathered data would provide

349

a national basis on which to plan services, assess management and, most of all, learn something about prevention.

References

1   Rutter, N and Metcalfe, D (1978) *Brit. Med. J.*, *2*, 1345
2   Wynne, J and Hull, D (1977) *Brit. Med. J.*, *2*, 1140
3   Burt, CL (1937) *The Backward Child.* London: University of London Press
4   Hauser, WA and Kurland, LT (1975) *Epilepsia, 1*, 66
5   Kurland, LT (1959) *Epilepsia, 1*, 143
6   Pond, DA et al (1960) *Psychiatrica, Neurologica, Neurochirurgia, 63*, 217
7   Rutter, M et al (1970) *Education Health and Behaviour.* London: Longman
8   International League Against Epilepsy (1970) *Epilepsia, 11*, 114
9   Rose, SW et al (1973) *Epilepsia, 14*, 133
10 West, PB and Ross, EM (1974) *The Prevalence and Incidence of Epilepsy*, Report to the British Epilepsy Association
11 Ross, EM et al (1980) *Brit. Med. J., 1*, 207
12 Crombie, DL et al (1960) *Brit. Med. J., 2*, 416
13 Brewis, M et al (1965) *Acta Paediatrica Scandinavica*, Supplement 24
14 Costeff, H (1965) *New Engl. J. Med., 223*, 1410
15 Millichap, JG (1968) *Febrile Convulsions.* New York: Macmillan
16 Pilling, D (1979) Manuscript in draft. London: National Children's Bureau
17 Lennox, WG and Lennox, M (1960) *Epilepsy and Related Disorders.* New York: Little Brown
18 Rutter, M et al (1970) *Education Health and Behaviour.* London: Longman
19 Gudmundsson, KR (1966) *Acta Neurologica Scandinavica*, Supplement 25
20 Sillanpaa, M (1973) *Acta Paediatrica Scandinavica*, Supplement 237
21 Ross, EM (1975) MD Thesis, University of Bristol
22 Van den Berg, BJ (1969) *Pediatric Research, 2*, 298
23 Nelson, KB and Ellenberg, JH (1976) *New Engl. J. Med., 19*, 1029
24 Rossiter, EJR et al (1977) *Austral. Paediat. J., 13*, 182
25 Wallace, SJ (1977) *Arch. Dis. in Childh., 52*, 192
26 Livingston, S et al (1965) *J. Amer. Med. Assoc., 194*, 3, 227
27 Harrison, RM and Taylor, DC (1976) *Lancet, 1*, 948
28 Cooper, JE (1965) *Brit. Med. J., 2*, 1020
29 Kiørboe, E (1961) *Acta Psychiatrica et Neurologica Scandinavica*, Supplement 150, 166
30 Ross, EM (1973) *Proc. Roy. Soc. Med., 66*, 703
31 Advisory Committee on the Health and Welfare of Handicapped Persons (1969) *People with Epilepsy.* London: HMSO
32 Ross, EM and Evans, D (1972) *Epilepsia, 13*, 7
33 Editorial (1979) *Brit. Med. J., 1*, 576
34 Holdsworth, L and Whitmore, K (1974) *Devel. Med. and Child Neurol., 16*, 746
35 Hopkins, A and Scambler, G (1977) *Lancet, 1*, 183
36 *Fit for the Future* (1976) Report of the Committee on Child Health Services. London: HMSO
37 *Special Educational Needs* (1978) Report of the Committee of Enquiry into the Education of Handicapped Children and Young People. London: HMSO
38 *Epilepsy in Society* (1971) London: Office of Health Economics

Chapter 34

FEBRILE CONVULSIONS AND SUBSEQUENT EPILEPSY*

J F Annegers, W A Hauser and L T Kurland

Introduction

The risk of developing epilepsy after febrile convulsions has been a subject of concern and debate for many years. A review of the literature discloses a risk as low as 2 per cent and as high as 57 per cent [1, 2]. High rates of subsequent epilepsy are reported for patients seen at speciality clinics [3, 4], while population based cohorts have shown much lower risks [5].

Methods

We have reviewed the medical histories of residents of Rochester, Minnesota, who had a diagnosis of febrile convulsions between 1935 and 1974. Data were collected regarding the characteristics of the febrile convulsions, such as the number and duration of seizures, presence or absence of focal features, and subsequent afebrile seizures. The expected number of cases of epilepsy was derived by applying Rochester's age and sex specific incidence rates for epilepsy [6] to the person-years of follow-up.

Results

Incidence

We identified 678 residents of Rochester who were diagnosed as having febrile convulsions over a 40-year period of time. The cumulative incidence rate of such febrile seizures up to age 5 was 2.3 per cent. Frequency was slightly greater in males than in females and the rates did not change throughout the 40-year time period.

Since 12 of the 678 cases had been identified retrospectively as a result of a diagnosis of epilepsy, head trauma, or because a sib had a febrile convulsion, they were excluded and only 666 were retained for the follow-up study.

*Supported in part by Research Grants GM 14231 and NS 523-27-E, National Institutes of Health, Bethesda, Maryland, USA

Epilepsy after Febrile Convulsions

The 666 patients were followed a total of 8291 person-years after the initial febrile convulsion. During the follow-up of the 666 patients, 29 were found to have epilepsy (that is, two or more afebrile seizures). In addition to the 29 patients with epilepsy, 5 others had seizures which did not meet our criteria for epilepsy (that is, single idiopathic seizures in 4 patients and in another patient seizures associated with encephalitis). The expected number of cases of epilepsy was 4.05. Since 29 were observed, the relative risk is 7.2. The relative risk of epilepsy after febrile convulsions declined with increasing age; it was 11.5 under 5 years, 6.6 from 5 until 9, and 3.9 after age 10. However, the risk remained significantly increased during each age interval throughout the follow-up period.

Characteristics of the Febrile Convulsion

A neurological abnormality was known or presumed to have existed in 25 of the 666 patients prior to the first febrile convulsion. Fourteen had mental retardation (IQ less than 70), 7 had cerebral palsy and 4 had both. These children had an especially high incidence of subsequent epilepsy which developed in 10 (40%) of the 25. The children with neurological deficits tended to have their first febrile convulsions at earlier ages and all those who developed subsequent epilepsy had the first episode of seizures prior to age 10.

Another risk factor for subsequent epilepsy was the atypical character of the febrile convulsion. In our study this included unilateral or focal origin, repeated episodes the same day, or Todd's paralysis. Among patients without cerebral palsy or mental retardation, the relative risk for those with atypical febrile convulsions was 13.2, as compared to 3.9 among those who did not have atypical attacks (Table I).

TABLE I Influence of Neurological Deficit and Atypical Character of Febrile Convulsions on Risk of Subsequent Epilepsy

Subjects		Patients	Epilepsy cases			95% confidence interval
			Observed	Expected	RR	
Without CP or MR						
Atypical character of	No	569	14	3.50	3.9	2.1–6.4
convulsion	Yes	72	5	0.38	13.2	4.3–30.6
With CP or MR						
Atypical character of	No	15	6	0.10	60.0	22.0–130.8
convulsion	Yes	10	4	0.07	57.1	15.5–146.2

CP = Cerebral palsy
MR = Mental retardation
RR = Relative risk

Children whose febrile convulsions lasted less than about 10 minutes had a lower risk of subsequent epilepsy than those with one or more convulsions lasting longer. This was also true after exclusion of patients with prior neurological deficits or seizures of atypical character. If all patients with prior neurological deficits or prolonged or otherwise exceptional febrile seizures are considered together as a high-risk group of 181 members, the relative risk for subsequent epilepsy was 21.2 contrasted with 2.9 in the low-risk group of 485 without deficits or exceptional seizures (Table II).

TABLE II Influence of Low-risk and High-risk Status* on Risk of Subsequent Epilepsy

Patient group	Patients	Epilepsy cases		RR	95% confidence interval
		Observed	Expected		
Low-risk	485	9	3.10	2.9	1.3–5.5
High-risk	181	20	0.95	21.1	12.9–32.5

*Low-risk: Without cerebral palsy or mental retardation ($\geqslant$ 10 minutes) or other atypical features of febrile convulsions.
High-risk: With any of above.

TABLE III Risk of Epilepsy After Febrile Convulsion: Summary of Population-Based Cohort Studies

Population-based cohort studies	No. cases of febrile convulsion	With subsequent epilepsy		Mean follow-up period, years*
		No.	%	
Herlitz (1941) [8]	424	14	3.2	7.8
Friderichsen and Melchior (1954) [9]	282	8	2.8	6
Frantzen and associates (1968) [10]	200	5	2.5	5
Van den Berg and Yerushalmy (1969) [11]	246	8	3.2	3.2
Nelson and Ellenberg (1976) [1]	1706	34	2.0	7
Present report	666	29	4.4	15

*The follow-up period at risk to subsequent epilepsy would be approximately 2 years (mean age at first febrile convulsion) less than mean age at last follow-up.

Summary

The cumulative incidence of epilepsy up to age 20 in the Rochester population is about 1 per cent. The risk of developing epilepsy by age 20 for all children who have experienced febrile convulsions is about 6 per cent. However, this risk figure

353

consists of a combination of 2.5 per cent for children without prior neurological disorder or atypical or prolonged seizures and 17 per cent for those with such complications.

The risks of subsequent epilepsy are considerably lower in this cohort than in some reports. Wallace (1977) [4] and Tsuboi and Endo (1977) [3] reported 17 per cent of patients with febrile convulsions go on to develop epilepsy. Their series, however, consisted of patients admitted to hospital or those attending a specialty clinic. Even higher rates were reported in the earlier studies: 30 per by Peterman [7], and 57 per cent by Livingston [2].

Table III gives the results of six other studies concerned with epilepsy following febrile convulsions. Note the similarity in results between these population-based studies. The higher percentage in our study seems to be largely due to the greater duration of follow-up.

References

1   Nelson, KB and Ellenberg, JH (1976) *New Eng. J. Med., 295,* 1029
2   Livingston, S (1954) *The Diagnosis and Treatment of Convulsive Disorders in Children.* Springfield, Ill.: Thomas, pages 75–82
3   Tsuboi, T and Endo, S (1977) *Neuropaediatrie; J. Pediat. Neurobiol., Neurol. and Neurosurg., 8,* 209
4   Wallace, SJ (1977) *Arch. Dis. in Childh., 52,* 192
5   Annegers, JF, Hauser, WA, Elveback, LR and Kurland, LT (1979) *Neurology, 29,* No. 3, 297
6   Hauser, WA and Kurland, LT (1975) *Epilepsia, 16,* 1
7   Peterman, MG (1952) *J. Pediat., 41,* 536
8   Herlitz, G (1941) *Acta Paediatrica Scandinavica Supplement 1, 29,* 110
9   Friderichsen, C and Melchior, J (1954) *Acta Paediatrica Scandinavica Supplement 100, 43,* 307
10   Frantzen, E, Lennox-Buchthal, M and Nygaard, A (1968) *Electroencephalography and Clinical Neurophysiology, 24,* 197
11   Van den Berg, BJ and Yerushalmy, J (1969) *Pediatric Research, 3,* 298

Part V   Neurosurgical Aspects

Chapter 35

EPIDEMIOLOGY OF HEAD INJURIES

Bryan Jennett

Head injury forms a major health problem in all Westernised nations. Only last year Kraus of California wrote: 'the epidemiology of head injuries is woefully incomplete, because no single report includes all patients, irrespective of severity, within a defined population' [1]. There are good reasons why there is such a dearth of reliable statistics about head injury. One is that there is no formal definition; the term does not even appear in the *International Classification of Diseases* (ICD). But more important is the wide dispersion of head injuries, which, in turn, reflects the wide dispersion of head injured patients throughout the health care system. Half the fatal cases never reach hospital, while many patients with the milder injuries do not consult a doctor unless or until complications develop. Even within the hospital head injuries go to neurosurgeons, accident and general surgeons, rehabilitationists and pathologists, each of whom sees part of the problem, but none of them the whole of it. No one person accepts responsibility for the total care of the head injured individual, nor does any one discipline regard head injury as its own problem.

There are various sources of information about head injuries. In Britain we are fortunate that statutory returns are made for all deaths, and also for discharges from all NHS hospitals; these include the cause of injury *and* the site (the N code of the ICD). Individual hospitals usually keep records of admissions and of accident and emergency (A/E) attenders. Sporadically the medical journals report accounts of series of patients from clinicians, usually neurosurgeons; these are obviously highly selected but the policy which has led to the selection of such patients is seldom stated.

In Britain, head injuries account for 1 per cent of deaths, 20 per cent of accidental deaths, and about 50 per cent of road traffic accident deaths; between 50 per cent and 60 per cent of head injury deaths are due to road accidents. More than half the deaths occur before the victim reaches hospital, a proportion that has also been found in two unpublished American surveys. International statistics relate only to accidental deaths as a whole, but these presumably will be reflected in the head injury figures. WHO reports indicate the wide range between different countries, with Scotland, England and Japan the least accident prone in respect of accidents as a proportion of all deaths, or of road accidents as a proportion of accidental deaths, or on a population basis. Some years ago a study of the vital statistics of head injury as reflected in statutorily collected material for England and Wales [2] indicated the lack of any statistics about accident and emergency attenders and the limitation of what could be discovered from registered deaths and routine discharge statistics. Awareness of these gaps, together with our own interest in certain more specific problems of the various kinds of head injury, led us to set up the Scottish Head Injury Management Study; this was initially supported by the Health Department and is now part of a wider MRC head injury programme in my department. This aims to collect data about head injuries as a whole—from deaths that never reach hospital to accident and emergency attenders who are sent home; it also includes the patients admitted to hospital, the few that go to neurosurgical wards and the much larger numbers who go into primary surgical wards (PSW), a term we coined to cover the various kinds of non-neuro-surgical wards, which in Britain, as in most European countries, cope with the majority of admissions head injuries [3].

In our survey of all Scottish hospitals, for sample periods during 1974, we found a relatively consistent pattern in the head injured patients between one part of the country and another. About 10 per cent of all A/E new attenders had a head injury (15% of trauma attenders); four out of 5 were sent home. Only 60 per cent had an X-ray of skull; 40 per cent required treatment to a scalp laceration; many had recently ingested alcohol [4]. Our survey enabled us to calculate annual attendance rates for different Health Board Areas in Scotland; and also to estimate the variations in annual attendance rates for different sections of the population, and for head injuries due to different causes; for example, we discovered that for Scottish adult males an assault is as common a cause of head injury leading to A/E attendance as is a road accident. However, the distribution of causes is quite different according to the severity of injury; for example, road accidents account for less than one-fifth of A/E attenders but for more than a half of patients who reach a neurosurgical unit in coma.

Many of our larger hospitals (say over 750 beds) admit a thousand or more head injuries a year, and this number is increasing. However, this increase is almost wholly due to milder injuries, patients with which are discharged in less than 48 hours; as the death rate has remained almost constant for several years the case mortality has fallen; this does not, of course, indicate any improvement in standards of care. Another consequence of the predominance of mild injuries among admissions to primary surgical wards is that although they make up 3 per cent of all acute admissions they contribute only 1 per cent of occupied bed days in acute wards. In certain wards, however, they form a very significant load; in male surgical wards head injuries account for more than 25 per cent of emergency admissions, considerably more common than the acute abdomen. Two-thirds of admissions and one-third of occupied bed days attributed to head injury were for patients with no signs of brain damage, no skull fracture and no major extracranial injury; another third of head injury bed days was attributed to patients with major extracranial injury and only minor head injury [5]. These figures, together with other studies we have made, are leading us to a view that an over-cautious attitude prevails in Britain, which leads to the unnecessary admission of many mild injuries.

There is some evidence that in the United States attendance rates at emergency rooms for head injury may be higher but that a smaller proportion are admitted. The admission rate, on a population basis, is certainly lower in the Charlottesville region of Virginia according to an unpublished study recently completed [6]. Another

357

study, in the Houston/Galveston Bay area of Texas, gave a figure exactly the same as ours in Scotland [7]. Preliminary results from New South Wales in Australia show a considerably higher rate, which is consistent with their considerably greater death rate from accidents [8].

When we consider the role of the neurosurgeon in the care of head injuries we find large differences between the United States and Britain, and between some cities within Britain. In Britain there are 7 times fewer neurosurgeons (per million population) than in the United States, and all are concentrated in large regionalised units. Only about 5 per cent of patients admitted to hospital after head injury in Britain reach a neurosurgeon in most of the country; this proportion is much higher in most of North America. However, we have one eccentric British city, Edinburgh, which operates an American-type of policy and this provides an opportunity for looking at the consequences of this, in comparison with Glasgow, which is more typical (in this respect) of the rest of Britain. The rate for A/E attenders for head injury is the same in the catchment areas for Glasgow and Edinburgh, and so are the overall admission rates to hospital; but the neurosurgical admission rate is almost nine times greater in Edinburgh, where 35 per cent of all hospitalised head injuries in the region (and 56% of those in the immediate environs of Edinburgh) go to the neurosurgical unit, where they constitute 50 per cent of neurosurgical admissions [9]. In Glasgow, as also in Aberdeen and Dundee, only 4 per cent of head injuries go to neurosurgery. That Aberdeen and Dundee admit as few cases as Glasgow, in spite of considerably more neurosurgical beds available, indicates the influence of local medical geography—in these cities many head injuries go into primary surgical wards in the hospital which houses the neurosurgical unit—making possible neuro-surgical consultation without the need for transfer.

Does it matter whether head injuries reach a neurosurgeon? For this we need out-come measures; those we have devised in Glasgow, and published some years ago, are now in world-wide use, which means that comparisons are becoming possible. We have certainly demonstrated that the highly selective policy operating in Britain may have unfortunate consequences. We have published reports indicating that over 50 per cent of deaths in neurosurgical units following head injury could have been prevented by better management. usually by more rapid diagnosis and treatment of early complications, such as intracranial haematoma [10, 11]. However, we have also shown that it is possible to reduce the incidence of avoidable factors without fundamentally changing the organisational policy [9].

An Australian neurosurgeon twenty years ago stated that a mortality of much more than 10 per cent for extradural haematoma reflected either low standards of medical education or poor organisation, or both [12]. His pupil, Jamieson, achieved this 'ideal' in the vast State of Queensland; and that is also the figure recently attained in Edinburgh [13]. In Glasgow in the mid-1970s our results were much less good, but we were then operating a highly selective admission policy due to financial restraints having closed neurosurgical beds; indeed 50 per cent of requests for the transfer of head injuries to the neurosurgeons from other hospitals were then being refused. In 1978, more beds were available and attempts were made to reduce avoidable delays; the result was that we reached the Brisbane/Edinburgh level for extradural haematomas, and indeed did better than them for the more serious sub-

358

dural haematomas. Yet we still admitted only 4 per cent of head injuries. I therefore reject the Edinburgh/American contention that satisfactory results can be obtained only by the primary treatment of large numbers of head injuries by neurosurgeons. If all British neurosurgical units were to admit all the head injuries who at present go to primary surgical wards, the neurosurgical facilities would have to be greatly increased which would be a very expensive exercise.

Another area of controversy is the value of treating brain damaged head injuries with certain 'aggressive' therapies, which usually means expensive ones. Here the Glasgow International Data Bank study is of interest [14]. This now holds over 1300 prospectively collected injuries from the United Kingdom, the United States and The Netherlands, well-matched for their initial severity. Treatments were different in different countries; for example, American patients more often had steroids or bony decompression or tracheostomy or mechanical ventilation. Yet the outcome six months after injury on the Glasgow Outcome Scale was remarkably similar [9].

The unnecessary admission of mild injuries in Britain and the unsuccessful intensive treatment of some severe cases in America, are examples of inadequate triage. I believe that we could significantly reduce mortality and morbidity from head injury by improved organisation and by better use of existing resources. This must include facing up to the implications of the recently developed CAT scanning; there is no doubt that this is strikingly successful in detecting the presence of intracranial haematomas soon after injury [15], and it is delay in the management of this particular complication that is the commonest cause of avoidable death and disability. The crux of the problem of head injury care is to reduce these preventable factors, which implies considering the logistics of dealing with the large number of patients with mild injuries, of whom a few will develop serious complications; also of ensuring continuity of care for the severely injured, some of whom will have multiple trauma and many of whom will require long-term rehabilitation.

Planning improved services for head injuries is not possible without the kind of information which epidemiological studies alone can provide. There is need also to make use of standardised methods of assessing initial severity and ultimate outcome, it is encouraging to find such widespread adoption of the systems we have evolved over recent years in Glasgow. There is also a welcome awareness of the need for epidemiological data; fortunately, this again appears to be largely using the methodology which we have evolved in Scotland, so that international comparisons should soon be possible. It is my belief that combined biomedical and health service research in this field will lead to the improved care of the large numbers of patients who in our industrialised western societies fall victim to trauma of the head.

References

1 Kraus, JF (1978) Epidemiologic features of head and spinal cord injury. In *Advances in Neurology* (ed Schoenberg, Bruce S) Volume 19. Raven Press, New York, p. 261
2 Field, JH (1976) *Epidemiology of head injuries in England and Wales.* Her Majesty's Stationery Office, London

3   Jennett, B, Murray, A, MacMillan, R, McFarlane, J, Bentley, Cecily, Strang, I and Hawthorne, V (1977) Head injuries in Scottish hospitals. *Lancet, ii,* 696

4   Strang, I, MacMillan, R and Jennett, B (1978) Head injuries in accident and emergency departments at Scottish hospitals. *Injury, 10,* 154

5   MacMillan, R, Strang, I and Jennett, B (1979) Head injuries in primary surgical wards in Scottish hospitals. *Health Bulletin, 37,* 75

6   Jane et al (1979) Personal communication

7   Grossman et al (1979) Personal communication

8   Sewell, M, Ring, I, Selecki, B, Simpson, D and Vanderfield, G (1979). Trauma to the central and peripheral nervous system in New South Wales. Part I. Interim Report

9   Jennett, B et al (1979) Head injuries in neurosurgical units in Scottish hospitals. *J. Neurol., Neurosurg. and Psychiat.,* in press

10   Rose, J, Valtonen, S and Jennett, B (1977) Avoidable factors contributing to death after head injury. *Brit. Med. J. 2,* 615

11   Jennett, B and Carlin, J (1978) Preventable mortality and morbidity after head injury. *Injury, 10,* 31

12   Hooper, RS (1959) Observations on extradural haemorrhage. *Brit. J. Surg., 47,* 71

13   Mendelow, AD, Karmi, MZ, Paul, KS, Fuller, GAG and Gillingham, FJ (1979) Extradural haematoma: effect of delayed treatment. *Brit. Med. J., 1,* 1240

14   Jennett, B, Teasdale, G, Galbraith, S, Pickard, J, Grant, H, Braakman, R, Avezaat, C, Maas, A, Minderhoud, J, Vecht, CJ, Heiden, J, Small, R, Caton, W and Kurze, T (1977). Severe head injuries in three countries. *J. Neurol., Neurosurg. and Psychiat, 40,* 292

15   Galbraith, S, Teasdale, G and Blaiklock, C (1976) Computerised tomography of acute traumatic intracranial haematoma: reliability of neurosurgeons' interpretations. *Brit. Med. J., 2,* 1371

Chapter 36

HEAD TRAUMA AND SEQUELAE IN THE OLMSTED COUNTY, MINNESOTA, POPULATION*

John F Annegers and Leonard T Kurland

Introduction

In his monograph published four years ago, Dr Jennett [1] wrote, 'To assess the overall incidence of late epilepsy by following up large numbers of head injuries, many of them mildly injured, would be difficult if not impossible'. We are pleased to report that we have been successful in such an endeavour.

Methods

The medical records of all Olmsted County patients with a diagnosis that might indicate a head injury during the 40 years, 1935-1974, were reviewed [2]. Since all levels of head injury were included in the search of the diagnostic indices, nearly 40 000 possible cases came to the attention of the reviewers. About 90 per cent were minor or superficial injuries and were not included in the current study.

The minimum criteria for inclusion as head trauma was an injury to the brain manifested by a record of loss of consciousness, post-traumatic amnesia or evidence of skull fracture. A total of 3587 such head trauma episodes were identified in this population.

The series includes head injuries ranging from concussions with only post-traumatic amnesia to brain contusions resulting in a vegetative state. Although more detailed subdivisions are possible, for purposes of this discussion, we will define three large groups by severity: severe, moderate and mild. Severe head injuries include those with (1) brain contusion, (2) intracranial haematoma, or (3) 24 hours or more of loss of consciousness or post-traumatic amnesia. Moderate head injuries include all those not in the severe group, but who had loss of consciousness or post-traumatic amnesia of half an hour or longer or a skull fracture. Mild head injuries include head injuries without a fracture but with documented loss of consciousness or post-traumatic amnesia of less than a half hour's duration.

Incidence

The age adjusted incidence rate for head trauma was 274 per 100 000 per year in males and 116 in females. So many factors alter the risk of head trauma in a given

* This investigation was supported in part by Research Grants GM 14231 and NS 523-27-E, National Institutes of Health, Bethesda, Maryland, USA.

population that it may not be entirely appropriate to apply our rates to those of other populations in the United States. However, if the rest of the United States has the same age and sex specific incidence rates as Olmsted County, the annual number of cases would now be of the order of 400 000.

Traffic accidents were the major cause of head trauma, with automobile, motorcycle and bicycle accidents accounting for 47 per cent of the total. Falls accounted for 29 per cent, 9 per cent occurred during recreational activities, 5 per cent were occupationally related, 4 per cent were assaults, and 7 per cent were 'other'.

Post-traumatic Seizures

There is only limited information on the risks of seizures after head injuries in civilian populations. The major problems have been:

1 lack of consistent definitions of head injuries;
2 most reports have been based only on cases seen at specific neurosurgical centres;
3 inadequate follow-up of patients after head injury; and
4 inability to compare the frequency of seizures following head trauma with those which occur spontaneously.

By studying head trauma and post-traumatic seizures in the Olmsted County population it is possible to alleviate many of these problems. Our series consists of all patients in the population with a diagnosis of head trauma during the 40-year period of time who met specific clinical criteria. The patients have been followed for various, but known, intervals of time, during which the expected number of seizures unrelated to the trauma could be estimated from Rochester seizure disorder incidence rates [3]. Thus, it is possible to calculate the magnitude and duration of the increased risk of seizures after head trauma.

Exclusions for Study of Post-traumatic Seizures

Not all of the 3587 head trauma episodes could be included in our cohort analysis of post-traumatic seizures. Among the exclusions are the 448 patients who did not survive for one month after the head injury. Patients who had prior epilepsy were also identified and excluded from our analysis. To prevent confounding by more than one head injury, our evaluation was limited to the follow-up of the initial head trauma episode. In the 188 instances a second or successive head injury occurred in the same person; these second episodes were not included. Ours is a study of sequelae after a risk factor; therefore, those patients who did not receive medical attention for head trauma, but for sequelae, were also excluded. There were 168 such patients; most of these arrived as outpatients, a few days after the head injury, because of headaches, blurred vision or other symptoms, whereupon the history of a head injury which met our criteria was obtained. Thus, we have 2748 patients who were seen for their first head injury, survived the acute effects and were not known to have had prior epilepsy or head injuries.

362

Results

Early Seizures

Among the 2748 patients, 58 had seizures while they were still suffering from the direct effects of the head injury. All but 5 of these occurred within the first week after the head injury. The 5 cases occurred during the second week after head injury, in patients who had a protracted course, with surgery, a recurrent subdural haematoma or infection. In this cohort, 2.1 per cent of head trauma episodes were followed by early seizures (Table I).

TABLE I Seizures after head trauma

Type of head injury	Percentage with early seizures	Risk of late seizure	
		To 1 yr	Up to 5 yr
Severe			
Children	30.5	5.6	7.4
Adults	10.3	7.7	13.3
Moderate			
Children	1.1	0.5	1.6
Adults	2.4	1.0	1.6
Mild			
Children	1.0	0.0	0.2
Adults	0.4	0.1	0.8

The rate of early seizures is greater in children under 15 years of age than it is in adults. This is particularly the case in the severe head injuries, where 30 per cent of children were found to have had an early seizure in contrast to 10 per cent in adults. Among those with mild head injuries, that is, without a brain contusion or haematoma or skull fracture or loss of consciousness or post-traumatic amnesia greater than 30 minutes, early seizures occurred in 1 per cent of the children under 15, and in 0.4 per cent of the adults.

Late Seizures

Through a review of subsequent medical records and follow-up letters, the 2748 patients were followed from recovery of acute effects of the head injury to determine the frequency of subsequent seizures. Follow-up was terminated by emigration from the south-eastern Minnesota area, additional head trauma episode, death or the development of subsequent seizures.

If the Rochester incidence rates are applied to the 28 176 person-years of follow-up, the expected number of new cases of one or more seizures is 11.3. However, there were 51 patients with one or more late seizures. This represents a 4.5-fold increased risk during the entire period of observation after head trauma. However, during the first year after head trauma, we observed 19 cases, for a relative risk of 11.5. During the next four years, there were 20 cases, for a relative risk of 4.5.

363

During the period 5 years or more after head trauma, 12 cases were observed, with 8.3 expected. The relative risk after 5 years of 1.4 was not significantly different from the expected occurrence of new cases.

Severity of Injury of Post-traumatic Seizures

Table I presents the cumulative risks of one or more late seizures after head trauma through the first year and through the first five years within the three severity groups for adults and children. The estimates were computed from the incidence rates of new seizures among the patients followed that year. Among those with severe head injuries, that is, brain contusions or haematomas or loss of consciousness or post-traumatic amnesia of 24 hours or more, 7.1 per cent can be expected to have the onset of late seizures within the first year after recovery from head injury. By five years after the head injury, 11.6 per cent will have the onset of post-traumatic seizures.

Compared with the severely injured group, the risk of post-traumatic seizures is considerably less in those with moderate head injuries, that is, only 1.6 per cent through five years. Among those with mild head injuries, the risk of 0.6 per cent through the first five years is not significantly greater than the occurrence of seizures in the general population.

Children have lower risks of post-traumatic seizures than adults at each level of severity of head injury. Not only is the absolute risk lower in children, but the relative risk of subsequent seizures is considerably lower because of the higher incidence of spontaneous seizures in children. Thus, although children are more likely to have early seizures, particularly with severe head injuries, the likelihood that they will develop post-traumatic seizures is less than in adults.

Brain Tumours after Head Trauma

In this study we considered all patients who survived their head injury but who did not have a previously diagnosed brain tumour. Thus, we have a total of 2953 patients, followed 29 859 person-years. The Rochester incidence rates of brain tumours were applied [4] to the age specific person-years of follow up to generate expected numbers. We observed four cases of all types of brain tumours while the expected number was 4.1, thus our data do not indicate any increased risk of brain tumours after head trauma. However, due to the small numbers, we cannot rule out low levels of increased risk. The four cases of brain tumours were not associated with more severe head injuries and the sites of the brain tumours and of the head trauma did not correspond.

References

1   Jennett, B (1975) *Epilepsy after Non-missile Head Injuries.* William Heinemann Medical Books Ltd (Year Book Medical Publishers Inc.), Chicago, Ill.

2   Kurland, LT, Elveback, LR and Nobrega, FT (1973) Proceedings of the International Epidemiological Association, August 1971, Primosten, Yugoslavia. *Savremena Administracija, Belgrade, January 1973*
3   Hauser, WA and Kurland, LT (1975) *Epilepsia, 16,* 1
4   Percy, AK, Elveback, LR, Okazaki, H and Kurland, LT (1972) *Neurology, 22,* 40

Chapter 37

PRIMARY INTRACRANIAL NEOPLASMS IN ROCHESTER, MINNESOTA, 1935-1977*

John F Annegers, Bruce S Schoenberg, Haruo Okazaki, Leonard T Kurland

Introduction

Incidence rates are crucial for many types of epidemiological investigations. Differences between places and over time may suggest specific aetiological agents or may not support suggested aetiological hypotheses. In addition, we frequently need incidence rates to analyse the frequency of new events in cohort studies of patients with suspected risk factors. Determining the incidence rates of intracranial neoplasms presents methodological problems because of the diversity of these tumours and the many different means through which they are diagnosed. In this chapter we present the Rochester data and discuss these issues. In addition we present a small case-control study on a type of pituitary adenoma where the secular trends in a specific age and sex group suggest a possible aetiological factor.

Methods

In this study, intracranial neoplasms are defined as all benign, and primary tumours of the brain and cranio meniges as malignant. Because of their close anatomical proximity, tumours of the pituitary gland, craniopharyngeal duct and pineal body are also included. This series does not include tumours metastatic to the brain from other sites, neoplasms arising from vascular tissue, retinoblastomas, chordomas, or spinal cord tumours. The system of brain tumour nomenclature used in this paper is based on the presumed cell type of origin and has been utilised in other epidemiological studies of primary intracranial neoplasms [1].

The medical records linkage system for Rochester, Minnesota was used to identify all patients with a diagnosis of a primary intracranial neoplasm [2]. These include clinical, surgical, autopsy, or death certificate diagnoses. The medical records of these patients were reviewed to determine if they satisfied diagnostic criteria for a primary intracranial neoplasm. A special check was made to determine that each patient so identified was a bona fide resident of Rochester, Minnesota at the time of diagnosis. Slides were reviewed by one of us (H.O.) for all individuals with a histologically confirmed diagnosis.

* This investigation was supported in part by Research Grant GM 14231, National Institutes of Health, Bethesda, Maryland, USA.

Results

Table I presents the distribution by tumour type of the 223 primary intracranial neoplasms identified in 222 people. The diagnosis was histologically confirmed for 204 (91%) of the tumours. The final column on this table presents the number of neoplasms that were diagnosed before death. A total of 78 different brain tumours (in 77 different people) were first diagnosed at autopsy, of which 58 were meningiomas.

Figure 1 shows the average annual age-specific incidence rates for all types of primary intracranial neoplasms. The two curves present: (a) the rate for all cases, and (b) the rate for brain tumours diagnosed before death. The curves deviate greatly in the older ages when autopsy diagnoses become frequent. This phenomenon was first described by Schoenberg and his colleagues [1] in comparing tabulations from Rochester, Minnesota with figures derived from the Connecticut Tumour Registry. The Connecticut Registry yielded data resembling the Rochester curve [3] for brain tumours diagnosed before death. The discrepancy is accounted for in large part by the comparatively high percentage of such tumours first diagnosed at autopsy in the Rochester population. Among those 75 years of age or more, 40 of the 52 tumours were first diagnosed at autopsy.

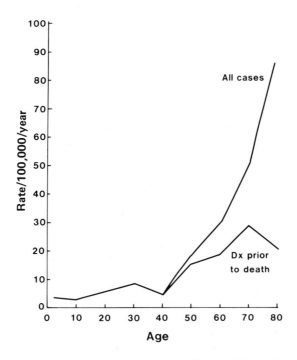

Figure 1 Average annual incidence rates for primary intracranial neoplasms in Rochester, Minnesota, USA 1935 through 1977, by age for both sexes

367

Tumour type	No.	No. with histological confirmation	No. diagnosed before death
Glioma	78	75	63
Meningioma	88	85	30
Medulloblastoma	2	2	2
Pituitary adenoma	29	21	25
Craniopharyngioma	5	3	5
Neurilemmoma	9	9	9
Germinoma	1	1	1
Sarcoma	4	4	4
Epidermoid	4	4	3
Unknown	3	0	3
	223*	204	145

* One patient with two types

It has been common practice to quote incidence rates including the autopsy-diagnosed cases [1, 4, 5]. Although such 'incidence rates' are useful for estimating the expected numbers of intracranial neoplasms to be diagnosed in cohort studies [6], they cannot be compared between places or over time. This is because such rates are a combination of incidence rates of symptomatic cases plus prevalence cases first discovered at autopsy. Prevalence cases at autopsy depend on two factors: (a) the autopsy rate, which obviously varies between place and over time, and (b) the number of deaths. The importance of these factors is illustrated by the effect they have on sex-specific incidence rates. Autopsy rates are usually higher in males, and male death age-specific rates are higher. The inclusion of cases diagnosed initially at autopsy in computing the incidence rates will give males a much higher probability of having had a brain tumour diagnosed than females. The proper denominator for autopsy-diagnosed cases—that is, the number of autopsies by age and sex over the entire study period—is not available for the Rochester population at present.

Table II shows the age-adjusted incidence rates by sex and tumour type for all cases and for cases diagnosed prior to death. The incidence rates including cases diagnosed at autopsy are somewhat higher than the incidence of brain tumours diagnosed prior to death. This is particularly so for meningiomas. This is presumably due to a greater number of autopsies among males. An alternative explanation would be that meningiomas are more symptomatic in females and, therefore, more frequently diagnosed before death. To answer this, of course, we would need the prevalence rates at autopsy. The latter explanation, however, could well be the case in pituitary adenomas where females are more likely to exhibit symptoms, e.g. amenorrhoea, galactorrhoea and infertility, than males.

The incidence rates of primary intracranial neoplasms diagnosed prior to death are somewhat higher in Rochester than in other population-based studies [1, 5].

TABLE II. Primary intracranial neoplasms, Rochester, Minnesota, USA, 1935-1977, age-adjusted* incidence rates (cases/100 000/year)

	All cases		Cases diagnosed prior to death	
	males	females	males	females
Glioma	5.1	4.8	4.0	4.1
Meningioma	4.9	5.8	1.2	2.6
Pituitary tumour	2.1	1.7	1.5	1.7
Others	1.9	1.9	1.6	1.7
Total	14.0	14.2	8.3	10.1

* United States 1950 population as standard

TABLE III Primary intracranial neoplasms, Rochester, Minnesota, USA, 1935–1977: method of diagnosis

	No.		
I. Diagnosis prior to death	145		
A. Diagnosis by surgery		106	
B. Clinical diagnosis confirmed at autopsy		18	
C. Diagnosis by symptoms and radiographic findings		18	
D. Incidental diagnosis prior to death		3	
1. X-ray			1
2. CAT scan			1
3. Incidental surgical finding			1
II. First diagnosis at autopsy	77		
A. With definite or possible symptoms		22	
B. Without symptoms		55	

This is presumably due to the greater access to specialised neurological and neuro-surgical care and to the more complete case ascertainment through the Rochester medical records linkage system.

The various methods by which the brain tumours were diagnosed are shown in Table III. Among the 145 cases diagnosed before death, 106 were diagnosed by surgery, 18 were diagnosed clinically before death and confirmed at autopsy, and 18 were diagnosed by symptoms and radiographic findings. Three cases diagnosed prior to death were actually incidental findings. These were diagnosed because of an X-ray for head trauma, a CAT scan for organic brain syndrome, and another was an incidental finding during surgery for an intracranial aneurysm. Among the 77 patients first diagnosed at autopsy, 22 had symptoms that were definitely or possibly due to the brain tumour, while 55 had no recorded symptoms.

369

TABLE IV   Primary intracranial neoplasms in Rochester, Minnesota, USA: case diagnosed prior to death only, average annual age-adjusted* incidence rates (cases/100 000/year)

	1935-1949	1950-1964	1965-1977
Both sexes	6.2	11.3	9.2
Males	4.8	10.5	8.2
Females	6.7	11.9	10.8
Glioma	2.2	4.7	4.3
Meningioma	1.5	2.8	1.4
Pituitary adenoma	1.1	0.9	2.0

* United States 1950 population, direct method, as standard

In Table IV we see the trends in incidence rates for cases diagnosed, prior to death, by sex and by tumour type. The rates were somewhat lower during the first 15 years of the study, presumably an artefact of poorer case ascertainment. From 1965-1977 there was a slight drop in the rates of all intracranial neoplasms despite advances in diagnostic and surgical technology. The age-adjusted rates by tumour type showed a significant deficit of meningiomas in the last time period and an excess of pituitary adenomas. The majority of pituitary tumours occurred in women of childbearing age. Because of the age and sex distribution of the pituitary adenoma cases, we embarked on a special study.

Pituitary Adenomas

To increase the size of the study population, we expanded the investigation to include all the residents of Olmsted County (which contains Rochester). From 1970-1977 we found 11 pituitary adenomas in females aged 15 through 44. This was an incidence of 7.0/100 000/year. The previous incidence in Rochester and that from other published reports in this age group is less than 1.0/100 000/year. It was apparent that there was an unusual occurrence of pituitary adenomas [6]. This increase could be due to an exposure to an aetiological agent such as oral contraceptives or due to advances in diagnostic and surgical techniques. For this reason, we performed a small case-control study on this group [7].

This study was limited to 8 patients whose tumours were confirmed surgically, and one in which an angiogram had indicated the presence of a pituitary tumour. Two tumours presumed by tomography were not included. *Each* case was matched to four controls from selected lists of all medical contacts of the Olmsted County population by age and year of diagnosis. Those lists constituted about 75 per cent of the population. The past histories of oral contraceptive use were compared and the results are shown in Table V. The relative risk and confidence interval were determined according to the matched quintuplets method of Miettinen [8]. This case-control study does not indicate the oral contraceptives are associated with pituitary adenomas; nevertheless, we could not rule out some association because of small numbers.

370

TABLE V Oral contraceptive use and pituitary adenomas

	Cases	Controls	Relative risk	95% Confidence interval
Oral contraceptives used prior to diagnosis:				
Any duration	5/9	26/36	0.5	0.1–2.2
1 year +	4/9	22/36	0.5	0.1–2.1
3 years +	1/9	8/36	0.4	0.1–1.7
Oral contraceptives used prior to onset of symptoms:				
Any duration	5/9	24/36	0.5	0.4–1.8
1 year +	4/9	18/36	0.6	0.6–2.6
3 years +	1/9	6/36	0.6	0.7–3.1

References

1 Schoenberg, BS, Christine, BW, Whisnant, JP (1976) *Amer. J. Epidemiol, 104,* 499
2 Kurland, LT, Elveback, LR, Nobrega, FT (1973) *Proceedings of the Sixth International Scientific Meeting on the Uses of Epidemiology in Planning Health Services,* 164. Belgrade. International Epidemiological Association
3 Schoenberg, BS, Christine, BW, Whisnant, JP (1978) *Neurology, 28,* 817
4 Percy, AK, Elveback, LR, Okazaki, H, Kurland, LT (1972) *Neurology (Minneap.), 22,* 40
5 Heshmat, MY, Kovi, J, Simpson, C, Kennedy, J, Fan, KJ (1976) *Cancer, 38,* 2135
6 Annegers, JF, Laws, Jr, ER, Kurland, LT and Grabow, JD (1979) *Neurosurgery, 4 (3),* 203
7 Coulam, CB, Annegers, JF, Abboud, CF, Laws, Jr, ER, Kurland, LT (1979) *Fertility and Sterility, 31 (1),* 25
8 Miettinen, OS (1970) *Biometrics, 26,* 75

Part VI   Miscellaneous

Chapter 38

EPIDEMIC MYALGIC ENCEPHALOMYELITIS

P O Behan and Wilhelmina M H Behan

Introduction

In this chapter we give a broad review of epidemic myalgic encephalomyelitis (EME) and report our preliminary findings in 12 patients with this disorder. Over the past 30 years, from many parts of the world there have been reports of epidemics of a clinically similar disease [1-4]. The commonest complaints of the patients affected have been muscle pains, weakness and exhaustion. One of the characteristic features has seemed to be that symptoms, especially weakness and tiredness, are prominent but physical signs are few and difficult to elicit. Because of this and the emotional lability and neuroticism that may occur, and because the aetiology is unknown, an entirely unjustified psychiatric basis for the disorder has been suggested [5].

Controversy has waged about a suitable name for this illness: in the past, a variety of names has appeared to describe it, including epidemic vegetative neuritis [6], persistent myalgia following sore throat [7], encephalomyelitis resembling poliomyelitis [8], acute infective encephalomyelitis [9], benign myalgic encephalomyelitis [10], Akureyri disease [11], Royal Free disease [12], Iceland disease [13], epidemic neuromyasthenia [14], and epidemic myalgic encephalomyelitis [15]. The latter term seems to encompass the most important features of the disease and is the term used here.

The first epidemic of EME was described in 1934 in Los Angeles. It appeared a few weeks after an epidemic of poliomyelitis [16] and indeed, was thought initially to be poliomyelitis. It soon became clear, however, that, although there were certain similarities, EME was an entirely different disease. Since then, as shown in Table I, there have been many other outbreaks from all over the world. The symptoms are many, as can be seen from Table II, but headaches, pain in the neck, back and limb muscles, lassitude, exhaustion and emotional lability form the kernel of clinical symptomatology in all outbreaks. Women tend to be affected more than men. One of the most curious of the epidemiological and clinical features is the great susceptibility of nurses and doctors to contract the disease. Several of the outbreaks have occurred among the staff of hospitals, of which that at the Royal Free Hospital is the most famous [12], and indeed, it should be noted that some of the outbreaks are virtually confined to medical personnel [12, 14, 16-18]. Although EME usually occurs in epidemics, there is compelling evidence to suggest that sporadic cases may appear [4].

The disease tends to occur acutely with headache and muscle pains, about a quarter of all patients having a mild elevation of temperature at this time. Pain in the muscles, usually in the neck, is the commonest presenting symptom. A high proportion of patients give a history of sore throat, cough, diarrhoea or vomiting from days to a couple of weeks prior to the onset of their illness. In some outbreaks,

TABLE I Outbreaks of 'Epidemic Neuromyasthenia' 1950–77

Year	Place	Number of cases	Nature of epidemic
1950	Louisville, Kentucky, USA	37	Student nurses
1952–54	Denmark	over 70	District
1952	Lakeland, Florida, USA	over 27	District
1952	Middlesex Hospital, London	14	Student nurses
1953	Coventry, England	over 13	Hospital staff
1953	Rockville, Maryland, USA	50	Student nurses
1954	Tallahassee, Florida, USA	450	District
1954	Seward, Alaska	175	District
1954–55	Johannesburg, South Africa	14	District
1955	Durban, South Africa	140	Hospital staff
1955	Berlin, Germany	7	Military
1955	Boscombe, England	2	Hospital staff
1955	Dalston, England	233	District
1955	Royal Free Hospital, England	292	Hospital staff
1955	Perth, Australia	Not recorded	District
1955	Gilfach Goch, South Wales	Not recorded	District
1955	Segbwena, Sierra Leone	45	District
1955	Thorshofn, Iceland	114	District
1955–56	North West London	34	District and Hospital staff
1955–56	Ridgefield, Connecticut, USA	70	District
1956	Coventry, England	7	District
1956	Pittsfield, Massachusetts, USA	7	District
1956	Punta Gorda, Florida, USA	over 150	District
1956	Newton-le-Willows, Lancashire, England	over 162	District
1957	Brighton, South Australia	over 60	District
1958	Athens, Greece	27	Nursing staff
1958–59	South West London	2	District
1959	North West London	7	District
1959	Newcastle-upon-Tyne, England	48	Student teachers
1960	Mississippi, USA	?	District
1961	Illinois, USA	?	District
1961–62	New York State	26	Convent
1948–65	Los Angeles, USA	approx. 330 (sporadic)	District
1964–65	Kentucky, USA	59	Factory and District
1964–66	North West London ·	approx. 370	District
1965–66	Galveston County, Texas, USA	55	District
1968	Fnaidek, Lebanon	?	?
1969–70	Edinburgh, Scotland	4 (sporadic)	District
1970	Great Ormond Street Hospital, London	over 145	Hospital staff
1970	Lackland Air Force Base, Texas, USA	221	Hospital staff
1975	New York State, USA	?	District
1976	South West Ireland	over 65	District
1977	Dallas–Fort Worth, Texas, USA	?	District

the onset seems to be insidious and the illness is ushered in by headache, fatigue, malaise and depression. In the majority of outbreaks, symptoms were present on average for three weeks before the patients were confined to bed.

TABLE II Symptoms of EME	TABLE III Physical Findings Reported in EME
Headache	Muscle tenderness
Pain in neck, back and limb muscles	Neck stiffness
Lassitude	Pareses
Exhaustion	Lymphadenopathy
Malaise	Increased tendon reflexes
Emotional lability	Muscle twitchings
Irritability	Sensory loss
Poor memory	Extensor plantar responses
Depression	Conjunctivitis
Difficulty in concentrating	Nystagmus
Dizziness	Cranial nerve palsies
Sore throat	Urinary retention
Diarrhoea	Respiratory failure

Physical signs (Table III) have been well documented in several of the outbreaks [1, 2, 4, 12] but it is clear that these were in the main difficult to elicit. Muscle tenderness and neck stiffness are commonly recorded as is localised muscular weakness. Apart from the description of the first outbreak, reports of detailed neurological examination are scanty. Urinary retention and the necessity for assisted ventilation have been described but these symptoms have been rare and fleeting. Disturbances of consciousness have never been found. Localised pareses may occur a week or two after the onset of the disease but the paralysis is usually mild and is often confined to a single muscle group or part of a muscle. Reflexes have been reported as increased, normal or hypotonic, and extensor plantar responses have been described as occurring transiently.

Lymphadenopathy is very common in the early stages while liver enlargement has been found in up to 10 per cent of cases: in the Royal Free outbreak the liver was palpable in 8.5 per cent of cases. In this outbreak cranial nerve palsies occurred also in 69 out of 200 cases. A characteristic feature of EME is its protracted course, one-third of the patients having the disease for years [4].

Table IV lists the laboratory findings that may be present. While an infective aetiology seems the most likely, the organism or organisms have never been identified. The large amount of laboratory studies that have been performed, including detailed virological investigations with animal inoculations (reviewed in detail by Henderson and Shelokov [2]) have essentially met with little success in determining the aetiology of the pathogenesis of this illness. In studying the literature, however, we were struck by the similarity of this illness to that of post-infectious encephalo-myelitis, where the aetiology seems to be that of an immunological reaction, triggered by a wide variety of different agents [19]. We have previously compared and contrasted these two diseases [20] and we now decided to study the immunological features of patients with EME searching for evidence of an aberrant immunological response.

TABLE IV Laboratory Findings Reported in EME

Urine:	Creatinuria
Peripheral blood:	Lymphocytosis
	Abnormal lymphocytes
Serum:	Increased lactic dehydrogenase, glutamic
	oxaloacetic transaminase concentrations
	Positive anticomplementary activity
Cerebrospinal fluid:	Rarely, increased cells and protein, and a
	positive Pandy test
Electromyography:	Reduced motor unit potentials on volition
Electroencephalography:	Minor non-specific changes

Materials and Methods

Patients. Twelve patients were admitted for detailed clinical and laboratory evaluation. There were eight females and four males whose ages were from 33 to 61 years, with a mean of 42 years. The duration of illness was from 3 to 20 years with a mean of 7 years.

Clinical Evaluation. All patients had a full documentation of the history of their illness, their previous medical history and any family diseases known and a note was made of any drugs taken. A detailed clinical and neurological evaluation was made. Urinalysis, full haematological examination, 24-hour creatinine clearance, liver function tests, serum protein electrophoresis and serological studies for syphilis were carried out. Chest and skull X-rays and ECGs were also done. EEG, visual evoked responses and a full neurophysiological evaluation, including nerve-conduction studies and electromyography were also performed. All patients had a lumbar puncture with examination of the cerebrospinal fluid including a search for oligoclonal immunoglobulins on specimens of concentrated CSF.

Immunological Studies

Protein Synthesis by Peripheral-blood Lymphocytes. The synthesis of protein by peripheral-blood lymphocytes *in vitro* was measured by the whole-blood technique [21]. This method is an assay of lymphocyte function. It estimates the uptake of tritiated leucine by peripheral-blood lymphocytes on stimulation with purified phytohaemagglutinin (PHA), over a 22-hour period. A dose-response curve to various concentrations of purified PHA (Burroughs Wellcome) was drawn for each patient.

Immunoglobulins. IgG, IgM, IgA, and IgE concentrations for each patient were determined by single radial immunodiffusion. The following reagents were used: for IgG and IgM 'Tripartigen' plates (Behringwerke); IgA, (Immunoplate 3′ (Hyland Lab); IgE, kit (Meloy Laboratory).

377

Detection of Autoantibodies. Rheumatoid factor was estimated by means of a 'Rheumaton' reagent 3 titration kit (Denver Laboratories). Antibodies to thyroglobulin were detected by a precipitin test in an Ouchterlony plate with a saline-solution extract of thyroid. When this test was positive, a titration was performed by means of the tanned-red-cell agglutination technique (Burroughs Wellcome). The following autoantibodies were also sought by standard immunofluorescence techniques: antinuclear (rat liver), mitochondrial (rat kidney), smooth muscle (rat smooth muscle), thyroid microsomal (human toxic thyroid), gastric parietal cell (human gastric mucosa), adrenal cortex (human adrenal), and salivary duct (human salivary gland). Anti-epithelial antibodies (intracellular and basement-membrane antibodies) were sought by indirect immunofluorescence using fresh oesophageal tissue from baboon as substrate.

Complement Studies. The functional efficiency of the complement system was determined in terms of the total haemolytic complement activity (CH_{50} units) by the technique of Kent and Fife [22]. Anticomplementary activity was assayed in the serum by Mayer's method [23]. The following components of complement were measured in EDTA plasma by means of the single radial immunodiffusion technique, in conjunction with monospecific antisera: Clq, C3, Factor B and C4. Commercially available plates (Behringwerke) were used to estimate C4 concentrations. C7 concentrations were measured by the reactive lysis method with activated C5/6 [24]; C3 and Factor B conversion products were sought by crossed antibody electrophoresis and immunoelectrophoresis [25]. The antisera used for the other determinations were prepared in our laboratory by standard techniques.

Virology. Viral isolation was attempted from throat swabs and faecal specimens. Antibodies to common viruses including infectious mononucleosis were sought and samples were sent to the Enterovirus Reference (Scotland) Laboratory for Coxsackie virus antibody estimation.

Results

All 12 patients gave a clinical history which was compatible with epidemic myalgic encephalomyelitis as previously described. In essence, they all complained of severe muscle pains, generalised malaise, exhaustion and weakness which was present most of the time but varied in intensity over the number of years they had had the disease. A detailed physical and neurological examination showed no abormalities. One very interesting feature was that the husband and two sons of one of the women patients developed similar symptoms to hers during one of her relapses. The husband had a skin rash in addition, and laboratory investigations revealed an increased serum creatine phosphokinase and the typical muscle biopsy findings of dermatomyositis; trial studies were unfortunately not done.

Laboratory tests
These results are shown in Tables V and VI. All urine tests were normal; three of

378

TABLE V Summary of Laboratory Findings in 12 Cases

		Number affected
Blood	Eosinophilia of 7–10%	3/12
	Abnormal lymphocytes	2/12
	Increased serum CPK (132) units /L	1/12
	Increased LDH (840–1580) units /L	9/12
EMG	Abnormal	5/12
EEG	Abnormal	4/12
VERs	Abnormal	2/12

the 12 patients had an eosinophilia of from 3–10 per cent and two of these patients also had large lymphocytes (immunocytes) in their peripheral blood. Kidney and liver function tests were all normal but one patient had an increased serum creatine phosphokinase (132 iu/L) and in 9 of the 12 patients the serum concentrations of lactic dehydrogenase were greatly increased, ranging from 840–1580 iu/L (normal 240–525 iu/L). On electromyography there were reduced motor unit potentials on volition in 5 patients and non-specific EEG abnormalities were present in 4. Visual evoked responses were abnormal in 2 of the 12 patients, with prolonged latencies. All routine tests on the cerebrospinal fluid were normal but in three specimens faint but definite oligoclonal bands were detected on electrophoresis of concentrated CSF.

Immunoglobulins. Abnormal concentrations of immunoglobulins IgM and IgA were found in six patients. In these six, the IgM was markedly increased in all; the IgA was conspicuously low in three and absent in three. The abnormal IgM values varied from 400–520 per cent of the mean normal adult concentration; and the abnormal IgA concentrations varied from 0 to 8 per cent of those of the normal adult mean.

Serological Abnormalities. Six patients had abnormal serological tests. An anti-nuclear antibody to a titre of 1/250 was present in two; smooth muscle antibody was strongly positive in two, two had positive rheumatoid factors, and one had gastric parietal cell antibody. No antibodies to intrinsic factor were found in any of the patients.

Complement Studies. Figure 1 shows the abnormal complement findings and the results of tests for anticomplementary activity.

Virology. Two patients had very high titres to Coxsackie A9, up to 1/1024 +. A preliminary trial run in which attempts were made to absorb out the IgG, showed specific IgM titres of 1/128 and 1/256. Two other patients had increased titres, 1/1024 and 1/512, to Coxsackie B1.

379

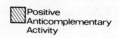

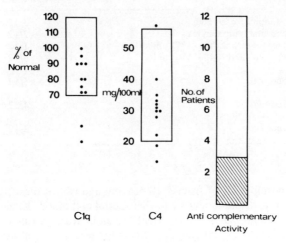

Figure 1 Complement components C1q and C4 and anticomplementary assay

Discussion

Outbreaks of the mysterious paralytic disease known as epidemic myalgic encephalomyelitis have occurred throughout the world for the past 30 years [3]. Several of these epidemics have been studied in detail: one of the best known was that which occurred at the Royal Free Hospital in London in 1955 in which more than 300 people were affected [12]. The outbreaks have predominantly affected young women and the clinical data suggest infection spread by personal contact [1]. In all epidemics, despite great variation in clinical symptomatology and findings, the kernel of the symptoms is that of muscle pains usually in the back of the neck, shoulders and limbs, associated with gross generalised fatigue and exhaustion. Psychiatric symptoms are common, in the main consisting of emotional lability, difficulty in concentration, lack of drive and 'psychic energy'.

As mentioned, while abnormal physical findings may be present, on the whole these are scarce and fleeting. It is therefore easy to understand that this symptomatology, in which there are no objective findings and which bears such a strong resemblance to severe neuroticism, depression or even some forms of schizophrenia, is such that psychiatrists have not been loth to suggest a psychological aetiology [5]. In this preliminary study, had detailed immunological studies not been undertaken, it would have been easy to concur with McEvedy and Beard [5] that the illness is entirely a manifestation of hysteria.

The presence of atypical lymphoblasts (immunocytes) in the peripheral blood of two of the patients is an important finding. Similar cells have been described in animals and human subjects undergoing immunological reactions, e.g. in the blood and lymphnodes of animals with host-graft responses [26] and in the blood of patients with systemic lupus erythematosus, infectious mononucleosis or other viral conditions [27, 28]. Identical cells have also been found in cases of post-infectious encephalomyelitis [19, 20, 29]. Their presence therefore suggests persistent antigenic stimulation perhaps caused by a virus. In this regard it is interesting to note that lymphocytes from children with EME grew and multiplied in tissue culture [30], a phenomenon strongly suggestive of a persistent virus. The presence of eosinophilia in the peripheral blood of three patients also suggests an allergic reaction.

Increased concentrations of IgM and decreased concentrations of IgA were found in half our cases: a similar pattern has been described in subacute sclerosing panencephalitis where the measles virus is persistent. Autoantibodies were also common: they most likely represent a disturbance in the immune system. Together with low or absent IgA, their finding suggests T cell depression but, in this small number of patients, our *in vitro* tests did not detect such a defect.

The complement results suggest involvement of this system and, together with the serum anticomplementary activity found, strongly suggest the presence of circulating immune complexes. In a previous study of acute cases of EME, positive anticomplementary activity of the serum and serum aggregates on immunoelectron-microscopy were reported [30].

How can one envisage the tissue damage being caused in EME? It has to be acknowledged that we have no definite evidence of a long-lasting virus infection in this disorder, but the chronicity of the illness, the disturbance in humoral immunity, the presence of circulating immunocytes and, finally, the finding of very high titres of antibodies to Coxsackie virus (with possible specific IgM), all point to the presence of such a persistent virus. Such an antigen could elicit the formation of immune complexes with resultant deposition in certain sites and subsequent tissue damage [31].

Increased serum lactic dehydrogenase concentrations were also found, in 9 of the 12 patients. This abnormality has been reported previously [4] and helps to confirm that there is muscle involvement. The neurological symptoms and signs, together with the abnormal CSF findings that have been described, and our demonstration of abnormal visual evoked responses and oligoclonal bands in the CSF, show that central nervous system white matter is also affected.

Coxsackie viruses demonstrate a characteristic myotropism which may be to cardiac and skeletal muscle: Coxsackie B viruses have been identified in the epidemics of myalgia known as Bornholm disease [32] but in the 1965 Coxsackie B5 virus outbreak in Europe both carditis and meningitis were found [33]. It has previously been suggested that enteroviruses may cause a chronic polymyositis in man because picornavirus-like particles have been demonstrated in muscle cells from such cases: Coxsackie A9 has been obtained from an adult with polymyositis [34] and a Coxsackie virus has also been isolated from an infant with congenital myositis [35].

It may thus be very significant that the husband and two sons of one of our cases developed an illness apparently similar to EME, during one of her relapses, and that muscle biopsy of the husband revealed the characteristic features of dermatomyositis. Activation of the complement system and the presence of circulating immune complexes has been described in polymyositis [36]. Here the muscle damage has been thought to be due to a vasculopathy secondary to immune complex deposition: in EME the pathogenesis may be that of a persistent virus with the formation of immune complexes and widespread deposition of these antigen-antibody aggregates in the blood vessels of central nervous system and muscle.

Acknowledgement

The invaluable assistance of Dr Gordon Parish in supplying epidemiological data and of Dr Eleanor Bell in performing antibody titres is gratefully acknowledged. Supported by the Muscular Dystrophy Group of Great Britain.

References

1   Acheson, ED (1959) *Am. J. Med., 26,* 569
2   Henderson, DA and Shelokov, A (1959) *New Engl. J. Med., 260,* 757
3   Parish, JG (1978) *Postgrad. Med. J., 54,* 711
4   Ramsay, AM (1978) *Postgrad. Med. J., 54,* 718
5   McEvedy, CP and Beard, AW (1970) *Brit. Med. J., 1,* 7
6   Fog, T (1953) *Ugesk. f, laeger, 115,* 1244
7   Houghton, LE and Jones, EI (1942) *Lancet, i,* 196
8   Ramsay, AM and O'Sullivan, E (1956) *Lancet, i,* 761
9   Geffen, D and Tracy, SM (1956) *Brit. Med. J., 2,* 904
10 Leading article (1956) *Lancet, i,* 789
11 Sigurdsson, B (1956) *Lancet, ii,* 98
12 Medical Staff of the Royal Free Hospital (1957) *Brit. Med. J., 2,* 895
13 White, DN and Burtch, RB (1954) *Neurology, 4,* 506
14 Shelokov, A, Habel, K, Verder, D and Welsh, W (1957) *New Engl. J. Med., 257,* 345
15 Leading article (1978) *Brit. Med. J., 1,* 1437
16 Gilliam, AG (1938) *Public Health Bulletin,* U S Treasury Dept., No. 240
17 Poskanzer, DC, Henderson, DA, Kunkle, EC, Kalter, SS, Clement, WB and Bond, JO (1957) *New Engl. J. Med., 257,* 356
18 MacRae, AD and Galpine, JF (1954) *Lancet, ii,* 350
19 Behan, PO and Currie, S (1978) In *Clinical Neuroimmunology.* WB Saunders Co. Ltd., London, Philadelphia and Toronto, page 49
20 Behan, PO (1978) *Postgrad. Med. J., 54,* 755
21 Pauly, JL, Sokal, JE and Han, T (1973) *J. Lab. Clin. Med., 82,* 500
22 Kent, JF and Fife, EH (1963) *Am. J. Trop. Med. Hyg., 12,* 103
23 Mayer, MM (1961) In *Experimental Immunochemistry* (ed EA Kabat and MM Mayer). Charles C. Thomas, Springfield, Illinois, page 133
24 Thompson, RA and Lachmann, PJ (1970) *J. exp. Med., 131,* 629
25 Laurel, CB (1965) *Analyt. Biochem., 10,* 358
26 Damashek, W (1963) *Blood, 21,* 243
27 Cooper, IA and Lirkin, BG (1965) *Aust. Ann. Med., 14,* 142
28 Hanna, C and Dowling, PC (1967) *J. Ark. Med. Soc., 62,* 453
29 Behan, PO, Geschwind, N, Lomarche, JB, Lisak, RP and Kies, NW (1968) *Lancet, ii,* 1009
30 Dillon, MJ, Marshall, WC, Dudgeon, JA and Steigman, AJ (1974) *Brit. Med. J., 1,* 301
31 Gerson, KL and Haslam, RHA (1971) *New Engl. J. Med., 285,* 78

32 Kibrick, S (1964) *Prog. Med. Virol., 6,* 27
33 Leading article (1967) *Brit. Med. J., 4,* 575
34 Tang, TT, Sedmak, GU, Siegesmund, KA and McCreadie, SR (1975) *New Engl. J. Med., 292,* 608
35 Freudenberg, E, Roulet, F and Nicole, R (1952) *Ann. Paediat., 178,* 150
36 Behan, WMH and Behan, PO (1977) *J. Neurol. Sci., 34,* 241

Chapter 39

MIGRAINE

W E Waters

In studying the epidemiology of migraine there are two significant problems, the relative importance of which depends on the discipline of the investigator conducting the study. The clinician interested in migraine may have much information on the patients, but does not know the total population from which they come. The clinician knows about the numerator but not the denominator. It is an important feature of epidemiology, indeed it is the essence of the subject, that one must have information on both. There is, in addition, a further difficulty for the clinician in that we now know that not all patients with migraine attend a doctor. Studies have suggested that it is only about half of sufferers with migraine who have consulted a doctor because of their headaches [1, 2]. The proportion of individuals with migraine who consult a neurologist is even lower than this, and they may be even more selected (that is, atypical of the general run of migraine sufferers in the population). The problem, from the point of view of the epidemiologist, is rather different. Here the details of the denominator, that is the population, will be known, but the problem is in identifying those individuals who have migraine. As only a proportion of migraine sufferers consult a doctor a review of medical records, however well kept, would give an inaccurate estimate of the prevalence of migraine. It is therefore essential that each individual in the population, or a statistically chosen sample, is questioned about symptoms that may indicate migraine. As the diagnosis of migraine depends largely on symptoms, rather than on physical examination or special investigation, it seems appropriate to screen the population with an administered or self-administered questionnaire. A number of such surveys have been done in the past 25 to 30 years. Details of headaches in various occupational groups in the United States have been given by Ogden [3] but these figures do not distinguish migraine from other causes of headache. One of the pioneering studies in the epidemiology of migraine was conducted in schoolchildren between the ages of 7 and 15 years in Uppsala, Sweden, by Bille [4]. In the last 15 years several surveys have been conducted in England and Wales on various population samples.

The Problem of a Definition

Nearly 100 years ago Gowers [5] wrote that 'Migraine is an affection characterised by paroxysmal nervous disturbance, of which headache is the most constant element. The pain is seldom absent and may exist alone, but is commonly accompanied by nausea and vomiting, and is often preceded by some sensory disturbance, especially by some disorder of the sense of sight. The symptoms are frequently one-sided, and from this character of the headache the name is derived'. This description includes most of the features that are now accepted in establishing the diagnosis of migraine. It is remarkably similar to a number of more recent attempts to describe the condition (e.g. World Federation of Neurology [6] ; Ad Hoc Committee on Classification of Headache [7]). The problem for the epidemiologist with such descriptions is that they are just descriptions, rather than explicit definitions. The various features characteristic of migraine are said to be 'commonly', 'often' or 'frequently' present, but it is not precisely stated whether they have to be present in order to establish the diagnosis and, if so, how many of the features have to be present. The three features that are usually considered most characteristic of migraine are: (1) the unilateral distribution of the headache, (2) the accompanying nausea or actual vomiting, and (3) some warning that the attack is coming, most characteristically a visual disturbance. It is, of course, possible in epidemiological surveys to make arbitrary definitions and say that in any subject with headache, and with a given number of these three features, the condition will be classified as migraine. This approach seems unsatisfactory and agreement would be difficult to produce between investigators. An alternative approach, which neatly sidesteps the problem of a definition, is for the epidemiologist to give the prevalence of head-ache, and the prevalence of each of the features of migraine (unilateral distribution, warning and nausea) without given the prevalence of migraine.

In the absence of physical findings and characteristic laboratory findings, the diagnosis of migraine is usually made after a normal clinical interview. In such conditions the clinician usually takes into account all the patient's symptoms and probably also other factors before making a diagnosis based on his overall impressions. It would therefore be theoretically possible for a clinician interested in migraine to see all subjects in a defined population and make a clinical diagnosis of each. This would be a laborious task, but a number of surveys have used a clinical diagnosis as an additional component of the study. The study in South Wales by Waters and O'Connor [1] used a questionnaire initially which was followed by a neurologist's clinical diagnosis of various randomly selected subgroups of the population. These subgroups were identified by the number of features of migraine elicited by the questionnaire. The results of this clinical validation of a questionnaire are shown in Table I. Rather than making an arbitrary decision about the number of features that are necessary to establish the diagnosis, this method therefore enables an estimate to be made of the prevalence of migraine, based on a clinical diagnosis.

Other studies have used a clinical interview in selected cases only where there have been problems in establishing the diagnosis from the questionnaire. An important aspect of the clinical validation of the questionnaire [1] is that the clinical interview was made 'blindly' without the neurologist knowing how the subject had replied to the questionnaire. Further, this study did not use the word 'migraine' in the questionnaire as it was felt that this might possibly introduce bias. A recently reported epidemiological study [2] simply asked the question 'Have you ever had migraine?' and classified the answers as 'Yes', 'No', 'Uncertain'. When samples of

385

TABLE I. Comparison Between Symptoms Elicited by Questionnaire and Clinical Diagnosis of Migraine [1]

Symptoms (from questionnaire)	Percentage diagnosed clinically as migraine
Unilateral headache only	12
Headache and warning only	50
Headache and nausea only	24
Unilateral headache with warning	58
Unilateral headache with nausea	32
Headache with warning and nausea	60
Unilateral headache with warning and nausea	88

these subjects were interviewed clinically it was found that 10 out of 12 men and 21 out of 23 women who had said 'Yes' to this question were diagnosed as having migraine. None of those who said 'No' were diagnosed clinically as having migraine, although only a relatively small number were clinically interviewed. When the group who said that they were uncertain whether they had migraine were seen clinically, one-third of the women but a very much smaller proportion of the men were diagnosed as having had migraine. This study [2] raises the possibility that the simplest way of determining prevalence is to ask the question 'Have you ever had migraine?', but in view of the difficulty that committees of doctors have in defining the condition it does seem rather inappropriate to put this onus on individuals in the general population. Further, it is not clear to what extent the doctors carrying out the clinical validation in that study knew of the subjects' replies to the questionnaire and there is, therefore, a possibility of bias in their clinical diagnoses.

The difficulty of an appropriate and comprehensive definition of migraine, along with other evidence, has led to the suggestion that migraine may not be a completely distinct clinical entity, but may perhaps be a continuum, or spectrum, with tension headache at one end and classical migraine at the other [8]. In this respect it might resemble the weight distribution of a population in which the definition of obesity is largely arbitrary. Another example would be the present concept of systemic blood pressure which is now regarded as a continuum, with hypertension having an arbitrary definition above certain pressure levels. Unfortunately, with migraine we do not have objective, and fairly reproducible, measurements such as weight and blood pressure. We rely, for the diagnosis of migraine, on a number of different symptoms which may be variable in different attacks, and this is a problem in trying to define migraine precisely. If one pursues the analogy between headache and migraine and blood pressure and hypertension further, it might be postulated that migraine, like hypertension, may have a number of different causes. It follows that, if indeed migraine is a continuum in the spectrum of headache, any consideration of the prevalence of the condition is purely arbitrary.

Nevertheless, the general feeling, at least among neurologists in this country, seems to be that migraine is a clinical entity and this concept dates at least from the time of the writings of Tissot in 1790 [9].

The Prevalence of Headache and Migraine

The prevalence of headache of all types is reasonably easy to ascertain if one accepts the subject's own answer to a question. In such studies it is most important to identify the period of time under consideration. Memory is likely to be best for fairly recent events but, if the selected time is too short, it will, of course, eliminate many sufferers who have infrequent headaches. Different surveys have used different time periods—sometimes one year, sometimes two years, and sometimes a lifetime prevalence. Data based on a lifetime prevalence seem particularly suspect, not only from the point of view of the subject's memory, but also because it can confuse the age effect with any cohort effect (that is, the condition may become more or less common in succeeding generations). Table II shows the prevalence of all types of headache in the year immediately preceding the survey and also the proportion with migraine, based upon a questionnaire validated by a neurologist [1]. It shows that both headache and migraine are more prevalent in women than in men and that in both sexes the prevalence declines with increasing age. These figures are very much higher than figures formerly quoted for the prevalence of migraine, but it must be remembered that many figures are based, not on any survey, but on clinical impressions derived from seeing patients, and not all individuals with migraine consult a doctor.

TABLE II. Prevalence of Headache and Migraine (based on clinically validated questionnaire) in Previous Year [10]

		Age Groups			
		21–34	35–54	55–74	75+
Headache	Men	74.0	69.0	53.3	21.7
	Women	92.3	82.6	66.2	55.2
Migraine	Men	16.8	16.4	12.6	4.9
	Women	30.1	26.0	16.6	10.3

One of the advantages of a questionnaire approach to migraine is that one can use exactly the same measuring tool, a questionnaire, to study migraine in different populations. What one may lose in accuracy of diagnosis is compensated by a likely reduction in bias. If there were important differences in the prevalence of the condition in different populations this may give possible clues to the cause of the condition. A number of studies have been conducted using the same method (Table III), but the results suggest relatively little differences in prevalence of headache, or in prevalence of individual features of migraine in widely differing populations in England and Wales [10]. Despite, or perhaps because of, the difficulty of defining migraine a study conducted among general practitioners in two areas of England is of interest because it asks doctors to diagnose migraine in themselves [11]. In the age-group 35–54 years, 13.5 per cent of the male general practitioners, and 26.4 per cent of the female general practitioners, thought that they had had migraine in the previous year. In this group of general practitioners it is interesting that about 7 per cent of the men and just over 11 per cent of the women had consulted a doctor because of their headaches, but only 1.1 per cent of the men and 4.2 per cent of the women had consulted a neurologist because of headaches.

TABLE III. Prevalence of Migraine (based on clinically validated questionnaire) in Previous Year (from Waters, various surveys)

	Men		Women	
	21–34	35–54	21–34	35–54
Pontypridd (South Wales)	16.8	16.4	30.1	26.0
London practice	22.3	19.2	31.5	28.1
Isles of Scilly	17.6	15.6	25.1	24.2

Epidemiology and the Testing of Hypotheses

In looking for the cause, or the causes, of migraine the characteristics of the sufferers have been described since these might provide clues to the aetiology. Until recently, most of the literature has been based on the clinical impression of doctors, or the study of medical records. The difficulty has been largely that of selecting controls to see if migraine sufferers really do differ from the general population or from those who do not have migraine. Epidemiological studies provide a particularly appropriate method of comparing individuals who have migraine with others who do not have migraine. These studies would be valid whether migraine was a separate entity or just an extreme in a continuous distribution as suggested above. A number of widespread clinical impressions have suggested that sufferers from migraine were more likely to be intelligent, of high social class, to have higher blood pressures and to have various ocular disorders. Epidemiological surveys have not provided support for any of these hypotheses [12]. More recently, Crisp and his associates [2] found a two-year prevalence of migraine of 29.1 per cent in women in Social Classes I and II, but only 14.6 per cent in Social Classes III–V. This difference was statistically significant. In men, the two-year prevalence was 17.6 per cent in Social Classes I and II, but only 6.9 per cent in Social Classes III–V. Perhaps due to the smaller numbers the differences in men were not statistically significant. It may be relevant that this was the study that asked subjects whether or not they had ever had migraine and that this may have possibly introduced some bias. In a comparative study of headache and migraine in two occupational groups Taylor and his colleagues [13] found that although there were no differences in the prevalence of headache, or in the prevalence of the individual features of migraine as judged by a questionnaire; 21 per cent of one occupational group, but only 6 per cent of another, claimed to have had migraine when they were subsequently interviewed. These differences in self-diagnosis of migraine between the two groups were statistically significant and, after standardisation for age, this study concluded that a comparative assessment of symptoms is always difficult but 'we believe that the replies to a standard questionnaire as described here are likely to be less biased than those to one in which the word migraine is used. This is all too often used like Lewis Carroll's Humpty Dumpty in *Through the Looking Glass*, who said, "When I use a word it means just what I choose it to mean—neither more nor less".'

There are a number of other hypotheses relating to characteristics of migraine sufferers that have recently been investigated. Psychological characteristics of migraine subjects have been described [2, 14]. There have also been many reports linking migraine with allergic disorders (especially asthma and hay fever) and with epilepsy. As Lance [15] has pointed out, any uncontrolled observation is suspect in view of the fact that migrainous patients are more likely to be referred for investigation if suffering from an associated illness, and various individual specialists may receive biased samples because of their particular interest. A number of studies have suggested that there is no primary relationship between migraine, epilepsy or allergy [15]. However, in an epidemiological study in which adults were asked if they were ever subject to bilious attacks, travel sickness or skin trouble (eczema) it was found that migraine sufferers reported these conditions significantly more often than other groups [16]. This difference persisted even after differences in age, and differences in the degree of neuroticism, were taken into account. Dietary factors have also been implicated and tyramine is thought to be particularly important [17]. However, a number of recently conducted double-blind cross-over trials have suggested that tyramine is unlikely to be important in more than a small minority of all attacks. Further data on the relationship of diet and migraine are needed.

This brief review of the role of epidemiology in testing hypotheses about the cause of migraine has shown that many firmly held clinical hypotheses are not supported by the epidemiological investigations. The epidemiological studies have

TABLE IV. Relation Between Intelligence of Migraine Sufferers (based on A.H.4 score of National Foundation for Educational Research in England and Wales) and Proportion Consulting a Doctor for Migraine [18]

Intelligence Score (A.H.4)	Men		Women	
	No. tested	Percentage Consulting Doctor	No. tested	Percentage Consulting Doctor
0–39	13	54	35	57
40–59	10	70	23	65
60+	11	73	14	71

suggested that patients with migraine who consult a doctor may be different in a number of respects from those migrainous subjects that do not consult a doctor. It may be obvious that this would apply to the severity and frequency of attacks, but data suggest that it applies also to intelligence (Table IV) [18] with the intelligent migraine sufferers being more likely to consult a doctor. These data show the desirability of biasing such studies on whole populations and not on possibly selected migraine patients.

In view of these largely negative epidemiological results, new clinical hypotheses about the cause of migraine are now required. The clinical hypotheses should then be tested by careful epidemiological studies. In conducting these studies it is important that there should be close collaboration between epidemiologists and clinicians interested in migraine in order that the results may be scientifically valid.

References

1   Waters, WE and O'Connor, PJ (1971) Epidemiology of headache and migraine in women. *J. Neurol., Neurosurg. and Psychiat., 34,* 148
2   Crisp, AH, Kalucy, RS, McGuiness, B, Ralph, PC and Harris, G (1977) Some clinical, social and psychological characteristics of migraine subjects in the general population. *Postgrad. Med. J., 53,* 691
3   Ogden, HD (1952) Headache studies: statistical data. *J. Allegery, 23,* 458
4   Bille, B (1962) Migraine in school children. *Acta Paediatrica, 51,* Suppl. 136
5   Gowers, WR (1888) *A Manual of Diseases of the Nervous System.* London: Churchill
6   World Federation of Neurology: Research Group on Migraine and Headache (1969) Editorial comment. *Hemicrania, 1,* 3
7   Ad Hoc Committee on Classification of Headache (1962) Classification of headache. *J. Amer. Med. Assoc., 179,* 717
8   Waters, WE (1973) The epidemiological enigma of migraine. *Internat. J. Epidem., 2,* 189
9   Tissot, SA (1790) *Oeuvres de Monsieur Tissot,* Vol. 13, Lausanne
10 Waters, WE (1974) *The Epidemiology of Migraine.* Bracknell: Boehringer Ingelheim
11 Waters, WE (1972a) Headache and migraine in general practitioners. *Proceedings of a Symposium held at Churchill College, Cambridge, 10-11 July, 1972.* Bracknell: Boehringer Ingelheim
12 Office of Health Economics (1972) *Migraine.* London: Office of Health Economics
13 Taylor, PJ, Pocock, SJ, Hall, SA and Waters, WE (1970) Headaches and migraine in colour retouchers. *Brit. J. Indust. Med., 27,* 364
14 Henryk-Gutt, R and Lindford Rees, W (1973) Psychological aspects of migraine. *J. Psychosom. Res., 17,* 141
15 Lance, J (1973) *Mechanism and Management of Headache.* London: Butterworths
16 Waters, WE (1972b) Migraine and symptoms in childhood: bilious attacks, travel sickness and eczema. *Headache, 12,* 55
17 Hanington, E (1974) *Migraine.* London: Priory Press
18 Waters, WE (1971) Migraine: intelligence, social class and family prevalence. *Brit. Med. J., 2,* 77

Chapter 40

PARKINSON'S DISEASE AND ENCEPHALITIS: THE COHORT HYPOTHESIS RE-EXAMINED

M G Marmot

Introduction

The epidemics of von Economo's encephalitis (encephalitis lethargica) that occurred mainly between 1918 and 1926 were followed by the emergence of post-encephalitic Parkinson's syndrome, which has been clearly distinguished clinically and pathologically from the idiopathic form of parkinsonism—the classical paralysis agitans described in 1817 by James Parkinson as the 'shaking palsy' [1].

Poskanzer and Schwab questioned this distinction on epidemiological grounds [2]. They noted that, at the Massachusetts General Hospital, the average age of onset of parkinsonism had been increasing over time. The increase was approximately 1 year of age each calendar year and was seen in those patients diagnosed as 'idiopathic' as well as those diagnosed as 'post-encephalitic'. This was consistent with the concept of a 'cohort' of people all exposed to a single agent at a particular time period—the development of Parkinson's disease having a variable latent period. Poskanzer and Schwab suggested that the vast majority of new cases of so-called 'idiopathic' Parkinson's disease were developing in this cohort as a result of exposure to von Economo's encephalitis. The implication is that 'idiopathic' and post-encephalitic parkinsonism are not two diseases but are ends of the one clinical spectrum. Poskanzer and Schwab predicted that, as this cohort of people died off, the incidence of Parkinson's disease would fall in the 1970s and 80s.

Similar increases in average age of onset of Parkinson's disease have been found in other series [3-5]. The 'cohort' explanation has been questioned, however, [1, 6, 7]. It has been pointed out that an increasing age of onset is compatible with a 'two-disease' explanation: (*a*) an idiopathic form affecting old people with no change in incidence rate over time, and (*b*) a post-encephalitic Parkinson's affecting younger people that was common in the 1920s and 1930s and has been gradually decreasing thereafter.

Duvoisin and Schweitzer (1966) [8] further doubt the cohort hypothesis because they felt that in England and Wales 'mortality rates (from paralysis agitans) have been stationary for the past 40 years or more (1921-1962) at most ages'. On this basis they conclude that there can have been no long-term residual effect of the epidemic of encephalitis lethargica. In recent years there have been interesting divergent trends in age-specific mortality rates from paralysis agitans. We have examined these trends in mortality in England and Wales and Scotland for the period 1931-1975. This provided the opportunity for a re-examination of the cohort and two-disease hypotheses of the aetiology of Parkinson's disease.

391

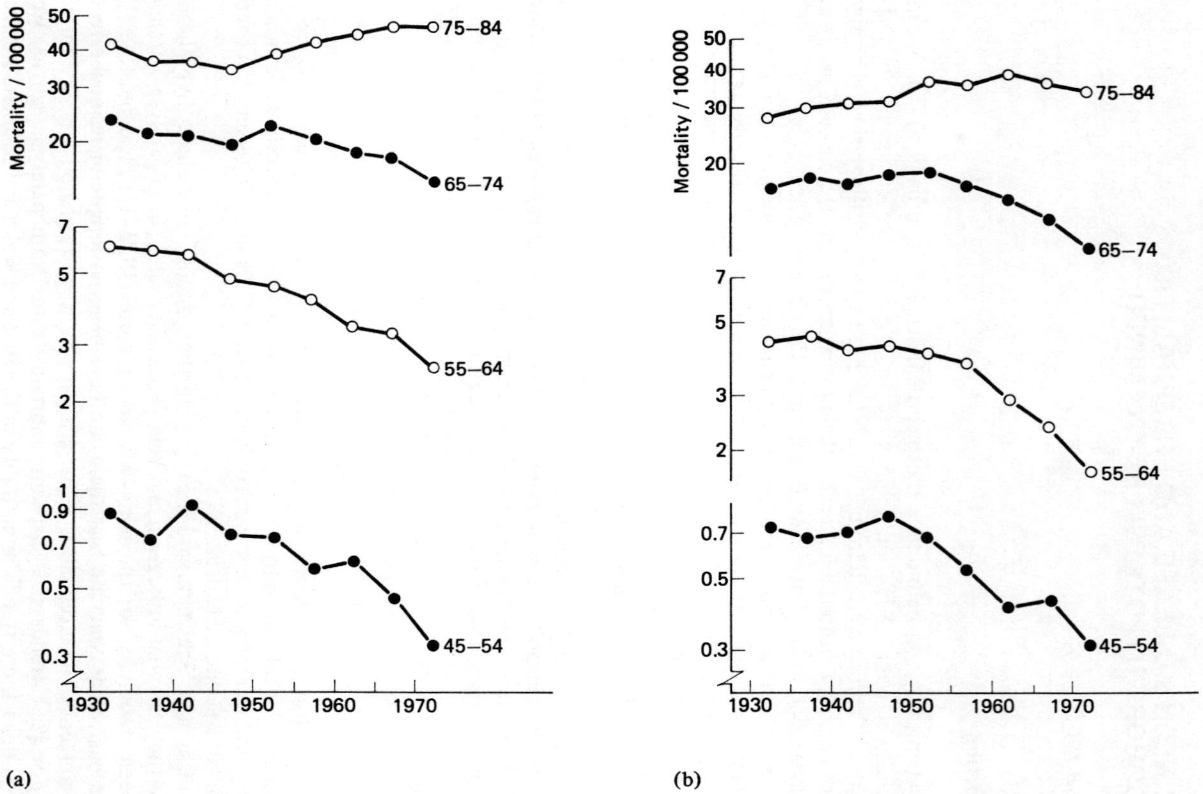

Figure 1 Paralysis agitans mortality, England and Wales: (a) males (b) females

392

Methods

The mortality data for England and Wales come from successive annual reports of the Registrar General. In the period 1931-1975 the *International Classification of Diseases* (ICD) was changed successively from the 4th to the 8th Revision. The ICD coding of paralysis agitans changed from 87c (4th and 5th Revisions) to 350 (6th and 7th Revisions) to 342 (8th Revision). Changes in ICD coding after the 5th Revision appear to have had little effect on paralysis agitans mortality [8]. The adoption of the 5th Revision in 1940, however, appears to have had substantial effect. In that year there was a change in the practice of assigning underlying cause of death. This was investigated by the Registrar-General's Office (Statistical Review 1939—Appendix B1). When death certificates were classified according to the 4th and 5th Revisions, there were 30 per cent fewer assigned to paralysis agitans under the 5th than the 4th Revision. This figure varied with age and sex. We have therefore used the Registrar General's figures to adjust downwards the mortality figures for 1931-39.

The Scottish data came from successive publications of the General Register Office and the estimates of the home population of Scotland were kindly made available by that office. In Scotland there was a similar change in coding practice between 1939 and 1940, although in Scotland the effect was to increase the number of deaths assigned to paralysis agitans (Report of General Register Office, 1940, Appendix VII). Accordingly the mortality figures 1931-39 were adjusted upwards.

The standardised cohort mortality ratio was used as a method of age-adjustment in the cohort analysis. This follows the procedure used by Beral [9]. The 'observed' number of deaths was the yearly average of deaths due to paralysis agitans over a 5-year period. The rates for the 'standard' population were taken as the average of mortality rates at a particular age of all the birth cohorts. These standard rates could then be applied to the population of each birth cohort to get 'expected' numbers of deaths and thus a standardised mortality ratio for each birth cohort.

The data on social class came from successive Decennial Supplements to Reports of the Registrar General's Office. For ages 15-64, social class mortality is reported as a standardised mortality ratio (SMR). Because of problems of matching deaths to population data, the Registrar General reports social class mortality at age 65-74 as a proportionate mortality ratio (PMR).

Results

Time-trends

Figure 1 shows for males and females the trends in age-specific mortality rates from paralysis agitans in England and Wales. The data are the average of successive quinquennia: 1931-1935, 1936-1940, etc. Plotted on a log scale, it can be seen that the secular trends are different at different ages. Among men aged 75-84 there has been an increase in mortality. Among younger men, there has been a decrease; the younger the age group the greater the relative decline. The picture for women is somewhat similar.

393

Encephalitis Lethargica

To appreciate more closely whether this pattern is consistent with a cohort pattern, the mortality experience of each cohort or generation should be followed through its life time. In particular, if we wish to know if the mortality experiences of each cohort are related to its exposure to encephalitis lethargica in 1918-1926, we should have information on the age distribution of encephalitis lethargica. The age distribution of one published series from 1920 is shown in Figure 2 [10]. These figures are for numbers of cases not incidence rates but they give a rough guide to the age-distribution of encephalitis lethargica. The peak age of occurrence is in the age range 20-40. A similar age distribution was reported from other outbreaks (Matheson Commission, 1929).

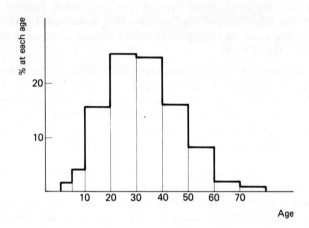

Figure 2 Age distribution of 864 cases of encephalitis lethargica 1918-1920

Cohort Analysis

Cohorts were then classified according to their age in 1920, and their subsequent mortality experience over the period 1931-1975 is shown in Figure 3 for England and Wales. The age-adjusted mortality is presented as a standardised mortality ratio for each cohort, 100 being the average for all cohorts. Those shown as minus 10 were born in 1930, which was close to the last reported year of any outbreak of encephalitis lethargica.

The picture for men and women is similar. Those who were aged 30-50 in 1920 had a higher mortality from paralysis agitans over the period 1931-1975 than those who were younger or older in 1920.

It could be argued that this excess mortality from paralysis agitans among cohorts apparently most heavily exposed to encephalitis lethargica might all have occurred in the early years after the epidemics when post-encephalitic parkinsonism was well recognised. That this is not the case can be shown by repeating the cohort analysis, examining only the later period of follow-up. When this was done for the

394

last 20 years (1956–1975) the results were substantially unchanged: the highest standardised cohort mortality ratio occurred in those aged 30–50 in 1920.

(a)

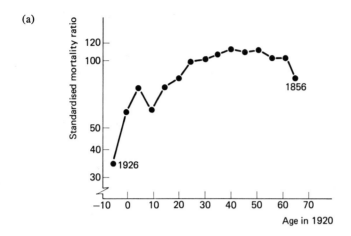

(b)

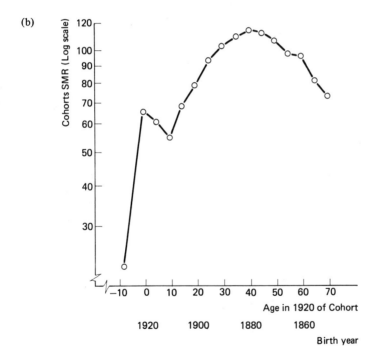

Figure 3 Lifetime Parkinson's disease mortality (1933–1973) of successive cohorts by age in 1920, England and Wales: (a) male; (b) female

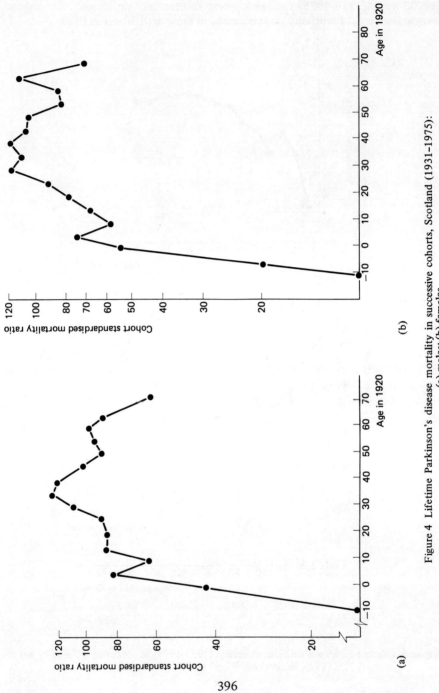

Figure 4 Lifetime Parkinson's disease mortality in successive cohorts, Scotland (1931–1975): (a) males; (b) females

The analysis of paralysis agitans mortality by cohorts in Scotland showed very similar results (Figs 4a, b). Among both men and women, cohorts aged 30–40 in 1920 showed a higher standardised mortality ratio over the period 1931–1975 than cohorts that were younger or older in 1920.

Social Class

The above analysis lends support to the view that a majority of cases of Parkinson's disease up to the present may be post-encephalitic in origin. The figures show that

(a)

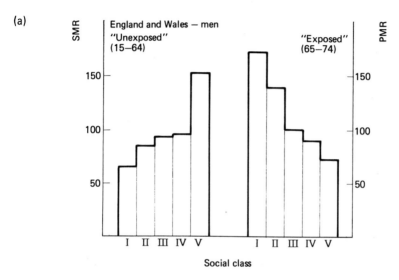

(b)

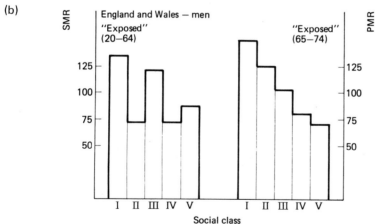

Figure 5 Parkinson's disease mortality by social class (males), England and Wales: (a) 1949–1953 (b) (1963)

among those less likely to have been exposed to encephalitis lethargica, particularly younger men and women, mortality from paralysis agitans is uncommon but does occur. If these younger cases are not the result of the encephalitis lethargica epidemic, they may be expected to show a different epidemiological pattern from the cases occurring in members of 'exposed' cohorts. Figure 5 shows the mortality from paralysis agitans among men in the different social classes in England and Wales. In the earlier period, 1949–1953 (Fig 5a), there was a clear gradient in mortality, higher in class I and lower in class V, among the older men, and a less clear gradient

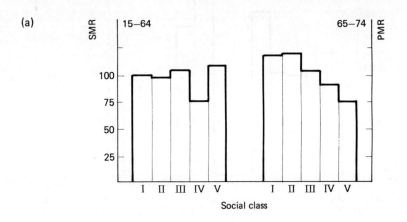

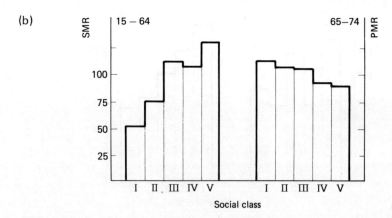

Figure 6 Parkinson's disease mortality by social class (females), England and Wales: (a) 1949–1953 (b) 1959–1963

398

among the men aged 20–64. These two age groups have been labelled 'exposed' as they both fell into the age range of peak exposure to encephalitis lethargica in 1920; for example, men aged 45–64 in 1950 would have been aged between 15 and 34 in 1920.

By contrast in the later period 1959–63 (Fig. 5b), there has been a marked change. Men aged 65–74 still show the clear upper-class predominance. Now, the younger men, aged 15–64, show a reversal of this trend, the mortality is lower in class I and higher in class V. The men aged 15–64 in 1959–63 would mostly have been less than 20 in 1920, hence younger than the peak age of exposure of encephalitis lethargica. These men appear to show a different mortality pattern.

The latest social class figures (1970–72) continue to show this contrast. In men aged 65–74, the PMR goes from 182 in class I to 100 in class V, but the gradient is not as smooth as in 1959–1963. In men 15–64, there continues to be a higher mortality in class V.

This same change in the social class pattern is seen for women (Fig. 6).

Discussion

In view of the decrease of one-half to two-thirds in the mortality from paralysis agitans at younger ages and the increase at older ages, the statement that 'the risk of dying with paralysis agitans is about the same today as it was in the 1920s' [8] does not give a complete description of the changes.

An analysis based solely on death certificate data is fraught with difficulties, especially with a chronic disease such as Parkinson's disease. The disease may not be diagnosed or, if diagnosed, may not be listed as the underlying cause of death. These 'errors' of classification may act differently at different ages and in different time periods. It seems more likely, however, that such differences would mask a cohort effect than be responsible for a spurious cohort pattern. For this latter to happen the errors would have to be cohort specific. It seems unlikely, for example, that doctors certifying deaths in 1950, should be biased towards favouring a diagnosis of Parkinson's disease for a 50-year-old and against this diagnosis for a 40-year-old or a 70-year-old; whereas in 1970 he should be biased towards this diagnosis for a 70-year-old and against it for a 50-year-old.

A simpler explanation of this apparent cohort pattern of mortality is that there has been a real change over time in the age of occurrence of Parkinson's disease. The clinical data, showing an increase in the average age of onset of Parkinson's disease, were held to be compatible, not only with a single disease occurring in an ageing cohort, but with the dying out of a younger population of post-encephalitic parkinsonians. This two-disease explanation is not compatible with the present findings. The increased mortality of the cohorts most heavily exposed to von Economo's encephalitis in the 1920s continued right through to the 1950s, 60s and 70s, a period when the majority of Parkinsonians were thought on clinical grounds to be idiopathic [1]. It seems possible then that the majority of so-called idiopathic Parkinson's disease occurring in these exposed cohorts is in fact post-encephalitic in origin.

399

Poskanzer and Schwab [2], pursuing the logic of their cohort hypothesis, predicted that as the exposed cohorts died off, the mortality from Parkinson's disease would decline. The present data, showing a decline in mortality at younger ages, support that prediction. Of course, treatment for Parkinson's disease has greatly improved in recent years. Well-controlled studies of the effect of this treatment on survival are lacking, but most clinical opinion holds that the new treatment improves the quality of survival for Parkinsonians without an appreciable effect on mortality.

The cases of Parkinson's disease occurring in people too young to be exposed to the 1920s epidemics do appear to have a different epidemiological pattern, at least as shown by the social class distribution. These younger cases now have the higher mortality in lower social classes seen with most other causes of death. It is not easy to determine if the class I predominance in mortality in the 65-74 age group is consistent with the social class pattern of occurrence of encephalitis lethargica. The review conducted by the Matheson Commission (1929) did not reach a firm conclusion on this point. Unpublished data made available by the Registrar General's Office showed that in 1931 the occupations with a high mortality from Parkinson's disease included clergymen, ministers, judges, employers and managers and teachers, and those with a low mortality included agricultural labourers, navvies and labourers. This is consistent with at least an equal social class distribution, if not a class I and II predominance.

The fact that the 'newer' cases of Parkinson's disease may be different epidemiologically from the older ones does not preclude a viral aetiology for them. If it is true that clinically-defined idiopathic Parkinson's disease may be a very late result of a viral infection, it is possible that these newer cases may be the end result of a viral infection that has been unrecognised clinically. It is possible that new epidemics of viral infection could be responsible for an upsurge in the occurrence of Parkinson's disease.

References

1 Duvoisin, RC, Yahr, MD, Schweitzer, MD and Merritt, HH (1963) Parkinsonism Before and Since the Epidemic of Encephalitis Lethargica. *Arch. Neurol., 9,* 232
2 Poskanzer, DC and Schwab, RS (1963) Cohort Analysis of Parkinson's Syndrome. Evidence for a single etiology related to subclinical infection about 1920. *J. chron. Dis., 16,* 961
3 Brown, EL and Knox, EG (1972) Epidemiological approach to Parkinson's disease. *Lancet, i,* 974
4 Leibowitz, U and Feldman, S (1973) Age Shift in Parkinsonism. *Isr. J. Med. Sci., 9,* 599
5 Kaplan, SD (1974) Age distribution of patients with Parkinson's Disease in 1960 and 1970 in 110 hospitals. *Neurology (Minneap.), 24,* 972
6 Kessler, II (1973) Parkinson's Disease: Perspective on Epidemiology and Pathogenesis. *Prev. Med., 2,* 88
7 Kurland, LT, Kurtzke, JF, Goldberg, ID, Choi, NW and Williams, G (1973) Parkinsonism. In *Epidemiology of Neurologic and Sense Organ Disorders.* Harvard University Press, Cambridge, Massachusetts, page 41

8 Duvoisin, RC and Schweitzer, MD (1966) Paralysis Agitans Mortality in England and Wales, 1855-1962. *Brit. J. Prev. Soc. Med., 20,* 27
9 Beral, V (1974) Cancer of the cervix—a sexually transmitted infection? *Lancet, i,* 1037
10 Strauss, I and Wechsler, IS (1921) Epidemic encephalitis (Encephalitis Lethargica). *Int. J. Publ. Hlth, 11,* 449

Chapter 41

SYRINGOMYELIA

J B Foster

Until a disease is defined as a nosological entity, epidemiological studies have little value. Such is the case with syringomyelia. In the Department of Neurology, Newcastle-upon-Tyne, we have recently had an opportunity of studying a sequential group of patients suffering from 'clinical syringomyelia'. We presented the results of these investigations in a monograph [1]. The cases were divided into five categories and broadly into two groups following the work of Gardner [2], that is, communicating and non-communicating forms of syringomyelia (Table I).

TABLE I Classification of the Varieties of Syringomyelia

---

1. Communicating syringomyelia (syringo-hydromyelia)
   (a) With developmental anomalies at foramen magnum and in the posterior fossa.
   (b) Associated with acquired abnormalities at the base (basal arachnoiditis, posterior fossa tumours and cysts).
2. Syringomyelia as a late sequel to trauma.
   (a) Serious spinal cord injury.
   (b) Mild to moderate spinal cord injury.
3. Syringomyelia as a sequel to arachnoiditis confined to the spinal cord.
4. Syringomyelia associated with spinal cord tumours.
   (a) Intramedullary
   (b) Extramedullary
5. Idiopathic syringomyelia.

Previous prevalence and incidence figures relating to this disorder must be misleading, for the nosology has not until now been clearly defined. Brewis and his colleagues [3] determined a period prevalence of 8.4 per 100 000 population in 1966. No prevalence figures are available for the 100 patients described in our monograph, but recently we have had the opportunity of studying a further 70 cases of syringomyelia, and data are available for 139 of these. A study of the epidemiology of the cases has just begun, and we present here some initial data available for 113 patients living in the Newcastle area (Fig. 1). The place of residence for each patient at the time of diagnosis has been defined, and we shall be completing a geographical survey of the birthplace of the individual patient and also a family study. Figure 2 illustrates the residence of patients outside the Tyneside area, also included in the study. There is apparently some clustering in the Morpeth area as shown in Figure 2, and in the Westerhope and East Rainton area on Figure 1.

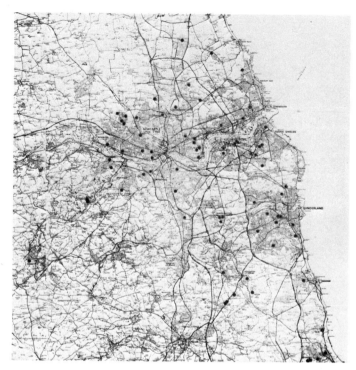

Figure 1 Places of residence of the Newcastle series

Of our 113 local patients we have estimated a period prevalence of 5.6 per
00 000 with an incidence of 0.4 per 100 000 per annum (Table II). The mean age
ɔf onset of our original 100 cases was 30 years. The mean age of onset for the 113
local patients was 33 years, with a range of 5 to 64 years. The male to female ratio
of the 113 local cases is 64 to 75, whereas the first 100 cases had an equal male and
female distribution.

TABLE II Epidemiological Data for the Newcastle Syringomyelia Survey

Data available for	139 patients
Data available for	113 local patients (population 2 000 000)
Period prevalence	5.6 per 100 000 (8.4 per 100 000 Carlisle study of Brewis et al, 1966) [3]
Incidence	0.4 per 100 000 per annum
Mean age at onset	33 years (range 5–64)
Male to female ratio	64 : 75

Figure 3 illustrates the pathology of the cases studied thus far. It is evident that
the greater number are cases of syringomyelia associated with the Chiari malformation, i.e. those most likely to benefit from surgical decompression. Smaller groups
include those without Chiari malformation, those with basal arachnoiditis, and
other forms of non-communicating syringomyelia associated with trauma and
posterior fossa tumour etc.

403

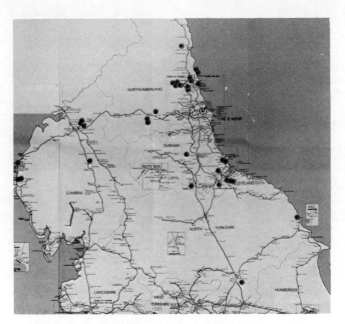

Figure 2 Places of residence of cases outside the Newcastle area

Newcastle syringomyelia study
pathology

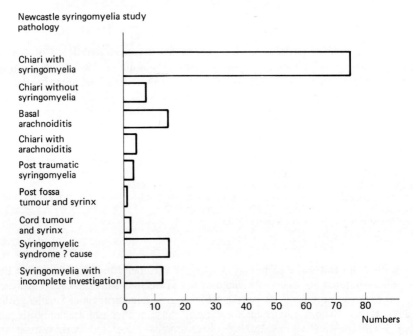

Figure 3 Pathology of the Newcastle cases

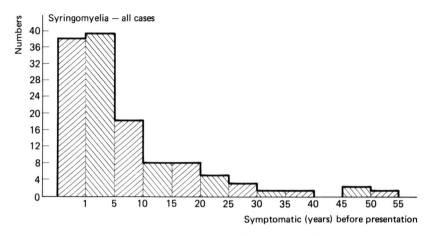

Figure 4 Symptomatic years before presentation

Figure 4 illustrates the symptomatic years before presentation. The majority of patients presented for diagnosis within 5 years of the onset of their symptoms. It is interesting to note that some had suffered symptoms for as many as 55 years before presentation. In Figure 5 we show the age of onset of the symptoms with a mean at 33 years. Figures 6 and 7 break down the two groups into those with Chiari (Fig. 6) and those with a negative myelogram (Fig. 7). There is little difference in these two groups except in numbers. The cases with arachnoiditis, i.e. cases showing a specific myelographic abnormality, and findings of arachnoiditis at operation, show a more even distribution for the age of onset, which suggests a different pathogenesis, perhaps perinatal trauma (Fig. 8). This possibility will be the subject of further enquiry.

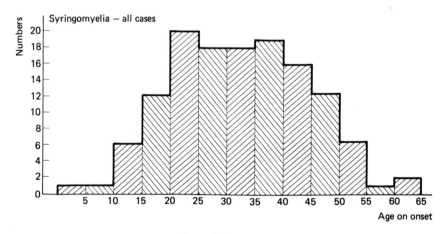

Figure 5 Age at onset

405

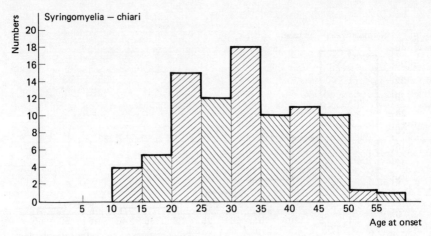

Figure 6 Age at onset of Chiari cases

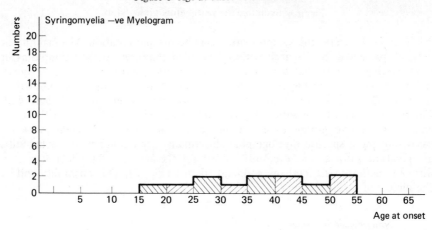

Figure 7 Age at onset of cases with negative myelogram

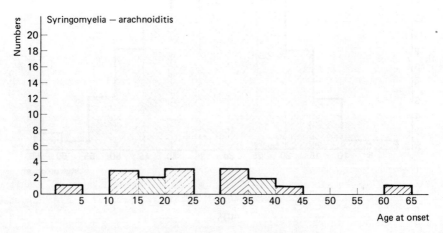

Figure 8 Age at onset of cases with arachnoiditis

Surgery

Of our original series, 62 patients were shown to have a Chiari malformation, i.e. cerebellar ectopia on myelography. Of these, 47 were operated upon. Five were cured and 30 were improved. In 11 there was no change. Of the 18 showing arachnoiditis, 12 were operated upon with very poor results. We felt that the demonstration of a Chiari malformation on myelography justified operation on such a patient, and we intend further to present operative results after the completion of the current study. Of the 34 patients not submitted to operation, 6 suffered from arachnoiditis, 13 showed normal myelography, suggesting that there may be a fifth form of syringomyelia (*see* Table I).

Epidemiology

It is thus conceded that syringomyelia is a relatively uncommon disease, and we have to recognise five different pathological categories (*see* Table I). Our own prevalence and incidence rates conform closely to those previously published [4-7]. The literature does not suggest that there is a preponderance of males over females, and indeed our initial results suggest rather the reverse. We have no figures to confirm the suggestion that syringomyelia is more common in individuals engaged in hard manual work [7-9] but in our original description we noted five patients whose symptoms had first appeared following trauma [1]. It has been suggested in the German literature that syringomyelia is more common in certain areas of central Europe [10]. The disorder is said to be more common in the South than in the North, in Austria and, in particular, around Vienna than in neighbouring Switzerland. Foci or concentrations of cases have been described in small villages in the Rhine valley [7], but these observations remain unexplained.

Genetics

We have no cases of familial syringomyelia in our series of 170 patients, but families have been described where syringomyelia has occurred in sibships [8-12]. In van Bogaert's two sisters, one case at postmortem was found to have an ependymoma, and the other cases mentioned in Table III did not have full radiological or operative confirmation except for the cases of Giménez-Roldán and his fellow workers

TABLE III Previous Reports of Familial Syringomyelia

Barré and Reys (1924) [8]	Brother and sister
Van Bogaert (1934) [9]	Two sisters
Wild and Behnert (1964) [10]	Monozygotic twins
Bentley et al (1975) [11]	(a) Brother and sister
	(b) Two sisters
Giménez-Roldán et al (1978) [12]	Father, son and daughter

[12] where full radiological investigation confirmed communicating syringomyelia in a father, son and daughter.

Thus, there is little known of the epidemiology of this rare neurological disorder, but recent attempts to re-classify the forms of cavitation of the spinal cord should be followed by epidemiological surveys, particularly concerned with cases of Chiari malformation, i.e. tonsillar ectopia and arachnoiditis. It is our intention to initiate such investigations in our Newcastle group of cases, this short chapter simply describing our, as yet, incomplete observations.

References

1 Barnett, HJM, Foster, JB and Hudgson, P (1973) In *Syringomyelia*. London: WB Saunders Co Ltd
2 Gardner, WJ (1965) *J. Neurol. Neurosurg. and Psychiat., 28,* 247
3 Brewis, M, Poskanzer, DC, Roland, C and Miller, H (1966) *Acta Neurol. Scand., 42,* suppl. 24
4 Wilson, SAK (1970) In *Neurology,* Vol. 2 (ed. Bruce, AN). New York, page 1389
5 Poser, CM (1956) In *The Relationship between Syringomyelia and Neoplasm*. Springfield, Ill.: CC Thomas & Alsen, V (1957). *Dtsch. Z. Nervenheilk, 177,* 156
6 Schliep, G (1978) In *Handbook of Clinical Neurology,* Amsterdam: Elsevier-North Holland Vol. 32, page 256
7 Hertel, G, Karmer, S and Placzek, E (1973) *Nervenarzt, 44,* 1
8 Barré, JA and Reys, J (1924) *Rev. Neurol., 1,* 521
9 Van Bogaert, L (1929) *J. Neurol. Psychiat., 29,* 146
10 Wild, H and Behnert, J (1964) *Münch med. Wschr., 106,* 1421
11 Bentley, SJ, Campbell, MS and Kauffmann, P (1975) *J. Neurol. Neurosurg. and Psychiat., 38,* 346
12 Giménez-Roldán, S, Benito, C and Mateo, D (1978) *J. Neurol. Sci., 36,* 135

Chapter 42

INCIDENCE AND LONG-TERM TREND OF AMYOTROPHIC LATERAL SCLEROSIS IN ROCHESTER, MINNESOTA*

S M Juergens, L T Kurland and D W Mulder

Introduction

At the 1976 Mansell Symposium, I had an opportunity to review the epidemiology of motor neurone disease [1]. Today my colleagues and I would like to update that report by describing, in brief, a study of the incidence and secular trend for more than half a century and the outcome of amyotrophic lateral sclerosis (ALS), a term we use as synonymous with motor neurone disease, in Rochester, Minnesota [2].

In contrast to most historical commentaries on disease, it cannot be said that ALS was described by Hippocrates. We are not aware of any documentation of its existence in Europe or America until 1850 with Aran's description of several cases [3]. It might be helpful to know whether ALS and its clinical variants existed before that date. Actually, the earliest case of which I am aware is based on native legend and refers to 'paralytico' (the form of ALS occurring on Guam) in a man from the village of Umatac, whose illness began about 1815, reportedly the result of a curse by the village priest on the man and his descendants because of repeated pilfering of mangos from the churchyard [4].

Since we have no evidence to the contrary, it seems reasonable to assume that ALS has existed for a long time, although its low incidence, insidious course and clinical features may not have enabled it to be distinguished from other wasting diseases until the era of Aran, Duchenne and Charcot.

We would like to explore what has happened to ALS incidence rates since 1850, or even earlier, but impressions based on case reports and clinical series are all that we have in the late nineteenth and early twentieth centuries. So we are forced, by the absence of any better data, to review official mortality reports and perhaps the only source in the world outside of Guam with reasonably accurate long-term incidence rates, namely that for the population of Rochester, Minnesota, and ask whether the frequency of the disease has been increasing or decreasing. Obviously, any appreciable change in the rates over time may help identify the cause(s) of ALS.

Motor neurone disease became a distinct rubric in the 6th revision (1948) of the WHO International Statistical Classification [5]. The rate in the United States, based on cases certified as the underlying cause (and estimated as about 70 per cent

*This investigation was supported in part by a grant (GM 14231), National Institutes of Health, Bethesda, Maryland, USA

complete), has been about 0.7 per 100 000 population [6, 7]; there is relatively little difference in the age-adjusted rates from several western European countries and Japan. There has been little or no change in the annual death rates for motor neurone disease in most of these countries over the succeeding 25 years [8].

Methods

Utilising the data resources described in Chapter 5 the incidence, trend and outcome for ALS in the Rochester, Minnesota, population have been determined for the 53-year period 1925 through 1977. For this study, we reviewed the unified records of Mayo Clinic, coded under a variety of categories suggesting ALS, including progressive muscular atrophy, progressive bulbar palsy and motor neurone disease. A resident was defined as one whose domicile was within the city limits of Rochester for at least one year before the onset of symptoms. More than 500 patient records were retrieved from the medical indexing file and reviewed for possible inclusion in the study. The autopsy records and death certificates were also examined, but these revealed no cases of ALS that were not already in the medical histories.

Results

Thirty-five residents of Rochester, Minnesota (18 males, 17 females), were identified as having the onset of ALS during the period 1925 through 1977.

The mean annual incidence rate per 100 000 population was 2.1 for males, 1.4 for females, and 1.8 for the sexes combined (Table I). The rate, adjusted by age to the United States white population of 1950, which is near the midpoint of the study period, was also 1.8 per 100 000 population.

TABLE I. Number and incidence per 100 000 population of ALS in Rochester, Minnesota, 1925-1977

	Number	Crude Rate	Adjusted Rate*	95% Confidence Interval
Total	35	1.8	1.8	1.3 – 2.5
Males	18	2,1	2.3	1.2 – 3.3
Females	17	1.4	1.4	0.7 – 2.2

* Adjusted to 1950 US white population
M : F ratio 1.6 : 1.

The numbers of males and females in the study were nearly the same, but Rochester has more females in the adult population. The rates by sex when adjusted to a standard population were 2.3 for males and 1.4 for females, resulting in a ratio of the incidence rates for males to females of 1.6:1.

410

The observed incidence rates increased with advancing age (Table III, Fig. 3). (Table II, Fig. 1), but because of the small sample size, no conclusion concerning trend can be made.

TABLE II. Number and average annual incidence per 100 000 population for ALS in Rochester, Minnesota, 1925 through 1977

Time	Population	No. of cases			Crude rate M & F	95% Confidence interval
		Total	Male	Female		
1925–54	23,976	9	6	3	1.2	0.6–2.4
1954–64	39,012	10	5	5	2.6	1.2–4.7
1965–74	56,629	10	5	5	1.9	0.9–3.5
1975–77	56,420	6	2	4	3.5	1.3–7.7
Total	36,665	35	18	17	1.8	1.2–2.5

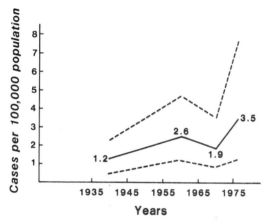

Figure 1 Average annual incidence rates for ALS in Rochester, Minnesota, 1925 through 1977. Thirty-five patients; 95% confidence interval indicated by dashed lines

TABLE III. Age-adjusted average annual incidence by age for ALS in Rochester, Minnesota, 1925 through 1977

Age (years)	No. of cases	Rate	95% Confidence interval
45 – 54	4	2.3	0.7 – 6.1
55 – 64	10	7.3	3.5 – 13.4
65 – 74	13	15.5	8.2 – 26.5
≥75	8	18,6	8.0 – 36.6

411

The age at onset of ALS in this population ranged from 48 to 88 years, with a median of 66 years (Fig. 2). Examining the patients by sex, there was no significant difference in age at onset. The median age at onset of the 18 males was 65.5 years, and the range was from 48 to 88 years. The median age at onset of the 17 females was 68 years, and the range was from 49 to 76 years.

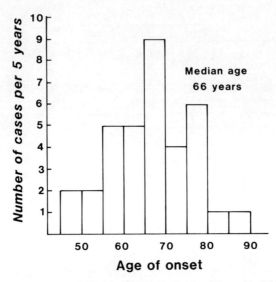

Figure 2 Ages at onset of ALS for 35 patients, Rochester, Minnesota, 1925 through 1977

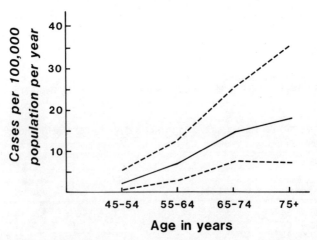

Figure 3 Average annual incidence rates by age for ALS in Rochester, Minnesota, 1925 through 1977. Thirty-five patients; 95% confidence interval indicated by dashed lines

The observed incidence rates increased with advancing age (Table III, Fig. 3). However, the series is small and, although suggestive, the rates in the age groups more than 54 years of age do not differ significantly. The rate in the group 45 to 54 years of age was significantly less than (P ≤ 0.01) that of the older groups.

The interval between the onset of symptoms and the first clinic visit ranged from 2 weeks to 62 months. The median interval was 7.5 months. Two patients waited more than 2 years before they had their symptoms evaluated (Fig. 4). No significant sex difference was demonstrated between age at onset for the interval from onset to first evaluation, although females tended to seek medical care a little sooner than did males.

The survivorship curve of the 35 patients (Fig. 5) demonstrated that the median (50%) survival was 22½ months. For the deaths observed to date, the range of time from onset to death was 9.5 months to 10 years. At 2 years after onset, the relative survival of those less than 65 years of age at onset was 72 per cent, while that for the older group was only 28 per cent. No patient in our series reported a family history of ALS.

There was no significant difference in median survival (21.2 vs. 22.6 months) or median age at onset (66.5 vs. 69 years) in patients who had onset of symptoms in the bulbar musculature as compared with those who had onset of symptoms in the extremities.

The clinical features at onset and during the course of illness were similar to those generally described for ALS.

Pathological Features

Of the 33 patients who died, 18 underwent autopsy. In 17, ALS was verified; in the other one, no sections were available for review. In these 17 autopsies reviewed by us, there were no neurofibrillary tangles or hyaline inclusions found, nor were abnormal findings noted in the posterior columns, Clarke's column or spinocerebellar tracts.

For 30 (91%) of the 33 deceased patients, the death certificates listed ALS as a cause of death. One report noted 'ascending paralysis of the lower extremities' as a contributory cause, and two had no mention of any neurological abnormality. Of the 30, 26 had ALS listed as the primary cause of death, and the others had it listed as a contributory cause. In view of the high correlation between certification of cause of death and the clinical diagnosis, it should be noted that most of the Rochester death certificates were completed by Mayo Clinic pathologists who had access to the patients' medical records as well as the pathological findings when autopsy was done.

The analysis of occupation and possible toxin and radiation exposure, prior trauma or illnesses, including paralytic poliomyelitis, failed to disclose any specific pattern. Three of the patients had had injuries within 3 years to the same extremity in which the disease was first noted, but coincidence seemed the most reasonable explanation.

413

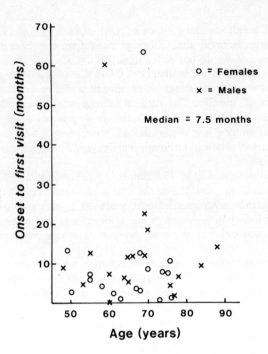

Figure 4 Interval from onset to first visit for 35 patients with ALS, Rochester, Minnesota, 1925 through 1977

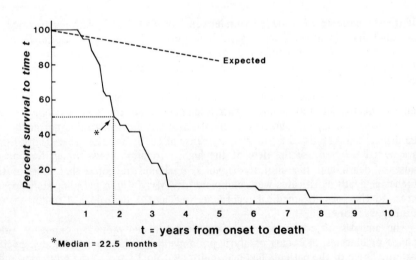

*Median = 22.5 months

Figure 5 Survival of 35 patients with ALS in Rochester, Minnesota, 1925 through 1977, compared with expected survival

In summary, we have noted a slightly greater incidence than reported from other centres (apart from the western Pacific islands), an older age of onset, and a shorter duration of disease.

Most published studies of ALS are based on patients who have diagnoses made at specialty centres. Referred patients who reside some distance from a specialty centre must, of necessity, live long enough to obtain appointments and be seen and be able to travel. Patients with rapidly advancing disease may not be included, and patients with an indolent course may be selected. The age of the patient may also introduce bias. If the patient is relatively young, his family or local physician may be more motivated to obtain a specialist's opinion. An elderly patient may have greater difficulty travelling to a specialty centre because of the limitations associated with age as well as the debilitation of ALS. Also, the family, physician, or patient himself may assume that his symptoms are part of the ageing process and will not seek a further opinion. Such would not apply to the Rochester patients, who would be seen locally and almost certainly be referred promptly to an experienced neurologist in the community.

Studies based on questionnaires from patient members of voluntary agencies have also been published. It is our opinion that patients who join such voluntary ALS organisations are more likely to be white, younger, to be from higher socio-economic levels and urban centres and to have a longer duration of disease than those who do not join. Patients who are severely debilitated early and with rapidly advancing disease are less likely to survive long enough to learn about the agency, join and participate in such studies. Those analysing such patient registry data should be alerted to such possible selection factors in their clientele. A similar bias in clinical series toward the selection of younger patients with a longer course has also been observed in other conditions, such as primary brain tumours and parkinsonism [9, 10].

Surveys based on death certificates may be less selective and provide evidence of a disease process that begins, on average, later in life than case series reported from specialty centres. The distribution of ages at death for ALS in the US for the years 1959 to 1961, revealed that the mean age was 64 years and the median age was 62 years. Assuming a 2 to 3-year duration from onset to death, the age at onset would then be approximately 60 years or between that noted in most clinical series and our population-based study.

The major findings of this study of ALS in Rochester, Minnesota, are a lack of evidence for any significant change in the age distribution at onset or of incidence rates over more than half a century, in contrast to reports based on clinical series [11]. Our results also reveal a much higher median age of onset and a strong suggestion of an increasing rate with increasing age. Other Rochester studies have shown similar patterns of increasing rates with age for primary brain tumours, other malignancies and parkinsonism which contrast with clinical studies suggesting a peak in the 6th or 7th decade of life [8].

Age distribution is a fundamental characteristic, reflecting disease mechanism; if the rates in Rochester provide a more accurate picture of this feature than do clinical series, it may help to focus attention on more plausible aetiological mechanisms which have been or will be suggested for motor neurone disease.

References

1 Kurland, LT (1977) *Motor Neurone Disease* (ed. FC Rose), Chapter 2. 14. Tunbridge Wells: Pitman Medical
2 Juergens, SM, Kurland, LT, Okazaki, H and Mulder, DW (1979) *Neurology* (in press)
3 Aran, FA (1850) *Arch. gen. de med., 84, 5,* 172
4 Kurland, LT, Mulder, PH and Mulder, DW (1954) *Neurology (Minneap.), 4,* 355
5 *Manual of the International Statistical Classification of Diseases, Injuries, and Causes of Death, Vol. 1* (1948). WHO: Geneva
6 Hoffmann, PM and Brody, JA (1971) *J. Chron. Dis., 24,* 5
7 Kurland, LT, Choi, NW and Sayre, GP (1969) *Motor Neuron Diseases* (ed. FH Norris, Jr and LT Kurland). Chapter 4, page 28. New York: Grune and Stratton
8 Kurtzke, J and Kurland, LT (1973) *Clinical Neurology, Vol. III* (ed. AB Baker). 1–80, Hagerstown, MD, Harper and Row
9 Nobrega, FT, Glattre, E, Kurland, LT et al (1969) *Excerpta Medica International Congress Series No. 175,* 474
10 Kurland, LT and Darrell, RW (1961) *Int. J. Neurol., 2,* 11
11 Aimard, G, Bady, B, Boisson, D et al (1976) (NIH Library Translation NIH-78-193) *Rev. Neurol. (Paris), 132,* 563

Index

419

424

426